# Trigeminal Neuralgias: A Neurosurgical Illustrated Guide

Marc Sindou • Andrei Brinzeu

# Trigeminal Neuralgias: A Neurosurgical Illustrated Guide

Springer

Marc Sindou
University of Lyon
Lyon, France

Andrei Brinzeu
University of Lyon
Lyon, France

Department of Neurosurgery
Neuroscience Research Center
Victor Babeş University of Medicine
and Pharmacy
Timişoara, Romania

ISBN 978-3-031-25111-5 ISBN 978-3-031-25113-9 (eBook)
https://doi.org/10.1007/978-3-031-25113-9



This Springer imprint is published by the registered company Springer Nature Switzerland AG
The registered company address is: Gewerbestrasse 11, 6330 Cham, Switzerland

# Preface

Trigeminal neuralgias are a group of diseases with common clinical manifestations marked by the great suffering incurred to patients. Their diversity means that a number of specialties have to deal with them, thus involving many disciplines such as neurology, neuro-imaging, ophthalmology, ENT, maxillofacial and dental surgery, and, of course, neurosurgery. Treating refractory trigeminal neuralgias is also within the competencies of the multidisciplinary Pain Centers.

During the past three decades, there were significant advances, not only concerning the mechanisms of the diverse forms of the disease, its diagnosis by new imaging methods, but also its specific pharmacological therapies and its various surgical treatments.

The aim of this book is to provide a practical guide for those specialists (or patients) dealing with trigeminal neuralgia, in particular in those situations where they may resort to surgery, i.e., refractory trigeminal neuralgia. These patients sadly reach the surgeon after much delay and undue suffering due to, at least in the experience of these authors, lack of knowledge about the surgical possibilities. The goal therefore is to help these patients and the treating physicians.

In the text, the authors have first addressed the definitions and descriptive classifications of the different forms of the trigeminal neuralgias, as established by the ad hoc international committees. Then they have attempted to give a background of anatomy of the trigeminal nervous system and surrounding structures for the good comprehension of the mechanisms of trigeminal neuralgias and ensuing clinical presentations.

Imaging is the key to etiologic diagnosis of trigeminal neuralgias and is therefore discussed in detail, the more so as this conditions the therapeutic choices which in the view of these authors should be tailored to the cause of the neuralgia.

In the last part, the book details, in an illustrative "surgeon's" way, the various interventions that may be offered to patients. Algorithms for therapeutic decision-making are proposed on the basis of current literature viewed through the lens of the experience of more than 5000 patients with trigeminal neuralgia treated surgically mainly by the senior author over the past 40 years.

Among the modern neurosurgical interventions, the Micro-Vascular Decompression (MVD) procedure is the sole anatomically and functionally conservative method for treating trigeminal neuralgias. MVD is now recognized as the gold standard for those neuralgias that are thought to be caused by a Neuro-Vascular Conflict, at present termed classical neuralgias. However, not all patients suffer from classical trigeminal neuralgia and not all might benefit from or can withstand microvascular decompression, thus making room for the lesioning techniques. These techniques can be performed percutaneously by several types of lesion makers: RF thermocoagulation, balloon compression or glycerol injection, and also by stereotactic radiosurgery. All these, as well as clinical and pharmacological data are included in the proposed decision-making algorithms.

Further research in genetics and biology on one side but more importantly on imaging and clinical outcome needs to be performed in order to reach the desired and now very much tangible targeted and personalized medicine for each particular patient and each neuralgia.

Lyon, France Marc Sindou
Timişoara, Romania Andrei Brinzeu

# Keywords

Trigeminal neuralgias · Primary trigeminal neuralgias · Classical trigeminal neuralgia · Idiopathic trigeminal neuralgias · Secondary trigeminal neuralgias · Hyperactive cranial nerve compression syndromes · Neuro-vascular conflicts · Magnetic resonance imaging · Anticonvulsant antalgic medication · Percutaneous lesioning procedures · RF-thermorhizotomy · Balloon compression · Glycerol neurolysis · Sterotactic radiosurgery · Microvascular decompression · Kaplan-Meier outcome probability

# Acknowledgments

First of all, the authors want to thank *Doctor Cristian Son* for his valuable help in the practical elaboration of this book. His special interest for Surgical Anatomy has been recognized and we strongly recommend he continue on this path.

The senior author of this book would like to express his considerable indebtedness to *Professor William Sweet* and *Professor Peter Jannetta* for their mentorships on the occasion of his training in Boston and Pittsburgh in the late 1970s, at dawn of his neurosurgical career.

Both authors wish to manifest their admirative appreciation to *Professor Giorgio Cruccu*, *Professor Joanna Zakrzewska*, and *Professor Turo Nurmikko* for their sustained interest in the fields of comprehension and management of facial pain.

A special acknowledgment goes to our Colleague and Friend *Professor Kim Burchiel*, a recognized leader in pain surgery and surgical management of trigeminal neuralgia. A chain of fruitful exchanges and critical discussions along the years revealed themselves to be beneficial to select surgical indications more accurately.

# Contents

# 1 Introduction: Definition of Trigeminal Neuralgia and Evolution of Concepts

The pain of trigeminal neuralgia is so intense that it was qualified since the beginning of its description as "suicidal," and because of this was one of the first neurological diseases treated by neurosurgical procedures, before the introduction of specific and effective medications (Fig. 1.1).

The first description of the previously called essential trigeminal neuralgia dates from the end of the seventeenth century, and was given by J.H. Fehr and J. Locke. As soon as 1756 André used the term "tic douloureux de la face" which became international to designate it clinically. In English-speaking countries the name of the condition is attached to Fothergill who presented a detailed study in 1776 under the term "prosopalgia." In France Trousseau demonstrated an astonishing pathophysiological intuition by designating it "epileptiform neuralgia"; the three described acts of the attack included discharge, reflex contracture, and vegetative phase.

The incidence of the disease is 5 new cases per year per 100,000 population (Sindou and Keravel 2009). Classical trigeminal neuralgia is rather a disease of mid-age and senescence, pain occurring 3 out of 4 times after the age of 50.

**Fig. 1.1** Authors' artistic representations of a patient with right trigeminal neuralgia in pain and of a right trigeminal nerve with its three division branches


M. Sindou, A. Brinzeu, *Trigeminal Neuralgias: A Neurosurgical Illustrated Guide*,
https://doi.org/10.1007/978-3-031-25113-9_1

## 1.1 Definition of Trigeminal Neuralgia

According to the International Headache Society, trigeminal neuralgia is defined as "a disorder characterized by recurrent unilateral brief electric shock-like pains, abrupt in onset and termination, limited to the distribution of one or more division(s) of the trigeminal nerve and triggered by innocuous stimuli. It may develop without apparent cause or be a result of another disorder" (IHS 2018).

Trigeminal neuralgia can reveal an underlying pathology and then corresponds to "secondary" neuralgia. When considered "primary," trigeminal neuralgia is often due to vascular compression with structural alteration(s) of the root; in this eventuality it is termed "classical" (Cruccu et al. 2016).

Easy in the typical form, the diagnosis can be difficult with atypical presentations. The diagnosis is essentially based on clinical criteria; it should also take into account the sensitivity to anticonvulsants. Careful clinical examination is mandatory and classification requires imaging.

## 1.2 Evolution of Concepts

The history of the medical treatment of trigeminal neuralgia begins in the seventeenth century with an extraordinary number of trials including: poisons (arsenic, hemlock), opiates, Galvano-therapy, and so on. The only positive results of these corresponded in fact to spontaneous remission of the pain. The hypothesis of a paroxysmal activity in the trigeminal nuclei formulated by Trousseau as early as 1853 was only pharmacologically validated with the introduction of diphenylhydantoin in 1942 by Bergouignan (Bergouignan and D'Aulnay 1951) then of carbamazepine in 1962 by Blom (1962).

The first attempts at neurosurgery were Gasserotomy by Victor Horsley (1891a, b), retrogasserian neurotomy by William Spiller and Charles Frazier (1901), and juxta-pontine rhizotomy by Walter Dandy (1925). Since then, new surgical techniques were developed, some lesioning either by percutaneous approach, proposed by William Sweet (Sweet and Wepsic 1974; Håkanson 1978; Mullan and Lichtor 1983), or by stereotactic radiosurgery pioneered by Lars Leksell (1971); some, conservatory, aiming to decompress the trigeminal nerve from its neurovascular conflict (Gardner 1962; Jannetta 1967) (Fig. 1.2).

**Key-Point**

Once recognized the neuralgia requires specific drug treatment, principally anticonvulsants. In the event of escape and/or intolerance to the medications, current surgical methods make it possible to obtain control of pain in most cases.

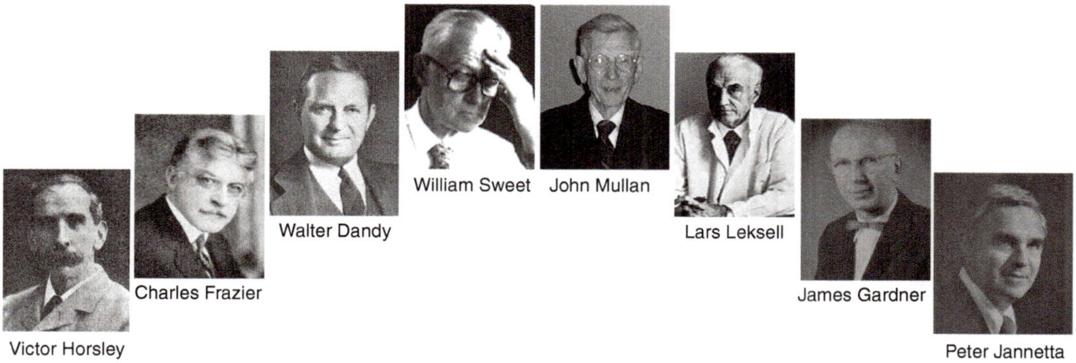


**Fig. 1.2** Portraits of the main pioneers in neurosurgery for trigeminal neuralgias: Victor Horsley (1857–1916): Sub-temporal Gasserectomy; Charles Frazier (1870–1936): Sub-temporal retrogasserian Trigeminal Neurotomy; Walter Dandy (1886–1946): Posterior fossa retrosigmoid approach for performing Juxtapontine partial rhizotomy, and the Observation of trigeminal root vascular compressions; William Sweet (1910–2001): Refining of the Percutaneous Radiofrequency-Thermorhizotomy; John Mullan (1925–2015): Percutaneous Balloon compression of the trigeminal ganglion; Lars Leksell (1907–1986): Stereotactic Radiosurgery of the trigeminal nerve with Gamma-knife; James Gardner (1898–1987): Concept of Vascular Decompression of the trigeminal root, and first successful attempts; Peter Jannetta (1932–2016): Codification of the Micro-Vascular Decompression procedure, and its popularization

# 2 Terminology and Classification of Trigeminal Neuralgias

The most admitted definitions and classifications of trigeminal neuralgias are those established in 2018 by the Classification Committee of the International Headache Society (IHS), under the vocable "The International Classification of Headache Disorders (ICHD), 3rd edition" (IHS 2018). The classification was based on a consensus with the International Association for the Study of Pain (IASP), and was largely influenced by Cruccu et al.'s article entitled "New Classification and diagnostic grading for practice and research" (Cruccu et al. 2016) (Fig. 2.1).


M. Sindou, A. Brinzeu, *Trigeminal Neuralgias: A Neurosurgical Illustrated Guide*,
https://doi.org/10.1007/978-3-031-25113-9_2

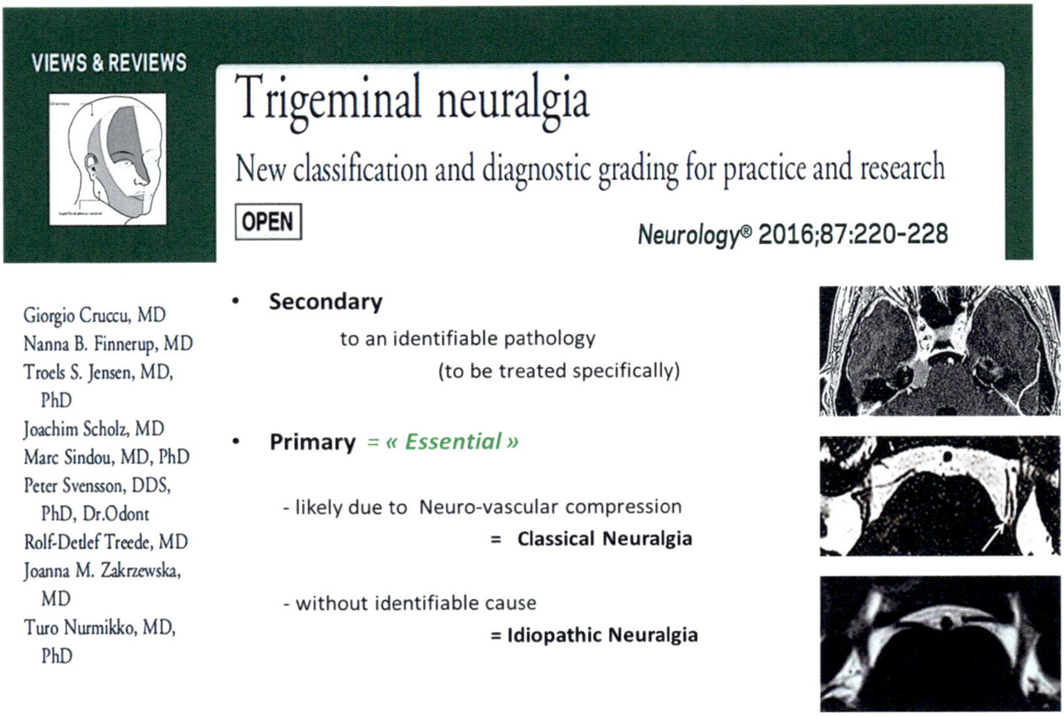


**Fig. 2.1** Classification of trigeminal neuralgias. Summary of the classification introduced by Cruccu et al. (2016), with illustrations from top to bottom of: right secondary trigeminal neuralgia due to a Meckel cave and petroclival meningioma, left classical neuralgia caused by a (likely responsible) neurovascular conflict from the superior cerebellar artery (arrow), and right neuralgia without any evidence on high-resolution MRI of causal factor, that is, corresponding to idiopathic trigeminal neuralgia

## 2.1 Criteria for Diagnosis of Trigeminal Neuralgia

### Diagnostic Criteria

(A) Recurrent paroxysms of unilateral facial pain in the distribution of one or more divisions of the trigeminal nerve, with no radiation beyond and fulfilling criteria B and C

(B) Pain has all of the following characteristics:
1. lasting from a fraction of a second to 2 min
2. severe intensity
3. electric shock-like, shooting, stabbing, or sharp in quality

(C) Precipitated by innocuous stimuli within the affected trigeminal distribution.

(D) Not better accounted for by another ICHD-3 diagnosis

NB. In the purely paroxysmal form, patient is pain-free between attacks, with a so-called refractory period immediately after attacks. In its atypical presentation, a background of continuous pain is associated with the painful paroxysms.

## 2.2 Classification on Presumed Etiology

### 2.2.1 Secondary Trigeminal Neuralgia

Trigeminal neuralgia caused by an underlying disease. Clinical examination often shows sensory changes in a significant proportion of these patients.

**Diagnostic Criteria**

(A) Recurrent paroxysms of unilateral facial pain, either purely paroxysmal or associated with concomitant continuous or near-continuous pain

(B) Underlying disease demonstrated and known to be able to cause neuralgia

### 2.2.2 Classical Trigeminal Neuralgia

Trigeminal neuralgia developing without apparent cause other than neurovascular compression.

**Diagnostic Criteria**

(A) Recurrent paroxysms of unilateral facial pain [Classical TN may be purely paroxysmal or with concomitant continuous pain]

(B) Demonstration on MRI (or during surgery) of neurovascular compression (not simply contact) with morphological changes in the trigeminal nerve root.

### 2.2.3 Idiopathic Trigeminal Neuralgia

Trigeminal neuralgia for which investigations do not show significant abnormalities.

**Diagnostic Criteria**

(A) Recurrent paroxysms of unilateral facial pain, either purely paroxysmal or associated with concomitant continuous or near-continuous pain

(B) Neither classical trigeminal neuralgia nor secondary trigeminal neuralgia has been confirmed by adequate investigation including electrophysiological tests and MRI

(C) Not better accounted for another ICHD-3 diagnosis.

This classification of the ICHD, established with the endorsement of the Neuropathic Pain Special Interest Group of the International Association for the Study of Pain by Cruccu and collaborators (2016), according to the most likely etiology after investigations (i.e., MRI) is the mostly adopted. The three groups described are secondary trigeminal neuralgia (related to other diseases of the nervous system—MS or tumors mostly), idiopathic trigeminal neuralgia, when no evident cause is found, and classical trigeminal neuralgia in patients in whom a vascular conflict of significance is found on the side of the neuralgia. Distinguishing patients with neurovascular conflict from other patients with trigeminal neuralgia may be criticized (Maarbjerg et al. 2015b) in the sense that trigeminal neuralgia may be multifactorial. However, this is the first classification system attempting to establish an etiologic basis for classification. Although not yet tested this may prove useful in the fact that patients with neurovascular conflicts could be identified and their treatment may be significantly different from that of other patients.

Knowledge on Trigeminal nerve anatomy is crucial for all of those who are dealing with the management of Trigeminal Neuralgia. The trigeminal nerve main function is to ensure sensory and some motor innervation to the face. The trigeminal nerve is composed of three branches, that join at the trigeminal ganglion, located within the trigeminal cave. These are known as the ophthalmic (V1), maxillary (V2), and mandibular (V3) nerves (Fig. 2.2).

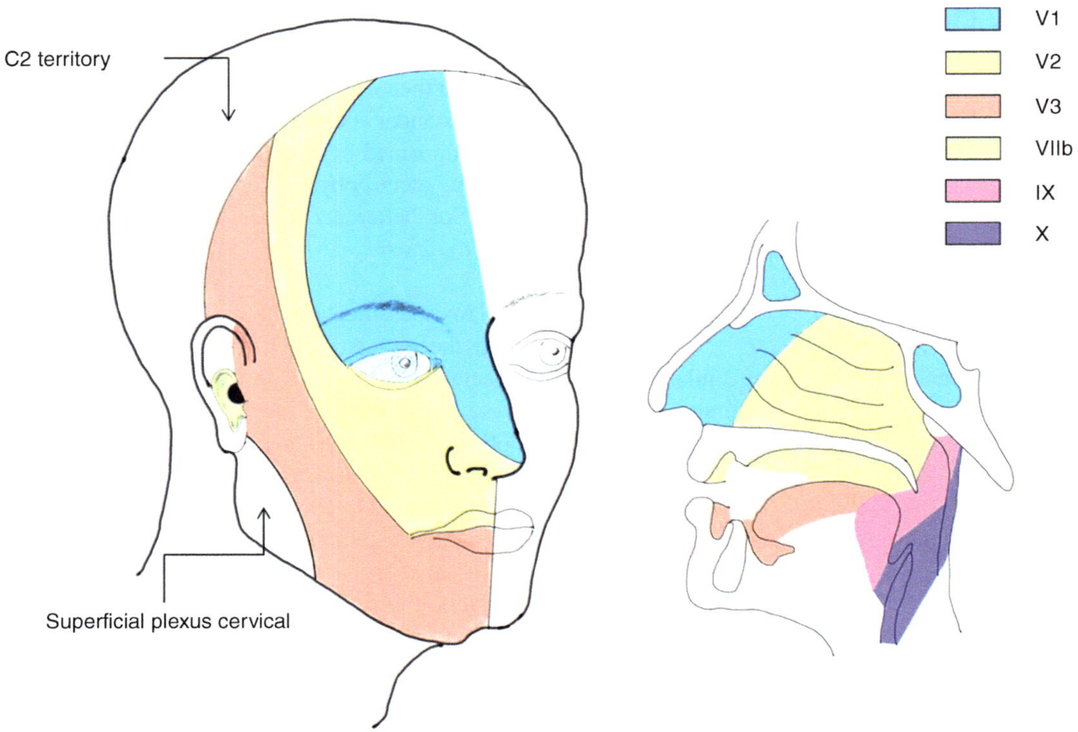


**Fig. 2.2** Cephalic sensory innervation and trigeminal divisions. The cutaneous territory innervated by the ophthalmic nerve division (V1) includes the anterior part of the temporal region, the forehead, the upper eyelid, and the dorsum of the nose. The mucous territory includes the frontal sinus, the sphenoidal sinus, and the nasal septum. V1 division also provides the sensation of the ocular and palpebral conjunctiva and particularly the cornea. The cutaneous territory of the maxillary division (V2) includes the midpart of the temporal region, the lower eyelid, the cheekbone area, the upper lip, the nostril, and the nasal vestibule. Its mucous territory includes the hard and soft palate, the Eustachian tube orifice, the upper pole of the tonsil, the maxillary sinus, the gum, the alveoli, and the maxillary teeth. The V3 nerve, which corresponds to the mandibular division, is the only mixed nerve of the three trigeminal branches. Its sensory cutaneous territory corresponds to the posterior temporal region, the anterior part of the outer ear, the anterior and superior walls of the external acoustic meatus, the lower lip, and the chin. Its mucous territory includes the anterior two-thirds of the tongue, the internal aspect of the cheek and roof of the mouth, the gum, the alveoli, and the mandible teeth. Its motor fibers innervate the masticatory muscles: the masseter, the temporalis, the medial and lateral pterygoids, the mylohyoid, the anterior belly of the digastric, and the tensor velum palatini muscles. Intermedius (VII bis); Glossopharyngeal nerve (IX); and Vagus nerve (X)

# Anatomy of the Trigeminal Nerve (TGN)

3

## 3.1 Descriptive Anatomy of the TGN

The trigeminal nerve (TGN) is the fifth cranial nerve and has three anatomical parts. The TGN is constituted of three nerves converging toward the trigeminal ganglion and is responsible for the sensation of the face.

The ophthalmic nerve (V1) enters the cranial cavity from the orbit via the superior orbital fissure and runs between the two layers of the dural lateral wall of the cavernous sinus. The maxillary nerve (V2) penetrates the skull base via the foramen rotundum. The mandibular nerve (V3) becomes endocranial through the foramen ovale, accompanied by the motor nerve responsible for the masticatory function (Fig. 3.1).

Noteworthy, the V2 (maxillary) and the V3 (mandibular) nerves do not belong to the cavernous sinus region itself, whereas the V1 (ophthalmic) nerve courses within the lateral wall of the cavernous sinus to transit from the superior orbital fissure to the trigeminal cave (Figs. 3.2 and 3.3).

Then the TGN extends from the trigeminal cave (TC), which is located in the middle fossa, to enter the cerebellopontine cistern in the posterior fossa through the porus trigeminus. Finally, the TGN penetrates into the ventral surface of the pons, with a large sensory and a smaller motor component (Fig. 3.4).

### 3.1.1 The Trigeminal Nerve in the Trigeminal Cave

The trigeminal cave of Meckel (TC) is the anatomical space where the trigeminal ganglion of Gasser (TGgl) and the retrogasserian portion of the sensory rootlets are located. There, the TGgl is crossed inferiorly by the motor nerve. The TC is formed by an expansion of the dura and the arachnoid of the posterior fossa that developed an anterior evagination laterally to the parasellar lodge, the latter being the so-called cavernous sinus.

The trigeminal cave contains cerebrospinal fluid which corresponds to the trigeminal cistern; this cistern is identifiable on high-resolution T2-MRI. The TC harbors the trigeminal ganglion—in its anterior part—and the triangular plexus of the trigeminal sensory root—in its posterior part. Both are surrounded by the trigeminal cistern at their superior part. There, the trigeminal motor root runs inferiorly to the triangular plexus and the TGgl to exit with the V3 mandibular sensory nerve through the foramen ovale, to innervate the masticatory muscles (Fig. 3.5).

The trigeminal ganglion has a semi-lunar shape with a convex anterior edge where the three peripheral nerves enter, and a concave posterior margin from which the sensory root emerges (Fig. 3.6). Between their emergence from the TGgl and the upper petrous ridge, rootlets form a trian-


M. Sindou, A. Brinzeu, *Trigeminal Neuralgias: A Neurosurgical Illustrated Guide*,
https://doi.org/10.1007/978-3-031-25113-9_3

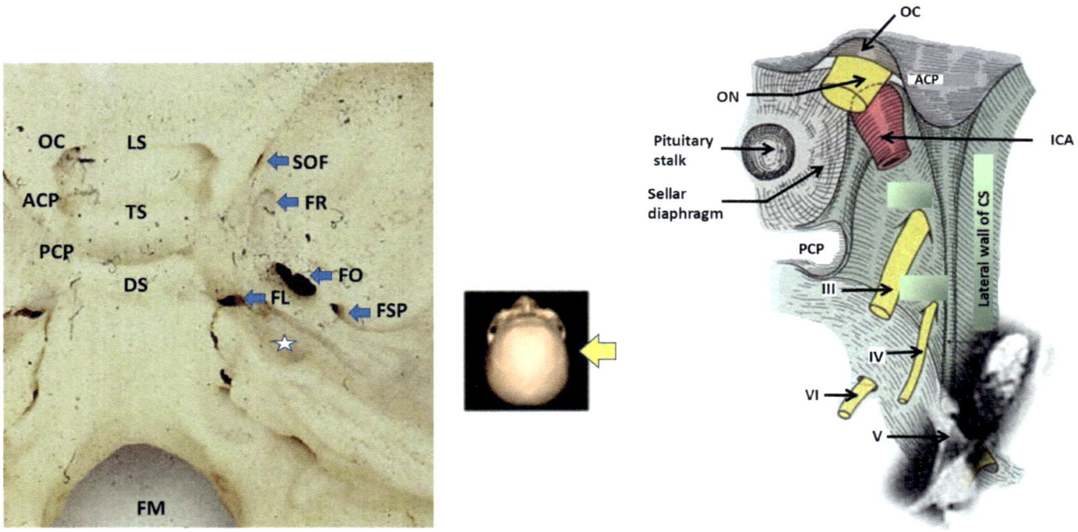


**Fig. 3.1** Superior view of the central skull base and the parasellar lodge with the Meckel's trigeminal cave laterally. The left image shows the following skull base foramina: the optic canal (OC), the superior orbital fissure (SOF), the foramen rotundum (FR), the foramen ovale (FO), the foramen spinosum (FSP), the foramen lacerum (FL). Image also shows the anterior (ACP) and posterior (PCP) clinoid processes, and the print of the trigeminal ganglion on the anterior aspect of the petrous pyramid (asterisk). *LS, TS, and DS* Limbus, Tuberculum, and Dorsum sellae, *FM* Foramen magnum; The right image shows the so-called cavernous sinus, which is an inter-periosteo-dural parasellar space, between the sellar lodge medially and the temporal fossa laterally. This lodge is crossed by the internal carotid artery (ICA) and the cranial nerves III, IV, and VI. *ON* Optic nerve; The right image also illustrates the trigeminal nerve (V), which enters the trigeminal cave, located laterally to the cavernous sinus. The trigeminal cave is a different anatomical space from the parasellar lodge. As shown on the superimposed MRI $T_2$-image, it contains cerebrospinal fluid which delineates the trigeminal ganglion within the trigeminal cistern

gle, named the triangular plexus (TP) (Fig. 3.7) because of its anastomoses. At the TP level, the sensory fibers have a somatotopic organization—similarly to the one of the ganglion level—before merging into the posterior root. Fibers of V3 are inferior-lateral, fibers of V1 are superior-medial, and fibers of V2 course in between.

Inside the trigeminal cave, the trigeminal ganglion and the triangular plexus are identifiable and dissectible. The TC can be accessed after its opening either by extradural or intradural (subtemporal) approach.

The findings from the histological studies of the trigeminal system at this level have been reviewed by Bernard et al. (2019). It was found that the cellular bodies of the sensory fibers, that is, the T-cells, are grouped in the TGgl. These cells send their axonal extensions toward the sensory nuclei in brainstem. Their peripheral (= dendritic) extensions form the fibers of the three nerves of the TGN (Emmons and Rhoton 1968).

Uryvaer et al. found fine "branches" (bundles of 50–150 microns in caliber) arising directly from the TGgl. and wrapped in an arachnoid covering corresponding to the trigeminal cistern (Uryvaev et al. 2008) These fine branches are supposed to innervate the dural walls of the trigeminal cave. Conversely, no connecting branches with the pericarotid plexus and the greater petrous nerve were seen.

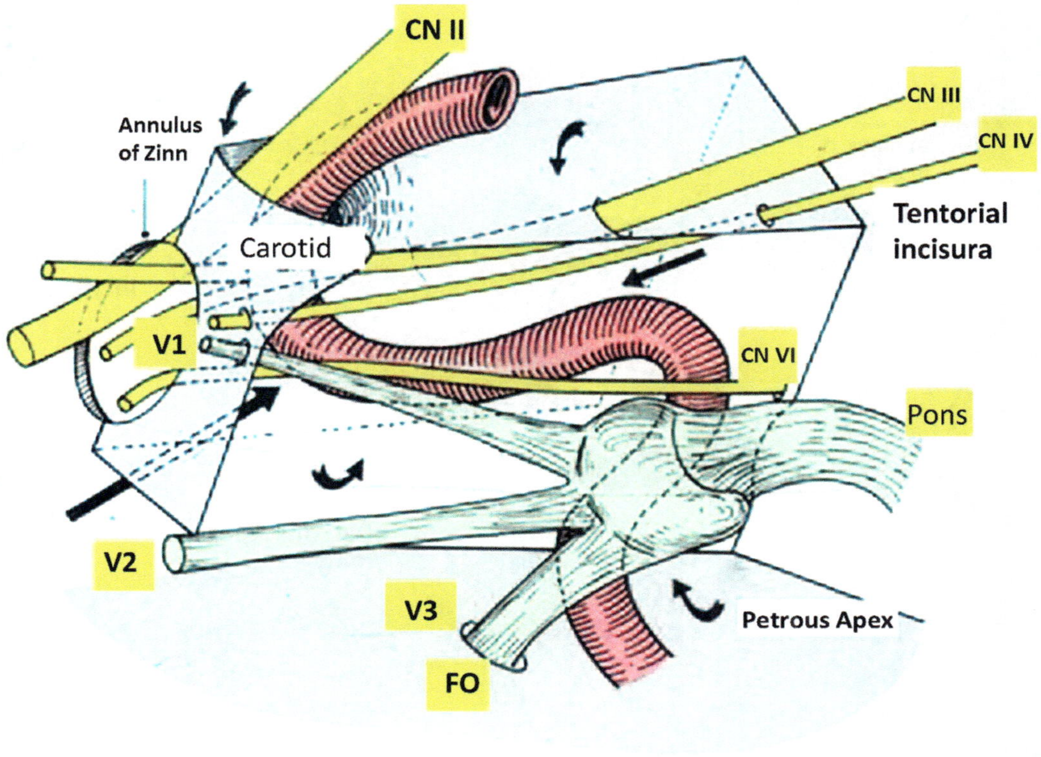


**Fig. 3.2** Spatial representation of the cavernous sinus (= parasellar lodge), and of the trigeminal cave and trigeminal nerve. The parasellar lodge and the orbital apex (seen laterally from left side) are both in continuity through the superior orbital fissure and the Annulus of Zinn. The trigeminal cave is an independent entity from the cavernous sinus. Black arrows indicate the various surgical entry points to the cavernous sinus. For abbreviations, see caption of Fig. 3.1

### 3.1.2 The Trigeminal Root in the Cerebellopontine Angle

The trigeminal root crosses the upper part of the cerebellopontine angle (CPA) over 2 cm length on average, to penetrate into the ventrolateral aspect of brainstem. The exit of root from the trigeminal cave is through the trigeminal porus, which is circumscribed by the upper petrous ridge, inferiorly, and the peripheral border of the tentorium, which contains the superior petrosal sinus, superiorly.

On crossing over the petrous ridge, the root is somewhat flat in the horizontal plane. In the CPA cistern it becomes cylindrical, approximately 5 mm in diameter in healthy nerves, then elliptical before attaining the pons (Fig. 3.8).

At entry into brainstem, at the so-called Trigeminal Root Entry Zone (TREZ), the sensory root divides into two components: (1) the pars major—the more voluminous—inferolaterally located and (2) the pars intermediaris formed by tiny rootlets, located in between the pars major

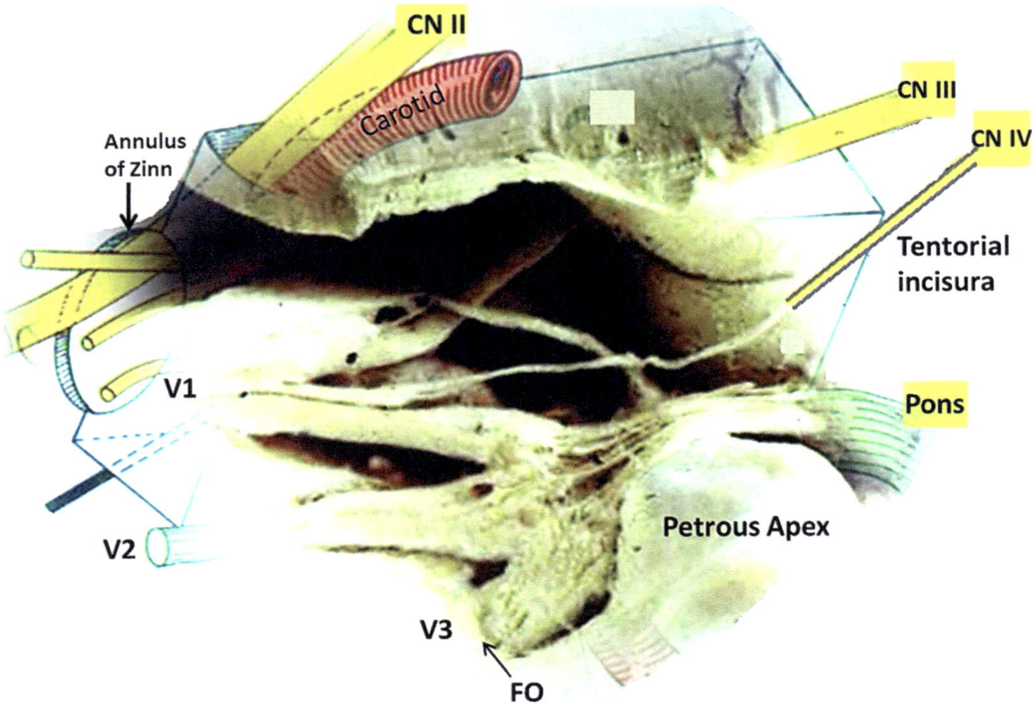


**Fig. 3.3** Contents of the cavernous sinus and Meckel cave. Spatial relationships of the cranial nerves in the central skull base region (seen laterally from left side). For abbreviations, see caption of Fig. 3.1

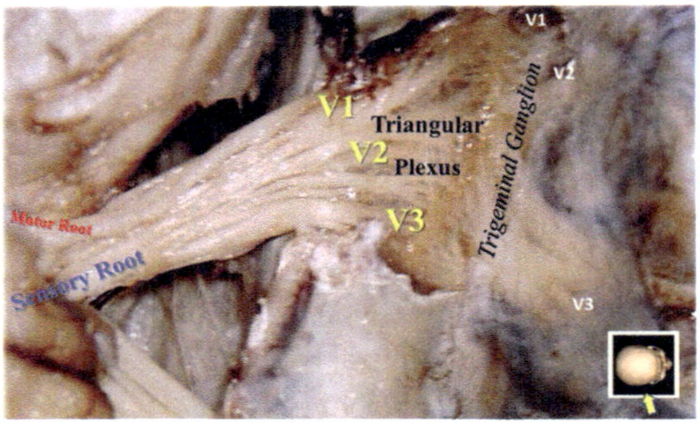


**Fig. 3.4** General view of the trigeminal nerve (TGN). Laboratory dissection of the (right) TGN; superior view after resection of the dural roof of the trigeminal cave

and the emergence of the motor root, superomedially, and named pars minor (Fig. 3.9).

In the cerebellopontine cistern the trigeminal root has several important anatomical relationships: rostrally, the superior cerebellar artery and the (tiny) trochlear cranial nerve coursing along the tentorium incisura and caudally, the cochleo-vestibular-facial nerve complex together with the anterior inferior cerebellar artery and its tributary: the labyrinthine artery. In its cisternal portion the trigeminal root is vascularized by small branches of the superior cerebellar artery. Posteriorly, the root is in close relationship with

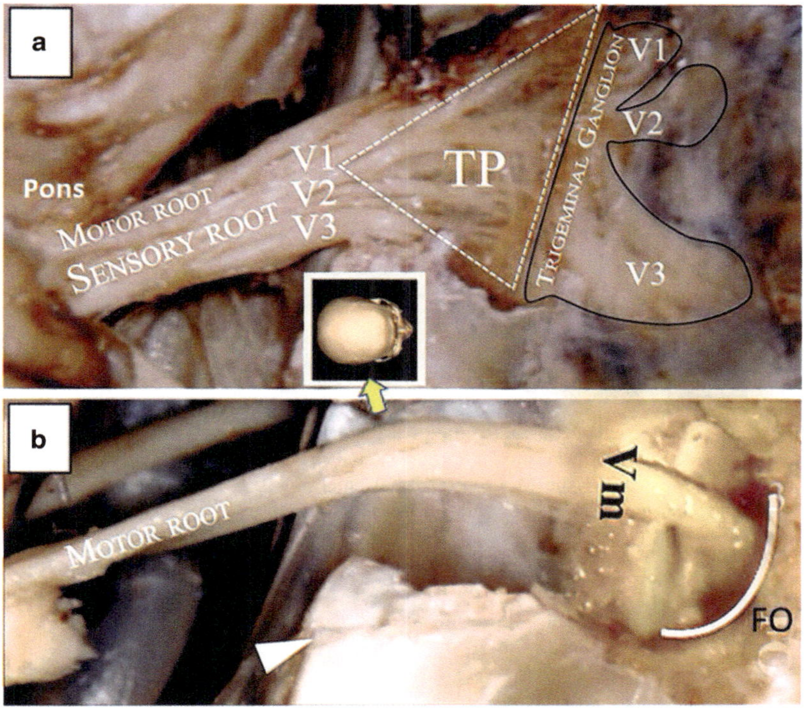


**Fig. 3.5** The motor root and nerve. Laboratory dissection of the (right) trigeminal motor root (superior view). (**a**) Motor root emerging from the pons at the superomedial border of the trigeminal root and situated medially along the cisternal portion of the root, then travelling below the triangular plexus (TP) and the ganglion to reach the foramen ovale together with the mandibular nerve (V3). (**b**) Motor nerve ($V_m$) after resection of the sensory root and trigeminal ganglion. See exit of $V_m$ through foramen ovale (FO)

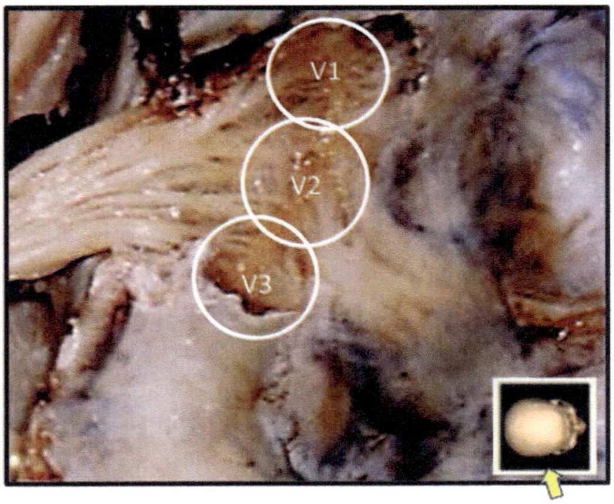


**Fig. 3.6** The trigeminal ganglion of gasser. Laboratory dissection of the (right) Gasserian Ganglion (G Ggl); superior view after resection of the dural roof of the trigeminal cave. The G Ggl has a semilunar shape and is trifoliated. It presents a convex anterior margin which receives the fibers of the peripheral branches and a concave posterior margin from which the axons of the sensory rootlets emerge. The Trigeminal G Ggl has a clearcut somatotopia with V1 medial and V3 lateral

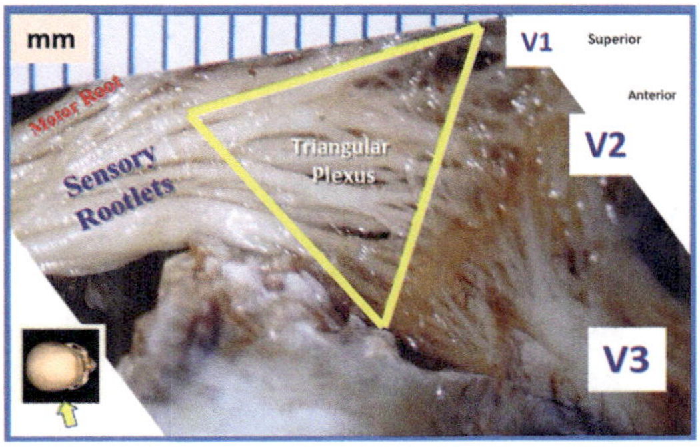


**Fig. 3.7** The triangular plexus. Laboratory dissection of the (right) trigeminal root at level of the triangular plexus. Superior view after removal of the roof of the trigeminal cave. The triangular plexus (yellow triangle) is exposed from the posterior margin of the trigeminal ganglion (anteriorly) to the crossing of the root over the petrous ridge (posteriorly). The triangular plexus is characterized by anastomoses between the sensory rootlets. In spite of its anastomoses the triangular plexus has still a clearcut somatotopia, with V1 medially, V3 laterally, and V2 in between

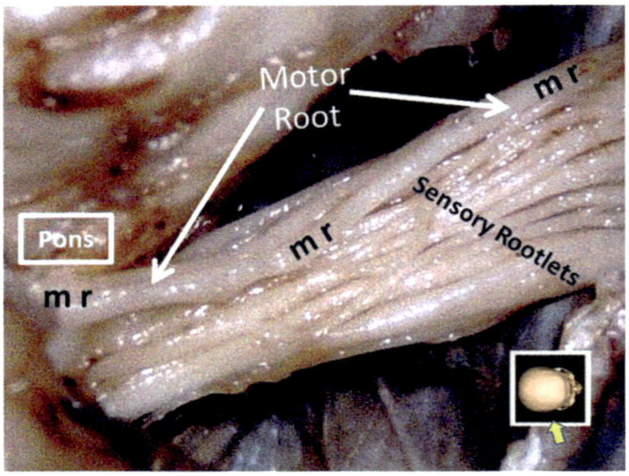


**Fig. 3.8** The cisternal portion of the root. Laboratory dissection of the cisternal portion of the root on right side. Superior view showing the Motor Root (mr) emerging from pons, and the sensory root with all its constituting rootlets

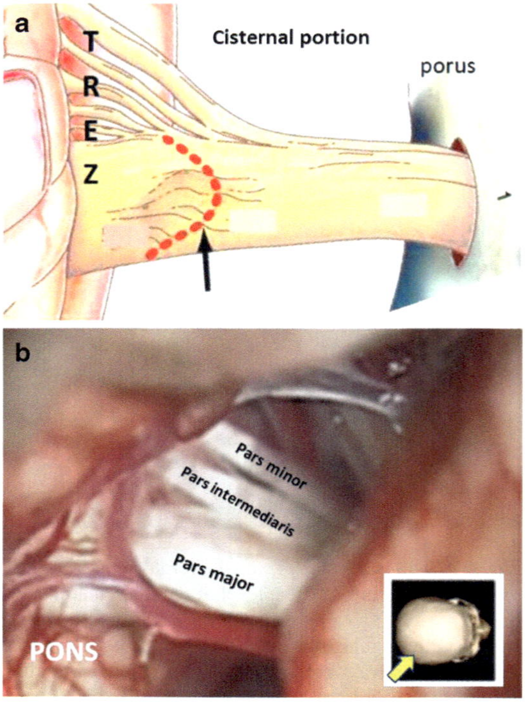


**Fig. 3.9** The juxta-pontine portion of the root. Posterior view of the juxta-pontine portion of the root on right side. (**a**) Schematic drawing of the Trigeminal Root Entry Zone (TREZ). Arrow indicates the Transitional Zone (dotted curve). (**b**) Microsurgical operative view of TREZ in the right cerebellopontine angle, with its different components: Pars minor, Pars intermediaris, and Pars major, at pons

the superior petrosal vein and its affluents, often stuck to the root.

### 3.1.3 The Trigeminal Root Entry Zone

There is a large agreement to consider the Trigeminal Root Entry Zone (TREZ) as a particularly "sensitive" zone (i.e., more excitable), so that vascular compression there is prone to elicit neuralgia. To our knowledge TREZ has not received any official taxonomic definition. However, for most authors TREZ corresponds essentially to that portion of the root which is of central myelin nature.

Obersteiner and Redlich stated that there was a transitional zone between the peripheral nervous system and the central nervous system in the brain, similarly to what has been described for the spinal cord (Obersteiner and Redlich 1884; Tarlov 1937a, b). In the peripheral portion, myelin sheaths are produced by Schwann cells and the supporting tissues include fibroblasts, collagen fibrils, and root sheath cells. In the central portion, myelin sheaths are produced by oligodendrocytes, and nerve fibers are partly separated from one another by astrocytes. Skinner measured the length of the central myelin portion of all cranial nerves and observed a dome shape of the central myelin-peripheral myelin transitional zone; he stated that the central myelin portion was longer in sensory nerves than in motor nerves (Skinner 1931). Tarlov stated that the central glial segment of a nerve presented essentially the structure of a fiber tract of the brain, its peripheral segment corresponding to a peripheral nerve (Tarlov 1937a, b). In a "stimulating" paper on the epidemiological plane, De Ridder et al. considered positively the correlation between the length of central nervous system segment, which differs among cranial nerves, and the incidence of the corresponding vascular compression syndromes (De Ridder et al. 2002). Peker et al. showed that central myelin occupied only the initial one-fourth of the trigeminal nerve length (Peker et al. 2006). More recently our group car-

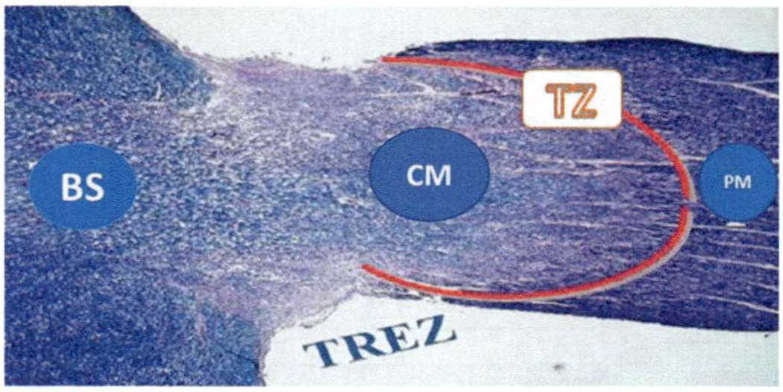


**Fig. 3.10** The central myelin portion of the trigeminal root. Photomicrograph of a longitudinal section of the trigeminal root at the Trigeminal Root Entry Zone (TREZ), stained with hematoxylin phloxine saffron and luxol fast blue which allow to differentiate the portion with central myelin (CM), produced by the oligodendrocytes, and the portion with peripheral myelin (PM), produced by the Schwann cells. Those two portions join at the Transitional Zone (TZ). *BS* brainstem

ried out structural studies of cranial nerves (V, VII, VIII, IX, X) in cadavers for enlarging anatomical knowledge and better understand pathophysiology of hyperactive cranial nerve syndromes (Guclu et al. 2011) (Fig. 3.10).

In our view, TREZ should include the transitional zone, the central myelin portion of the root, and the adjacent region of brainstem where root fibers have subpial paths on their way from or to their respective nuclei (Fig. 3.11).

These structures are likely to be considered as a whole harboring anatomical-physiological higher sensitiveness and excitability, likely explaining respective incidences of the cranial nerve hyperactive syndromes (Fig. 3.12).

**Fig. 3.11** Schematic representation of the TREZ. The root entry zone (for sensory nerves), similarly to the root exit zone (for motor nerves), can be considered as constituted of three elements: (1) the transitional zone (TZ) of Obersteiner–Redlich (OR), (2) the central myelin portion of the root, (3) the adjacent region of the brainstem where the afferent fibers are travelling

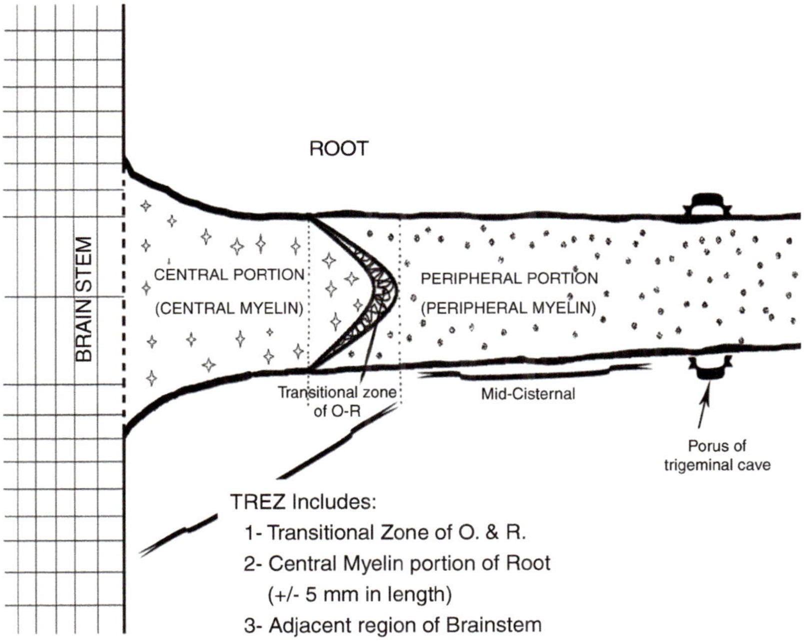

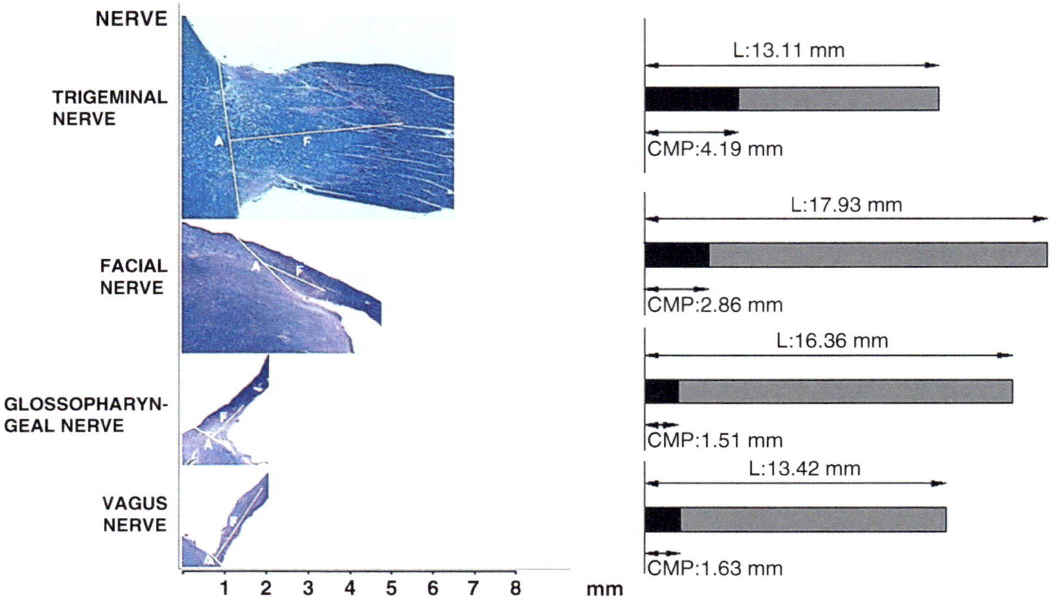


**Fig. 3.12** Length of the central myelin portion for the various cranial nerves, in the cerebellopontine angle (Guclu et al. 2011). Left: photomicrographs of the trigeminal, the facial, the glossopharyngeal and the vagus nerve roots, in longitudinal section. To establish comparison of lengths all the nerve roots are represented at same magnification scale. Right: mean values of the lengths of the central myelin portions (CMP) and of the corresponding entire intracranial portions (L), for each CN studied

## 3.2 Functional Anatomy of the TGN

The primary function of the trigeminal nerve is sensory input from the face and head cavities. Tactile and thermo-algesic fibers of the three divisions originate in the primary neurons situated in the trigeminal ganglion. From here the centrifugal fibers of the pseudo-unipolar sensory neurons run to the pons. Inside the brainstem two sensory nuclei receive the fibers from the trigeminal ganglion: in the pons, the principal trigeminal nucleus receiving the large tactile fibers, and in the medulla oblongata and upper cervical spinal cord, the spinal nucleus of the trigeminal tract which receives the small fibers related to nociception and temperature sensation (Haskel et al. 1995).

A somatotopic organization of the sensory fibers has been recognized not only in the trigeminal ganglion but also in the trigeminal root, particularly in its retrogasserian portion, named the triangular plexus (Bernard et al. 2019). There, the fibers from V3 (mandibular afferent fibers) are situated in a lateral position, with the V1 (ophthalmic) afferent fibers in a medial position, and the V2 (maxillary) afferent fibers taking an intermediate position (Fig. 3.13). These fibers then traverse the major sensory root of the trigeminal nerve to reach the pons. This cisternal portion of the nerve has an elliptical cross-section with the fibers having still relatively somatotopic and not yet functional organization with the V1 fibers situated supero-medially, the V3 fibers infero-laterally, and the V2 fibers somewhat intermediate to these.

This view of a somatotopic organization of the retrogasserian trigeminal root is corroborated by data from anatomical and surgical studies. Microsurgical dissection studies in cadavers (Emmons and Rhoton 1968; Gudmundsson et al. 1971; Joo et al. 2014) showed that the three trigeminal topographical divisions are well-delineated in the root at least immediately

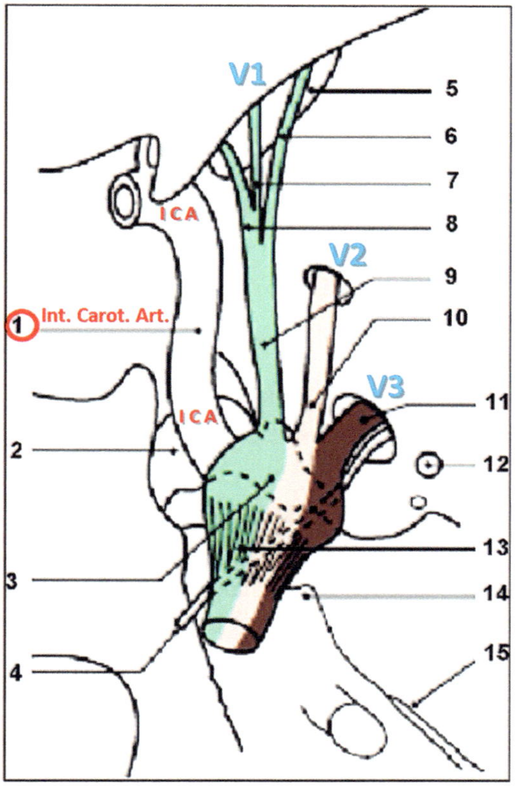


**Fig. 3.13** Location and somatotopia of the trigeminal nerve (Schematic representation, in upper view, on right side). The trigeminal nerve is located inside the trigeminal cave of Meckel, which is situated laterally to the cavernous sinus lodge where the internal carotid artery (1) passes after entering the foramen lacerum (2). There, the trigeminal ganglion of Gasser (3) occupies the anterior part of the trigeminal cave, lying over the motor branch (4) which runs along the inferior wall of the cave. The ganglion receives the following sensory peripheral branches: first, through the superior orbital fissure (5): the lacrymal (6), frontal (7) and naso-ciliary (8) branches, forming the ophthalmic nerve (9) which corresponds to the first trigeminal division (V1); second, entering the cranial cavity through the foramen rotundum, the maxillary nerve (10), which corresponds to the second division (V2); third, through the foramen ovale, accompanied by the (efferent) masticatory motor nerve, the mandibular nerve (11), which corresponds to the sensory third division (V3). As a surgical landmark, when approaching the trigeminal cave extradurally, the foramen ovale is situated medially to the foramen spinosum (12) where the middle meningeal artery penetrates into the cerebral middle fossa. Note the clear-cut somatotopia, not only at level of the gasserian ganglion but also at level of the triangular plexus (13). Posteriorly, the trigeminal root enters the posterior cerebral fossa crossing over the upper ridge of the petrous apex (14), inferiorly to the superior petrosal sinus (15)

posteriorly to the trigeminal ganglion, that is, in the so-called triangular plexus. Also, during percutaneous radiofrequency-thermo-rhizotomy, it was observed that direct stimulation of the root at triangular plexus level—for strict placement of the electrode in the sensory rootlets corresponding to the trigger zone—elicits sensory responses under the form of paresthesias somatotopically distributed (Sweet and Wepsic 1974; Sindou and Keravel 1979; Karol et al. 1991; Kanpolat et al. 2001; Peris-Celda et al. 2013). Furthermore, subsequent thermo-lesioning, when performed infero-laterally in the triangular plexus or in the neighboring cisternal portion of the root, produces hypoesthesia mainly in the V3 and more or less in the V2 territories, and when performed more supero-medially, preferentially in the V2/V1 territories. This somatotopic organization is also in accordance with the neurophysiological studies by Sindou et al., who—for guiding the targeting of thermo-rhizotomies—performed direct stimulation of the sensory root with EMG-recordings together with video-recordings of the face (Sindou et al. 1994; Tatli and Sindou 2008). According to the placement of the probe in the trigeminal root (as described above), stimulation provoked not only paresthesias in the expected V1, V2, or V3 territories but also twitches in the orbicularis oculi, levator labii, or orbicularis oris muscles, respectively. These clinically observable phenomena were considered trigemino-facial reflexes, and were subsequently used for intraoperative neurophysiological guidance because of their localizing value (Sindou 1999).

On penetrating the pons, the root undergoes a functional rearrangement with three distinct components: the pars minor (superomedial), with a motor function, the pars major (inferolateral), sensory and mostly thermo-algesic, and in between, the pars intermediaris considered as specially harboring the corneal sensory fibers (Fig. 3.14).

At the juxta-pontine level, the sensory fibers tend to locate according to their destiny and therefore function (Fig. 3.15). The thermo-algesic fibers regroup in the pars major to then follow the descending tract down to the spinal

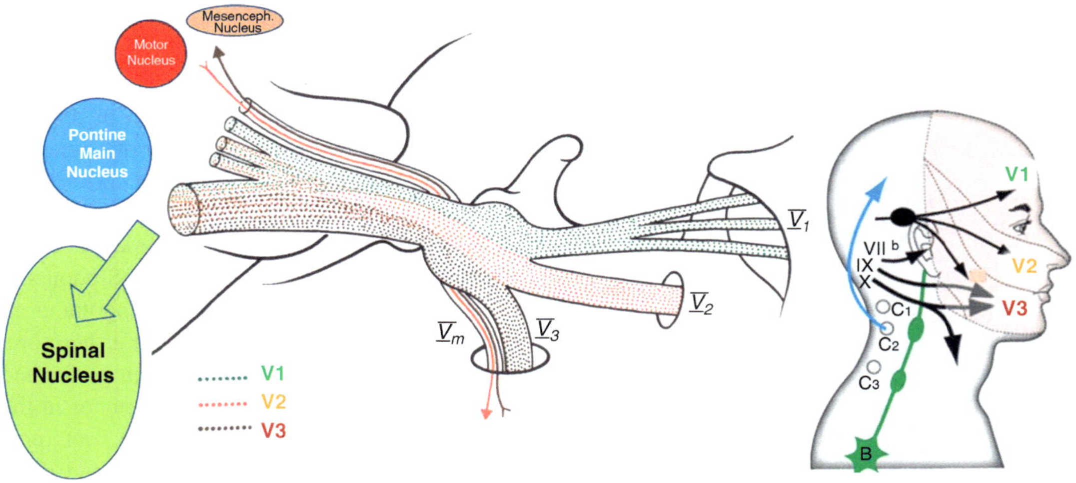


**Fig. 3.14** Somatotopia of the trigeminal fibers (lateral view, on right side). At the triangular plexus and the initial retrogasserian portion of the sensory root, the axonal fibers issued from the ganglionic bipolar T-shaped cells have a clearcut somatotopic organization. In the root the fibers from the mandibular nerve cells ($V_3$) predominate infero-laterally, those originating from the ophtalmic nerve ($V_1$) supero-medially, and those from the maxillary nerve ($V_2$) in between. This arrangement is clearer in the retrogasserian than in the juxta-pontine portion of the root, where the fibers are redistributed according to their destination in the brainstem, by means of anastomoses between the three contingents from the three branches, beginning in the triangular plexus. This is how the thermo-algesic (mainly nociceptive) fibers place with an inferolateral predominance, forming the pars major, to then travelling through the descending tract to the spinal nucleus, located in the spinal cord-medullary junction. The epicritic and proprioceptive fibers are more supero-medially situated, to reach the main pontine nucleus; these fibers can be individualized and termed as the pars intermediaris. Noteworthy, the superomedial "third" of the pars major and the pars intermediaris contain the sensory corneal fibers. This repartition explains the analgesic effect—without complete tactile anesthesia and without corneal anesthesia—obtained after partial section of the pars major in the selective juxtapontine rhizotomy procedure. The motor root emerges from the pons in a supero-medial position to the sensory root constituting the pars minor of the Vth cranial nerve, then crosses the trigeminal cave below the gasserian ganglion, to become satellite of the mandibular nerve at exit through the foramen ovale. The proprioceptive and myotatic fibers of the Vth—most from the masticatory muscles—after having travelled retrogradely in the pars minor, form the mesencephalic tract in brainstem to terminate into the mesencephalic nucleus. The cells of this nucleus send fibers onto the (pontine) motor nucleus, thus playing a role in relaying information for the regulation of the Vth motor nerve

trigeminal nucleus at the spinal cord—medullary junction (Fig. 3.16). Also classically, the epicritic and proprioceptive fibers would preferentially transit in the pars intermediaris to reach the pontine principal nucleus.

Despite such functional rearrangement clinical and surgical observations show—at this level of the root—a still relative somatotopic organization of the fibers. After partial juxta-pontine rhizotomy, by definition performed just at the entry of the nerve in brainstem, it was observed that a section of only the inferolateral portion of the pars major allows preservation of the sensory function in V1 and more or less V2 (Dandy 1925; Terrier et al. 2018).

Regarding the cornea innervation, the corneal reflex, which is the substratum of a protective autonomic and somatic function including blinking and lacrimation, obeys to nociceptive mechanisms. Electrophysiological and histological studies have shown that cornea is innervated by A delta and C fibers. Classically, it is considered that corneal fibers run into the pars intermediaris. Differently, Terrier et al. on their surgical experience assume that all corneal fibers run along the dorsomedial third of the pars major (Terrier et al.

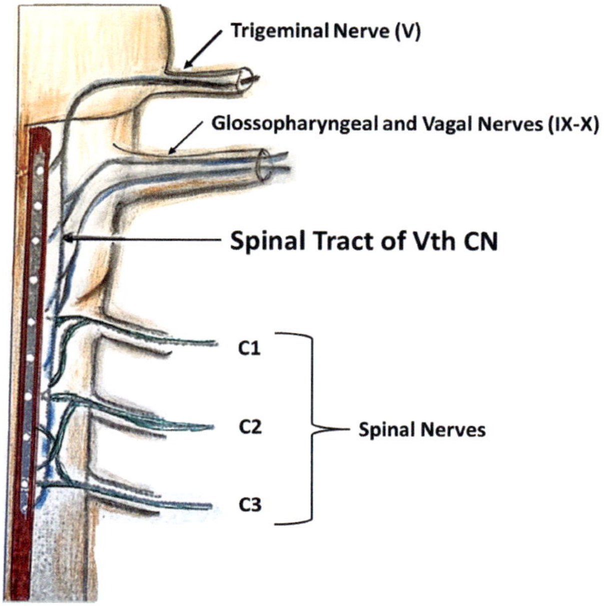


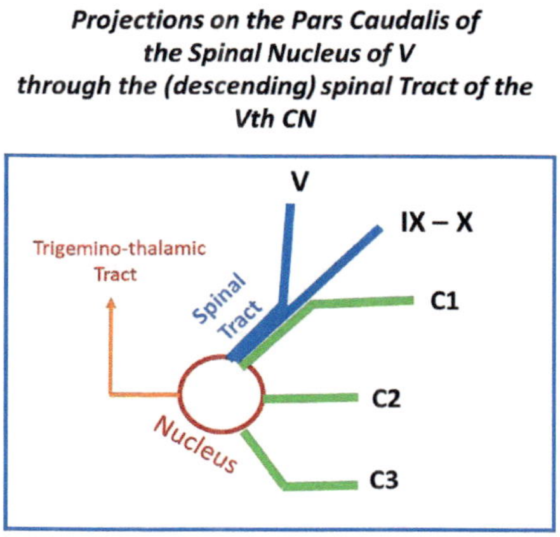


**Fig 3.15** Schematic drawing of projections onto the trigeminal tract and spinal nucleus. The sensory axons of the trigeminal nerve project onto the brainstem trigeminal nuclear complex which is composed of the main pontine nucleus and the spinal nucleus. The later comprises the interpolaris and the caudalis subnuclei. The large fibers, devoted to discriminative touch, project onto the pontine main nucleus. The small myelinated and the unmyelinated fibers, mostly thermal and nociceptive, go to the spinal nucleus through the descending spinal tract. Both are located as far as the third segment of the spinal cord, in a dorsolateral situation covered by the spino-cerebellar tract. The nociceptive fibers from the VIIth, IXth, and Xth cranial nerves, and also the fibers from the upper cervical spinal nerves, join the descending spinal tract and the caudalis part of the spinal nucleus. A rostro-caudal somatotopic organization of the subnucleus caudalis has been described, corresponding to an "onion-rings" pattern (Drake and McKenzie 1953; McKenzie 1954), the lips and lower nose territory being highest in the subnucleus, the most lateral regions of the face being more caudal in the subnucleus. To be noted, the caudalis part of the nucleus is in continuity with the gray of the dorsal horn of the spinal cord, and is hypothesized playing some role in the pain control. Also of paramount importance, the spinal nucleus is a region of convergent projections from the entire cephalic extremity. Then the fibers arising from the spinal nucleus project to a large number of encephalic structures, especially the reticular formation and the thalamus (similarly to the ascending spino-reticular tracts)

2017, 2018). Whatever that is, limiting the rhizotomy to the inferolateral two-thirds of the pars major would likely be the way to avoid corneal ulcer caused by sensory impairment.

Actually, the exact transition point between the two types of organization: somatotopic versus functional, is still uncertain, and remains to be further studied. Good knowledge of the morphological and functional anatomy of the TGN has important surgical implications.

In brainstem the afferent axons terminate on the trigeminal nuclear complex, which is composed of the principal (=main) sensory nucleus, located in pons, and the spinal trigeminal nucleus, caudally located. The later comprises three subnuclei: oralis, interpolaris, and caudalis. Within brainstem, the trigeminal afferent fibers separate into (1) ascending axons, which project onto the principal nucleus, and (2) descending axons, which form the well-circumscribed spinal tract that—whilst descending—distributes collateral branches to the several trigeminal spinal subnuclei for sensory information. Inside the spinal subnuclei, especially the subnucleus caudalis, the face is considered to be represented as a series of concentric bands, in other words with an "onionskin-shape" organization. The fibers corresponding to peri-oral region would terminate highest in the caudalis subnucleus, the fibers of successively more lateral regions of the face suc-

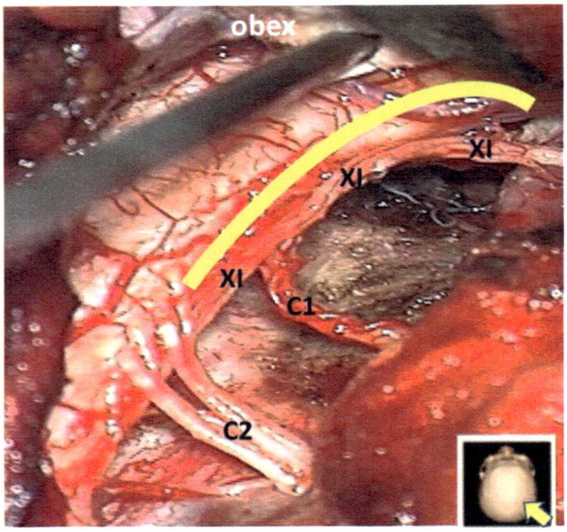


**Fig. 3.16** Location of the (caudalis) spinal nucleus, together with the trigeminal descending tract. Operative view of exposure of the dorsolateral aspect of the cranio-vertebral junction (on right side), after hemilaminectomy of $C_2$, $C_1$, and bony resection of the adjacent margin of the foramen magnum, and opening of the corresponding dura-mater. Landmarks: obex, dorsal rootlets of $C_2$, ventral rootlets of $C_1$ (dorsal rootlets of $C_1$ are most often absent), spinal rootlets of the accessory cranial nerve (XIth); Situation of the trigeminal spinal nucleus is at 3–4 mm in depth, covered by the overlying spino-cerebellar tract. Location extends in length from the $C_2$ dorsal root up to the axial level of the obex. Width is from the lateral margin of the dorsal column and cuneate nucleus, medially, and the line of exit of the rootlets of the spinal component of the XIth nerve, laterally; Projection to surface pia-mater corresponds to the dorsolateral nucleus line (yellow curve line)

cessively in more caudal parts of the subnucleus. According to our (speculative) view on the central (hyperactive) mechanisms of the trigeminal neuralgias, including those of the classical category—induced by the (peripheral) neurovascular insults of the root—such representation of the face seems concordant with the (frequent) topographies of the neuralgias and their trigger-zones.

**Key-Point**

*Importance of the somatotopic organization of the TGN*:

Good knowledge of the morphological and functional anatomy of the TGN has important surgical implications.

The TGN presents gross anatomical, microanatomical, electrophysiological, and histological particularities dominated by its somatotopic organization, not only at level of the ganglion and the triangular plexus part of the retrogasserian portion of the root, but also—although to a lesser degree—in its cisternal and TREZ portions.

Regarding classical trigeminal neuralgias, the somatotopic organization of the fibers explains the concordance between the location of the neurovascular conflict with its resulting insult and the distribution of the pain.

Also, the somatotopic organization permits targeting the lesioning-techniques to obtain a selective analgesia/hypoesthesia corresponding to the trigger zone(s) and covering the trigeminal division(s) involved, whilst sparing the rootlets not related to the clinical manifestations.

# 4 Anatomy of the Neighbouring Vessels and Structures Surrounding the Trigeminal Nerve

## 4.1 Arteries

In our series an artery was found in 93% of the patients, mostly alone, sometimes in association with a vein. A vein, alone or in combination with an arterial compression, was found in 27.6% of the cases, respectively in 7% and 20.6%. The arterial agents found in our 579 patients' series are summarized in Table 4.1. *Agents* were the superior cerebellar artery (SCA), alone or in association with one or more other vessels, in 88% of the cases (Fig. 4.1); a loop of the anterior-inferior cerebellar artery (AICA), alone or in association, in 25.1% of the cases (Fig. 4.2); and a vertebrobasilar megadolicho-artery (VBA), alone or in combination, in 3.5% of the cases (Fig. 4.3) (Sindou et al. 2002).

In another personal study the situation of the NVC in relation to the root—respectively the TREZ, the cisternal portion, or at exit from porus—was investigated in 100 consecutive cases (Brinzeu et al. 2018a). Site was TREZ, cisternal portion, juxta-porus portion, in respectively 28%, 67%, 4% for the SCA ($n = 75$); 67%, 33%, nil for the AICA ($n = 12$); and 75%, 25%, nil for the VBA ($n = 4$). To be mentioned, pure venous conflicts were nine in number, with equal repartition between cistern and juxta-porus portion.

**Table 4.1** Neuro-vascular conflicts from arterial origin found at surgery[a]

| |
|---|
| • *Superior cerebellar artery* (alone or in association with other vessel, arterial or venous) in 88% of the patient series |
| • *Anterior-Inferior cerebellar artery* (alone or in association with other vessel, arterial or venous) in 25.1% of the patient series |
| • *Megadolicho-Vertebro-Basilar artery* (alone or in association with other vessel, arterial or venous) in 3.5% of the patient series |
| NB: The sum of the percentages, superior to 100%, is explained by the high number of patients with multiple conflicts in a same individual: in one-third of the patients in the series |

[a]Data from personal series of 579 patients who underwent MVD for. Classical Trigeminal Neuralgia over the 1992–2002 period (Ref.: Sindou et al. 2002)

Location of the arterial compression in relation to the circumference of the root was superior for the SCA (mostly at the TREZ or the cisternal portion), half being superomedial and half superolateral. The SCA was generally found bifurcating in two branches, with important laxity and few collaterals or perforators, so that they could be rather easily mobilized and transposed (Sindou et al. 2002). As regards AICA, location was almost always inferior to the TREZ, with frequently short perforators to the pons.


M. Sindou, A. Brinzeu, *Trigeminal Neuralgias: A Neurosurgical Illustrated Guide*,
https://doi.org/10.1007/978-3-031-25113-9_4

**Key-Point**

*Neurovascular conflicts are in majority from elongated arteries neighboring to the root.*

Compression can be of more or less important degree: a mere contact with the root (grade I), a displacement of the root (grade II), or a deformation of the root with engrooving and focal demyelination (grade III).

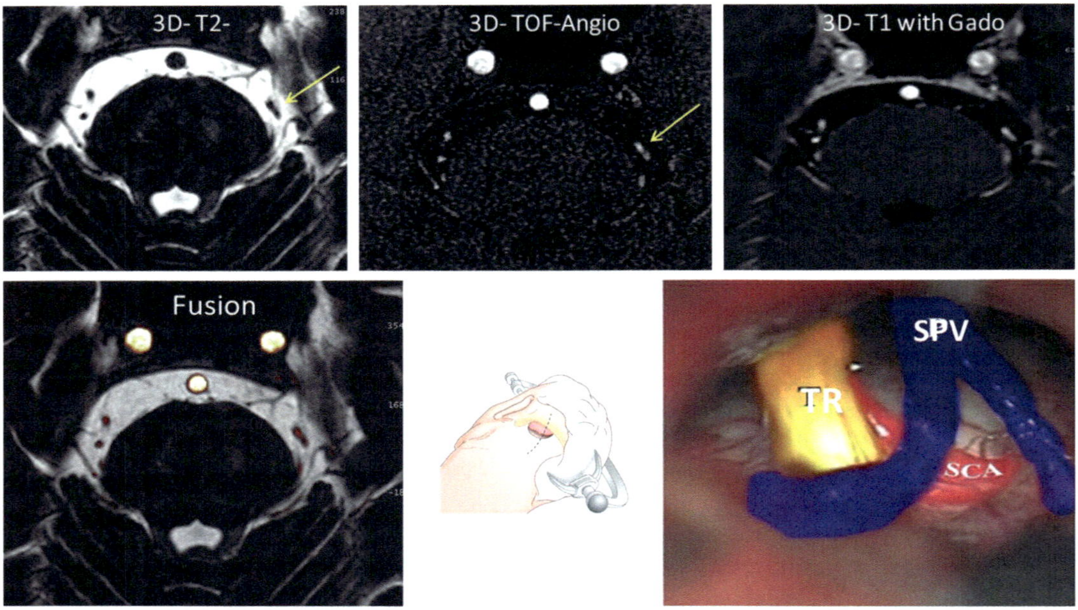


**Fig. 4.1** Left classical trigeminal neuralgia due to Neuro-Vascular Conflict (NVC) from the *Superior Cerebellar Artery* (SCA) situated in a superomedial position on the trigeminal root (TR). The NVC could be predicted on high-resolution MRI using the three sequences: 3D-T2, 3D-TOF-Angio and T1 with gadolinium, in association, and also fusion. Note preservation of the superior petrosal vein (SPV). See Imaging Assessment for interpretation

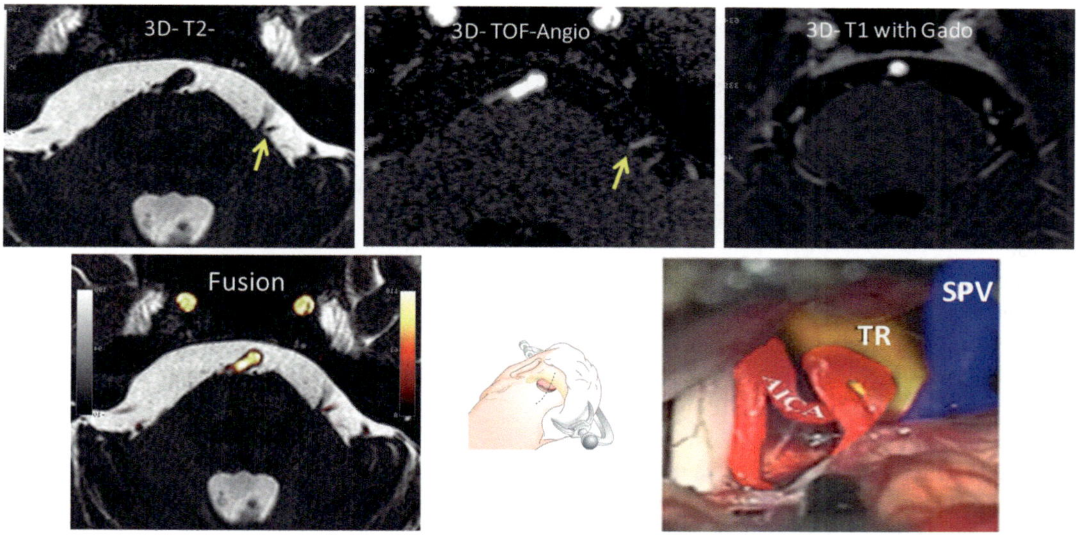


**Fig. 4.2** Left classical trigeminal neuralgia due to Neuro-Vascular Conflict (NVC) from the *Anterior-Inferior Cerebellar Artery* (AICA) situated in an inferior position on the trigeminal root (TR). The NVC could be predicted on high-resolution MRI using the three sequences: 3D-T2, 3D-TOF-Angio and T1 with gadolinium, and fusion. Note preservation of the superior petrosal vein (SPV). See Assessment for interpretation

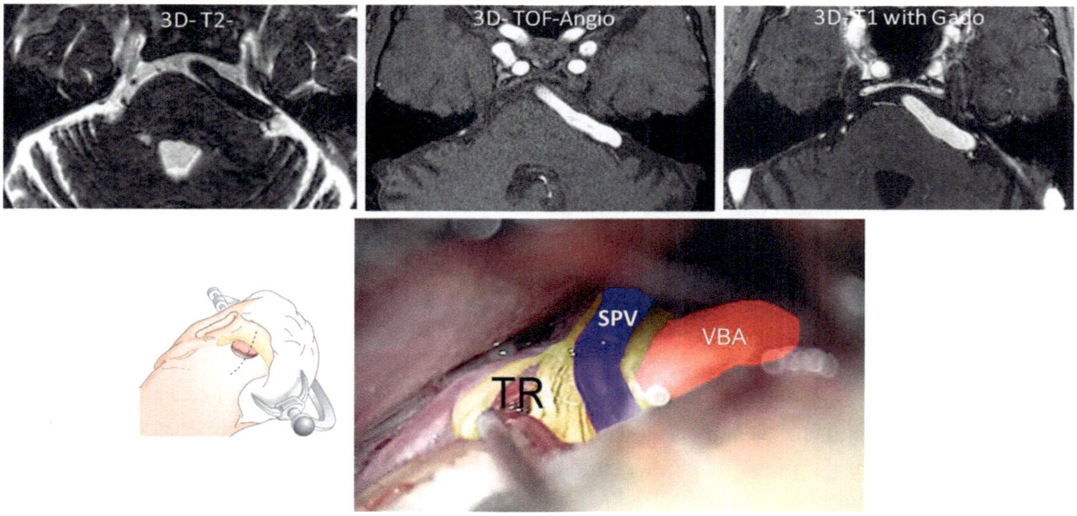


**Fig. 4.3** Left classical, atypical, that is, paroxysmal pain with a background of permanent pain, due to neuro-vascular conflict. Conflict was severe compression and stretching of the trigeminal root (TR) by a *megadolicho-VertebroBasilar Artery* (VBA), as shown on corresponding high-resolution MRI. Note the superior petrosal vein (SPV) parallel to the root

## 4.2 Veins

Implication of venous compression has long been and still is a matter of debate. However, several studies have brought some solid evidence of their implication, either in combination with arterial conflict or as the sole responsible factor.

According to a literature review which regrouped 31 publications harvested from the Pubmed system during the 1995–2014 period, rates of venous involvement were reported ranging from 13 to 58% with an average of 25.3% (Dumot and Sindou 2015). Such diversity can be explained by the difficulty to assure the compressive effect of the venous vessel, or to be certain of the real role of the vein when found associated to an arterial conflict.

In those publications veins were described as the only conflicting vessel in 4.4–18% (13.5% on average). In cases with multiple conflicts—estimated at 8–40% for the patients with classical TN, 38% in our own series (Sindou et al. 2002)—veins were involved alongside arteries in 7.2–56% (20.3% on average).

In a personal study aiming to be an inventory of the various types of vessels that we considered implicated in neurovascular conflicts the incidence of venous contact/compression was as high as 38% (Sindou et al. 2002). Types of implicated veins are summarized in Table 4.2. In 29.1% the venous compression was associated to an arterial compression and in 8.9% the vein was the sole compressive vessel. In half of the later, the conflicting factor was the Inferior Transverse Vein (Matsushima et al. 1983) and was located at exit of the root from the porus of the trigeminal cave. In approximately half of the 38% (17.6%) the vein exerted a marked compression on the root.

In our study, venous compressions were not only at TREZ (17%), but also at the mid-cisternal portion of the root (40%) or the porus (33%) (Dumot and Sindou 2015). This large distribution of locations justifies a systematic exploration of the entire root, from brainstem to trigeminal cave.

**Table 4.2** Types of veins found implicated in neurovascular conflicts at surgery[a]

- *Veins found implicated in 136 cases (i.e., 23% of the overall series of 579 pts)*
  - Vein alone: in 35 pts (26% of the 136)
  - Vein and artery (mixed): in 101 pts (74% of the 136)
- *Superficial SPV System: Total 81 (60% of the venous conflicts); vein alone in 22 and vein and artery (mixed) in 59*
  - Trunk of superior petrosal vein: 20 (14.7% of the 136); 5 alone and 5 mixed
  - Mesencephalic V.: 9 (6.6% of the 136); 2 alone and 7 mixed
  - Cerebellar V.: 2 (1.5% of the 136); 1 alone and 1 mixed
  - Pontine V.: 48 (35.3% of the 136); 13 alone and 35 mixed
  - Unspecified tributaries: 2 (1.5% of the 136); 1 alone and 1 mixed
- *Deep SPV System: Total 55 (40% of the venous conflicts); vein alone in 13 and vein and artery (mixed) in 42*

[a]Data from personal series of 579 patients who underwent MVD for classical trigeminal neuralgia (Sindou et al. 2002)
*V* vein, *sSPV System* superficial superior petrosal venous system, *dSPV System* deep superior petrosal venous system. Percentages are in parentheses

**Key-Point**

*Criteria for retaining a vein as a compressive factor*

- On imaging including T2-sequence, TOF – Angio and T1 + Gadolinium, vein making a cross-compression rather than having a parallel course.
- On intraoperative exploration, from brainstem to porus of Meckel cave, vein making a cross-compression rather than having a parallel course, especially if there is a greyish discoloration of the root at level of the compression.

Denomination of veins on imaging and at surgical exploration is often difficult because of their high variability (Matsushima et al. 1983; Rhoton 2000). For practical use, we developed a simplified denomination of the veins in relation to the trigeminal root adapted to the currently used Keyhole approach via the infratentorial-supracerebellar route (Dumot and Sindou 2015).

Almost all the veins in relation with the trigeminal root (TR) drain toward the superior petrosal sinus (SPS). These veins form the superior petrosal venous system (SPVS). From a surgical point of view, we classified these veins into two topographical systems: one superficial, the other deep (Fig. 4.4).

The first system includes the superior petrosal vein and its tributaries. Located posteriorly to the TR, we termed it the superficial superior petrosal venous system (sSPVS) (Fig. 4.5). The superior petrosal vein (SPV) is formed by the confluence of three main affluents: the mesencephalic vein emerging from the cerebello-mesencephalic fissure, the cerebellar vein coursing on the hemispheric cerebellar surface, and the pontine vein emerging from the cerebello-pontine fissure. These veins constitute a barrier to access the TR. The SPV generally drains directly to the superior petrosal sinus (SPS).

The second system, inconstant, is located deeper; it lies next to the porus of the trigeminal cave. We termed it the deep superior petrosal venous system (dSPVS) (Fig. 4.6). Its main constituting vein has a transverse course in relation to the TR, more often inferiorly. The corresponding veins generally drain to the superior petrosal sinus, either directly or indirectly through the Meckel cave.

Sacrificing veins of the sSPVS during approaches should be as much as possible avoided. Superior petrosal vein (SPV) and affluents, especially when of large caliber, should be respected to prevent from cerebellar swelling and parenchymal

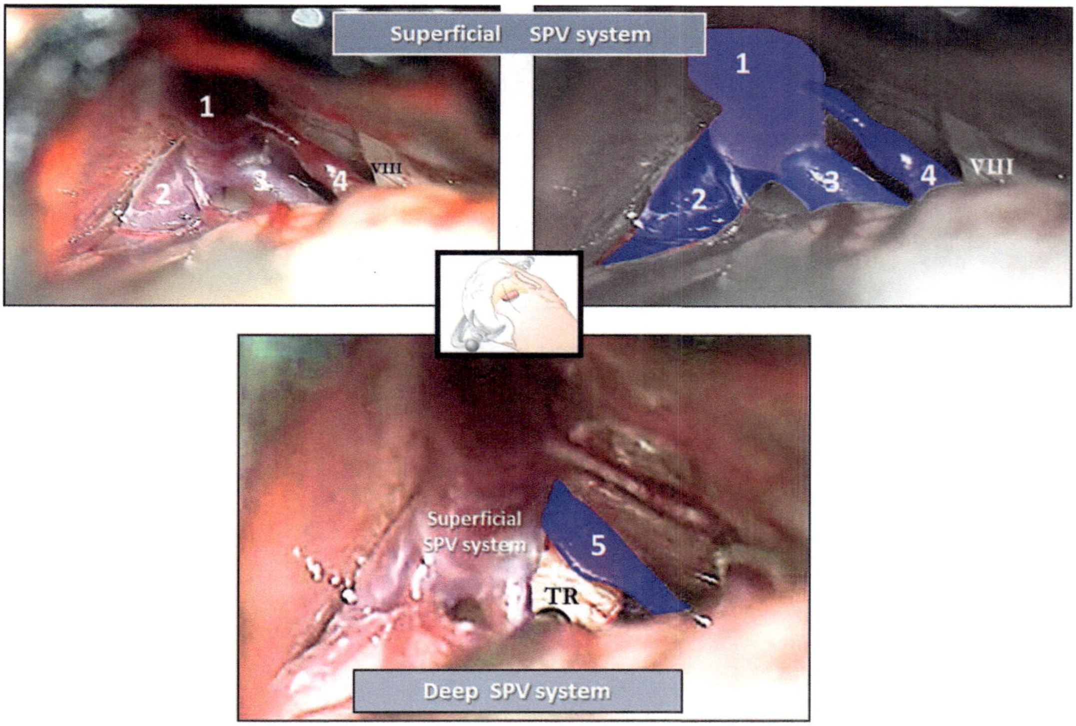


**Fig. 4.4** Anatomy of the Superior Petrosal Venous (SPV) system: superficial and deep. Operative view through an infratentorial supracerebellar route, on the right side. The system comprises the superficial SPV system and the deep SPV system. The superficial SPV system is formed by the confluence onto the superior petrosal vein (1) of: the mesencephalic (2), the pontine (3), and the cerebellar (4) veins. The SPV directly drains into the superior petrosal sinus. The deep SPV system is less constant. It is generally represented by a more or less big vein which has a transverse course (5), most often coursing on the inferior aspect of the trigeminal root (TR) at exit of the root from the trigeminal porus of the Meckel cave

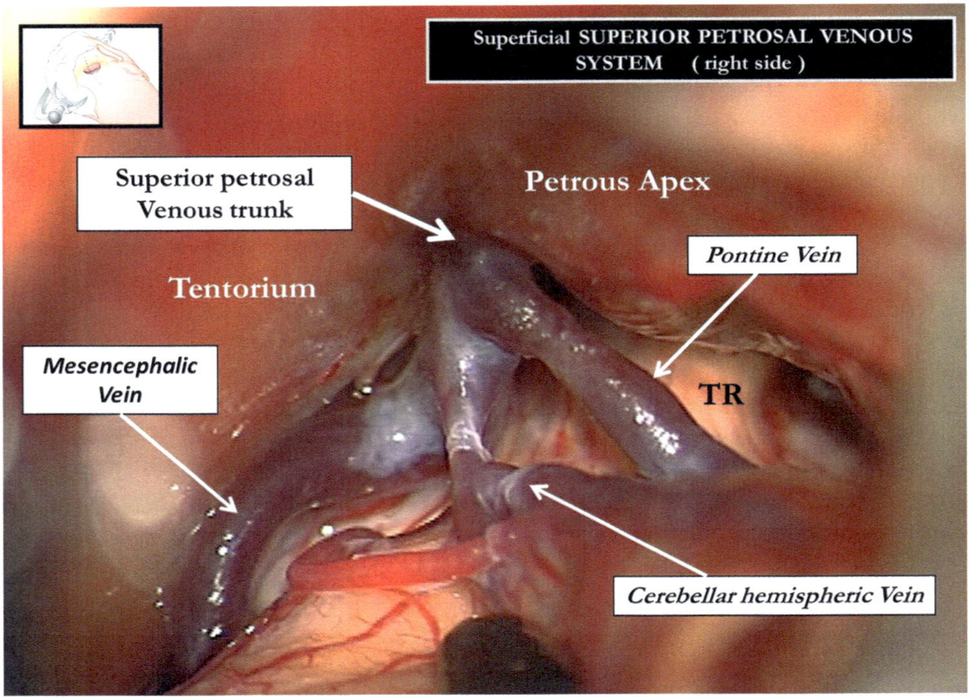


**Fig. 4.5** The superficial superior petrosal venous system as seen through right infratentorial-supracerebellar approach. Operative view shows a superior petrosal vein with a short trunk (SPV) draining to the superior petrosal sinus. The three main affluents of the SPV are clearly identifiable: the mesencephalic vein emerging from the cerebello-mesencephalic fissure, the cerebellar hemispheric vein coursing over the cerebellar surface, the pontine vein emerging from the cerebello-pontine fissure. *TR* trigeminal root in the depth

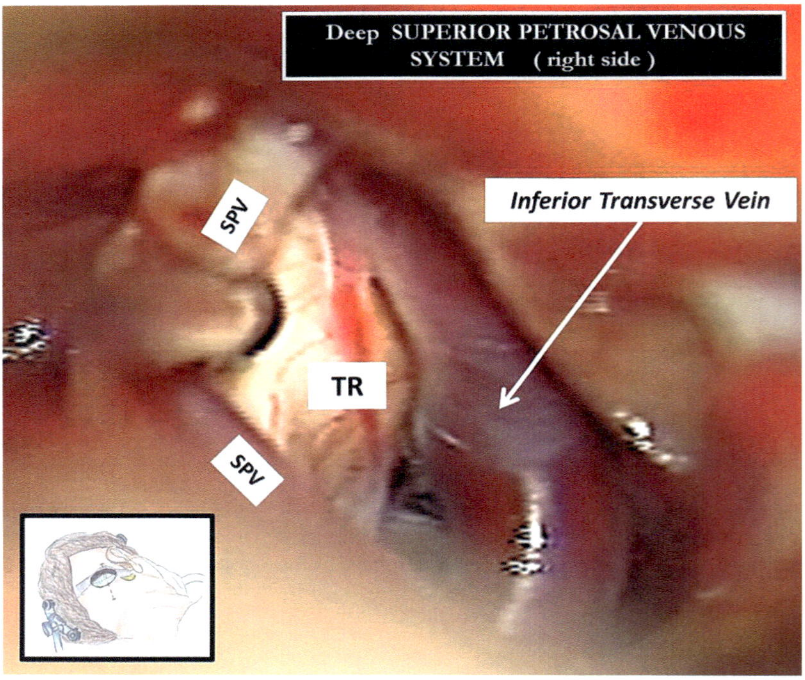


**Fig. 4.6** The deep superior petrosal venous system as seen through right infratentorial supracerebellar approach. Operative view shows, below the retracted superior petrosal vein (SPV), in the depth, a transverse vein coursing on the inferior aspect of the trigeminal root (TR) at exit from porus of Meckel cave

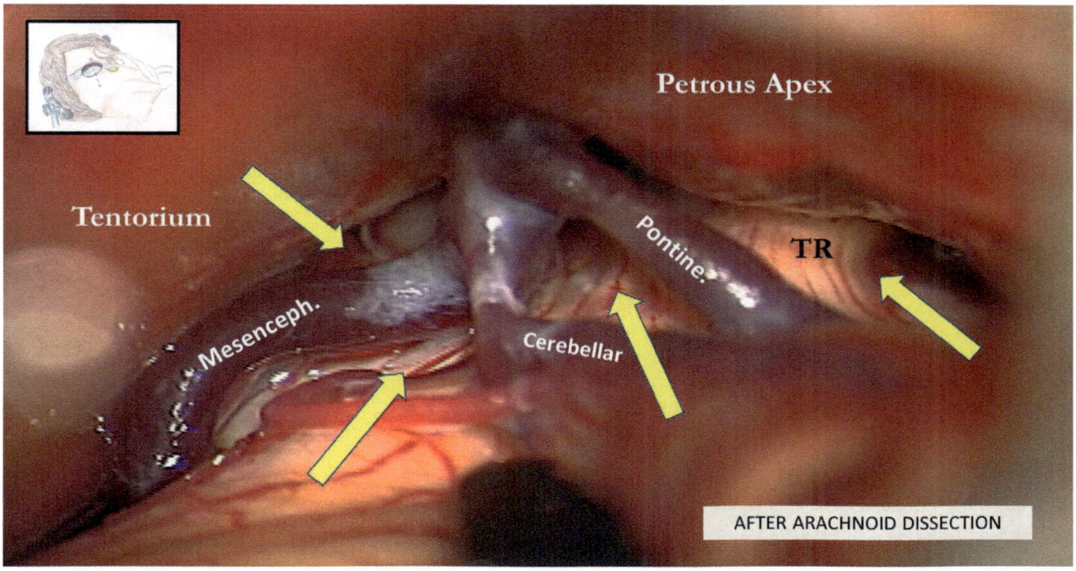


**Fig. 4.7** Operative view through infratentorial-supracerebellar approach on the right side showing superficial petrosal venous system in relation to the trigeminal root (TR) . *Triangular "access windows"* can be identified in between the affluents of the SPV, from rostral to caudal: below the tentorium and above the mesencephalic vein (arrow); in between the mesencephalic vein and the cerebellar vein (arrow); in between the cerebellar vein and the pontine vein (arrow); below the pontine vein (arrow). All of these triangles should be exposed—by large arachnoid opening (= fenestrations)—to allow complete exploration of the TR

infarction. For doing so, the trunk of the SPV as well as its tributaries must be dissected free from all arachnoid membranes. The trigeminal root can then be accessed through the several triangular windows of the sSPVS (Fig. 4.7). From superior to inferior, these windows are located as follows:

- above the mesencephalic Vein and below the tentorium incisura, to reach the peripenduncular cistern and the cerebellomesencephalic fissure where the SCA and branches are coursing, along the trochlear nerve;
- in between the mesencephalic V. and the cerebellar V., where to expose the TREZ, with its pars minor and intermediaris, at upper part of the cerebellopontine fissure;
- in between the cerebellar V. and the pontine V., to expose the TREZ, especially its pars major, at the lower part of the cerebellopontine fissure;
- below the pontine V., to access the ventrocaudal aspect of the TREZ and the AICA when looping there.

When exploring the TR at porus, dissection is often confronted to veins stuck to the root by arachnoid adhesions. Those veins belonging to the dSPVS, predominantly course transversally on the root after exit from Meckel cave (Figs. 4.8 and 4.9).

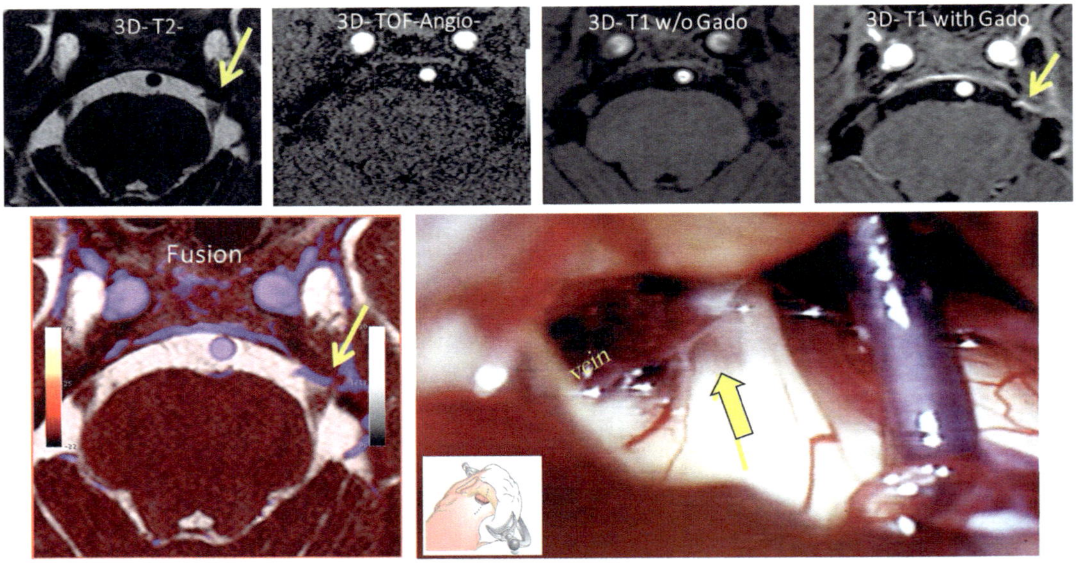


**Fig. 4.8** Neuro-Vascular Conflict (NVC) at porus of trigeminal cave. High-definition MRI associating the three following sequences allow to predict (pure) venous NVC. 3D-T2 sequence shows a likely cross-compression of the left root at exit from trigeminal cave (arrow). 3D-TOF-Angio sequence does not evidence any conflict at the site. Same applies with 3D-T1 w/o gadolinium, whereas the sequence 3D-T1 with gadolinium shows enhancement corresponding to the cross-compressing vessel visible in T2 (arrow). Such features testify of the venous nature of the vessel. The operative view demonstrates the (small caliber) cross-compression vein with a marked greyish zone at level of the compression (arrow), which corresponds to local demyelination of the root

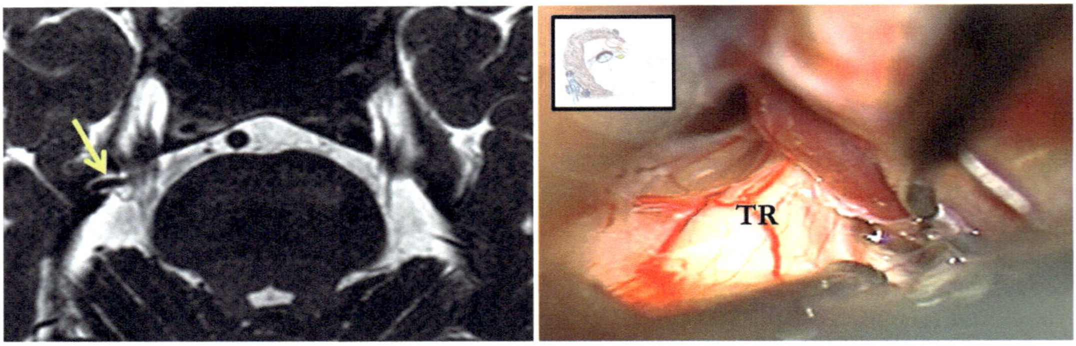


**Fig. 4.9** Patient with right classical trigeminal neuralgia due to pure venous neuro-vascular conflict from inferior transverse vein. Conflict was suspected on high-resolution MRI (arrow on T2 sequence). Keyhole approach should be designed so as to explore the entire trigeminal root (TR) from brainstem to trigeminal porus of Meckel cave. An effect of "*cross-compression*" type by the vein is paramount to retain the vein as (likely) responsible

## 4.3 Surrounding Structures

When considering the mechanism(s) of the classical TNs, the existence of additional factor(s) should be risen as favorizing the vascular contact/compression and making it symptomatic. As a matter of fact, a number of MRI studies show that an image of vascular <<relationship>> may be found in a rather high percentage of individuals without any trigeminal neuralgia (Klun and Prestor 1986; Peker et al. 2006; Miller et al. 2009a, b; Magown et al. 2019). Or on the asymptomatic side in patients with TN, in 30% of the patients in a personal series of 100 cases studied with high-resolution MRI (Brinzeu et al. 2018a).

Beside genetic predisposition, that still remains to be further investigated for recognition (Burchiel 2016), anatomical abnormalities or particular features can be suspected to play a role by their own or as associated factor to the potential vascular conflict.

Among several of these, the size of the cerebellopontine angle cistern, the shape of the petrous upper ridge and angulation of the trigeminal root on crossing over the ridge at exit of the trigeminal cave, and also the atrophy of the root, the presence of local arachnoiditis, as summarized in Table 4.3.

### 4.3.1 Role of the Size of the Cerebello-Pontine Angle Cistern

Several publications attracted attention on the favorizing role of a cerebellopontine angle cistern of small capacity in the genesis of TNs (Mueller and Levy 1963; Rasche et al. 2006; Horínek et al. 2009; Parise et al. 2010, 2013; Ha et al. 2012). Studies based on volumetric measurements showed that patients with TN tended to have smaller cistern than normal subjects, and that cistern was smaller on the affected side than on the contralateral side.

**Table 4.3** Root alterations associated to the neurovascular conflict found at surgery[a]

| |
|---|
| • *Root squeezed between petrous bone and pons due to small posterior fossa* |
| – 23 out of the 579 patients of the series (4%) |
| • *Angulation of the trigeminal root on crossing over the upper petrous ridge* |
| – 70 out of the 579 patients of the series (12%) |
| • *Local arachnoiditis (thickened arachnoid) adhesive to the root* |
| – 105 out of the 579 patients of the series (18%) |
| • *Global atrophy of the trigeminal root* |
| – 243 out of the 579 patients of the series (42%) |

[a]Data from personal series of 579 patients who underwent MVD for classical trigeminal neuralgia over the 1992–2002 period (Sindou et al. 2002)

Also, Parise et al. showed that in patients suffering from TN nerves were shorter on the affected side (Parise et al. 2013). In brief, cisterns of small capacity with the trigeminal root, more or less squeezed in between pons, cerebellum, and petrous pyramid, favor impaction of vessel(s) into the root, this corresponding to the concept of the so-called crowded posterior fossa (Fig. 4.10).

### 4.3.2 Role of the Upper Petrous Ridge

The shape of the petrous ridge, namely its sharpness at porus of Meckel cave, and angulation of the TGN at crossing over the upper ridge can be an alternative or a supplementary factor that may cause or contribute to the neuralgia (Fig. 4.11).

In a study on 42 patients, the averaged bony angle of the petrous ridge was found to be more acute on the neuralgia side (86°) than on the asymptomatic side (90°) ($p = 0.06$), and highly significantly sharper (86°) than that of the control group (98°) ($p = 0.004$) (Brinzeu et al. 2018b).

In same study, in patients with grade II or III of compression the median angle of the nerve on crossing over the upper ridge was found at 140° on average on the side of the neuralgia versus 149° on the asymptomatic side ($p = 0.003$). When the neurovascular conflict was the superior cerebellar artery which is naturally in a position that pushes down the trigeminal root in the cerebellopontine cistern, the median nerve angulation was more pronounced (139.5°) than with the non-SCA conflicts (i.e., the AICA or venous agents) (143°) ($p = 0.03$) (Brinzeu et al. 2018b). These "logical" anatomical features should be taken into account when dealing with TN patients.

Angulation of the TGN on crossing over the upper petrous ridge, with subsequent stretching of the root, can also be found in patients with so-called sagging phenomenon of brainstem and cerebellum in the posterior fossa (Fig. 4.12). This sagging phenomenon is frequently encountered in elder patients with important global atrophy, so that those structures are submitted to ptosis with traction of the trigeminal nerve(s) on the

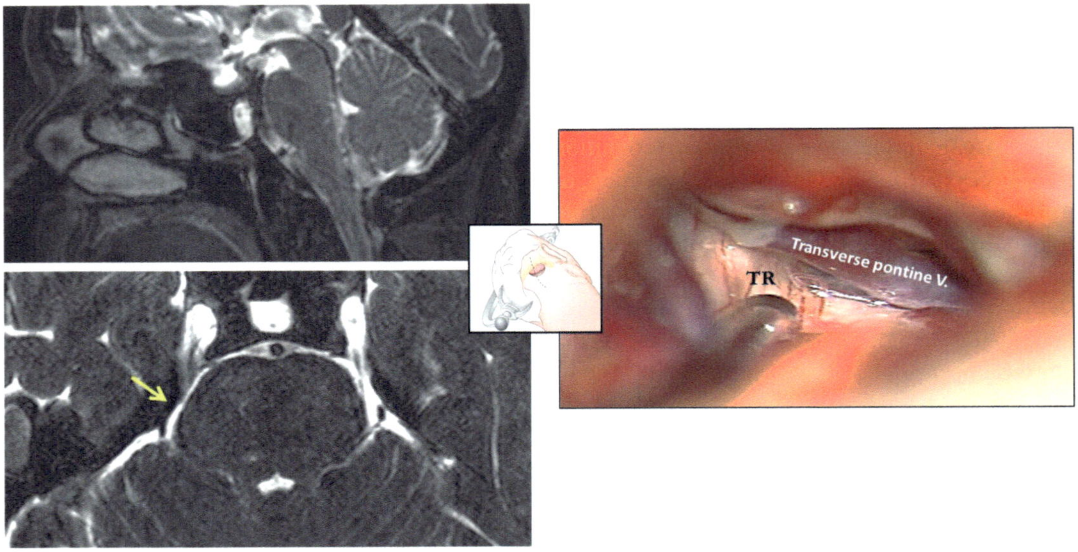


**Fig. 4.10** Illustrative case of right trigeminal neuralgia linked to neuro-vascular conflict by an inferior transverse vein cross-compressing the trigeminal root (TR) . The *small size of the posterior cerebral fossa* (PCF) likely plays a role in the genesis of the neuralgia. Note on MRI the reduced capacity of the cerebello-pontine angle cistern on the right side (arrow), also at surgery. Pain was relieved after decompressive craniectomy with enlargement of the PCF by duroplasty, and additional sacrifice of the conflicting vein

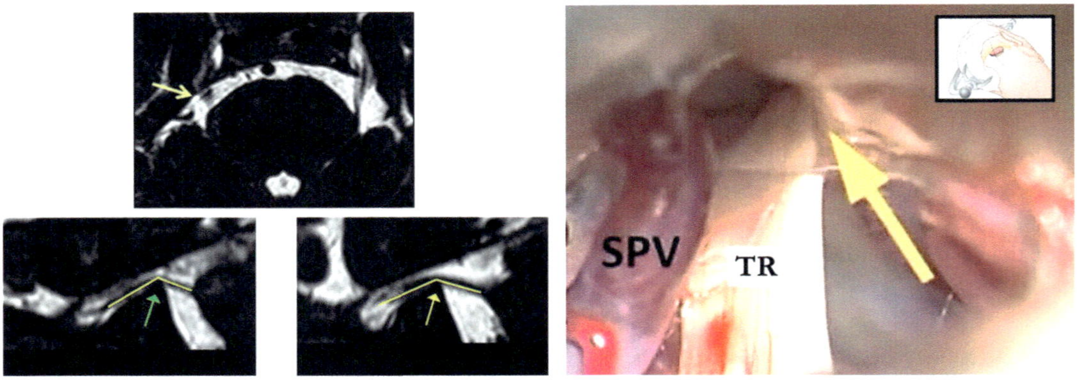


**Fig. 4.11** Illustrative case of right trigeminal neuralgia linked to an *angulation of the trigeminal root* (TR) on crossing over the petrous ridge at exit of root from the porus of the trigeminal cave (arrow). Note on MRI the more marked angulation of the root on the right side at crossing over the petrous ridge (green arrow). Also note on the operative view the ribbon-shaped and the greyish aspect (= demyelination) of the root at level of the angulation (arrow). In this case the Superior Petrosal Vein (SPV) was not considered conflicting the root

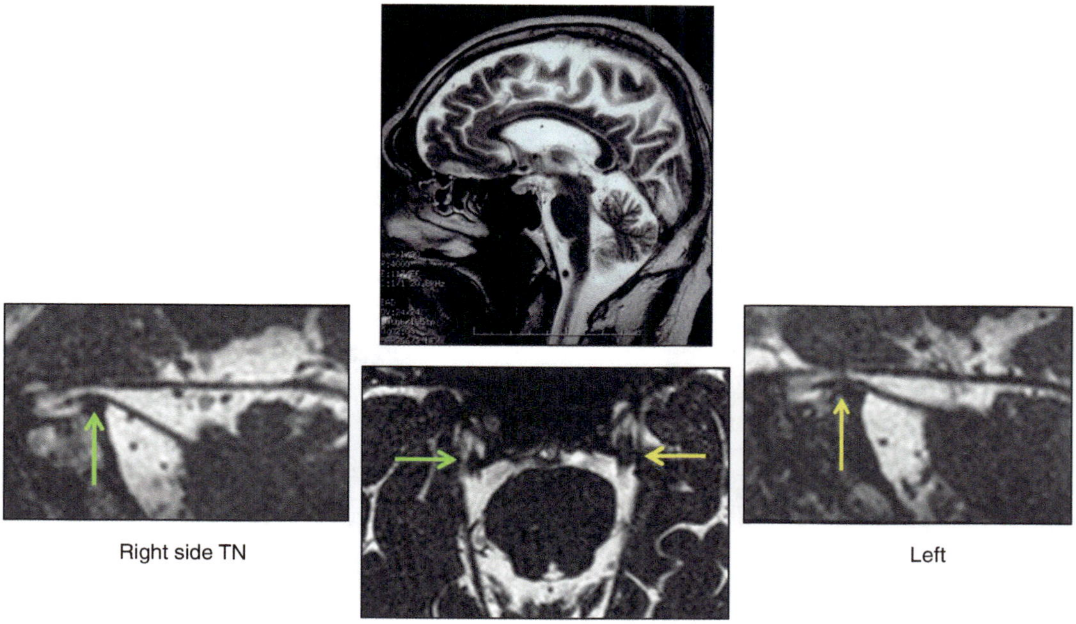


**Fig. 4.12** Stretched trigeminal roots with angulation on crossing over the upper petrous ridge (arrows) as often encountered in patients with important atrophic brain and cerebellum, and well visible on the MRI pictures. Such "*Sagging phenomenon*" has been frequently noticed by the senior author on the occasion of posterior fossa exploration in elder patients suffering from trigeminal neuralgia. A greyish aspect of the nerve at the point of angulation, corresponding to local demyelination, was frequently observed in those patients (Brinzeu et al. 2018b). Hypothesis is that the (most often atrophic) nerves undergo—under the sagging-phenomenon—traction by the gravity of the brainstem and cerebellum This phenomenon might be a factor influencing the pathogenesis of the neuralgia and could explain the failure or the incomplete effect of the MVD procedure, even when a neurovascular conflict is found, especially in elder patients

petrous ridge. At the point of the angulation, the root—most often atrophic—is ribbon-shaped, with a greyish aspect likely to correspond to local demyelination (Brinzeu et al. 2018b).

### 4.3.3 Influence of Focal Arachnoiditis

The presence of thickened arachnoid membranes responsible for adhesions and coalescence of nerve structures and neighboring vessels is not so uncommon finding in patients with classical TN (Fig. 4.13). Such focal "arachnoiditis" was found in 13% of the patients in a series of 375 patients who were operated on for MVD (Mazzucchi et al. 2019). In these 13% the clinical presentation of the neuralgia was typical in 59% of the patients and atypical in 31%, which corresponds to the percentage of the whole series (Sindou et al. 2007). Study of outcome in the group with the focal arachnoiditis showed a poorer outcome with a probability of being pain-free at 15 years of follow-up in only 42%, versus 80% for the whole series. However, the pain-free probability was of 75.2% when the NVC was of a high grade of compression versus only of 33% when the NVC was of a low grade (Mazzucchi et al. 2019).

Our (retrospective) study, unfortunately from a practical point of view, did not evidence any evocative sign of focal arachnoiditis on preoperative imaging. At present state of imaging technology, preoperative MRI cannot reliably predict focal arachnoiditis, and therefore help to forecast pejorative prognosis.

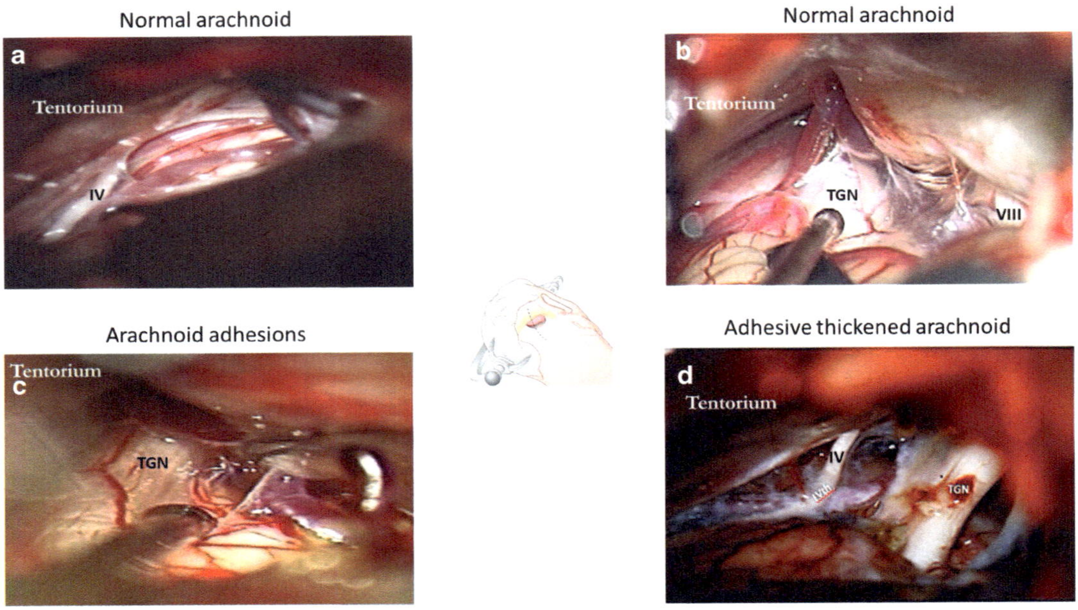


**Fig. 4.13** The various aspects of the arachnoid seen in the trigeminal root region (operative views, all on right side). (**a**) Thin and transparent arachnoid membrane, that is, normal, incised through an infratentorial—supracerebellar route. Incision is at the dorsolateral aspect of the mesencephalic peripeduncular region, just below the course of the (tiny and fragil) trochlear nerve (IV). The two branches of the right superior cerebellar artery are seen through the arachnoid opening. (**b**) Normal arachnoid, thin and transparent, surrounding the trigeminal nerve root (TGN), and not adhesive to it, on exposure of the root via a latero-cerebellar approach. Note the cochleo-vestibular nerve (VIII) exiting from the petrous internal auditory meatus. (**c**) Trigeminal nerve root (TGN) surrounded by arachnoid adhesions. Freeing the root from all stuck membranes—from brainstem to porus of the trigeminal cave—is an important preliminary step of the surgery. (**d**) Intraoperative image illustrating a case of strong focal arachnoiditis. The arachnoid membrane was thick, hard at dissection, and adhesive to the trigeminal nerve root (TGN), and also to the trochlear nerve (IV)

### 4.3.4 Presence of Global Radicular Atrophy

In many patients suffering from trigeminal neuralgia, especially elder patients, the trigeminal root (TR) is frequently globally atrophic, whether root is with or without vascular compression. As a matter of fact a certain degree of global atrophy was noted in 42% of our surgically explored patients; atrophy was marked to severe (i.e., equal or more than half of what would be considered a normal diameter in approximately half of those 42%) (Sindou et al. 2002). Global atrophy can be easily seen on T2-sequence of high-resolution MRI. At surgery, roots may present with a greyish aspect testifying a more or less degree of demyelination compared with healthy TRs, as seen under the operative microscope (Fig. 4.14). We did interpretate such global atrophy as a stigma of neuropathic alteration of the whole root.

In a statistical correlative study with the outcome following MVD, the influence of such global atrophy of the root on long-term (15 years) pain relief was evaluated (Sindou et al.

2007). Although probability of relief was lesser in the group with a severely atrophic root, difference did not reveal statistically significant ($p = 0.36$).

In addition, study of the influence of age on probability of long-term outcome after MVD showed that the group of the elder patients, that is those above 70 years of age, more propitious to harbor root atrophy, had a higher rate of pain relief than the younger group. However, differences did not reach statistical significance.

**Key-Point**

*Anatomic factors associated to the neurovascular conflict should not be neglected.*

Among those: small size of the posterior fossa, angulation and stretching of the root on crossing over the upper petrous ridge, a sagging phenomenon, focal arachnoiditis.

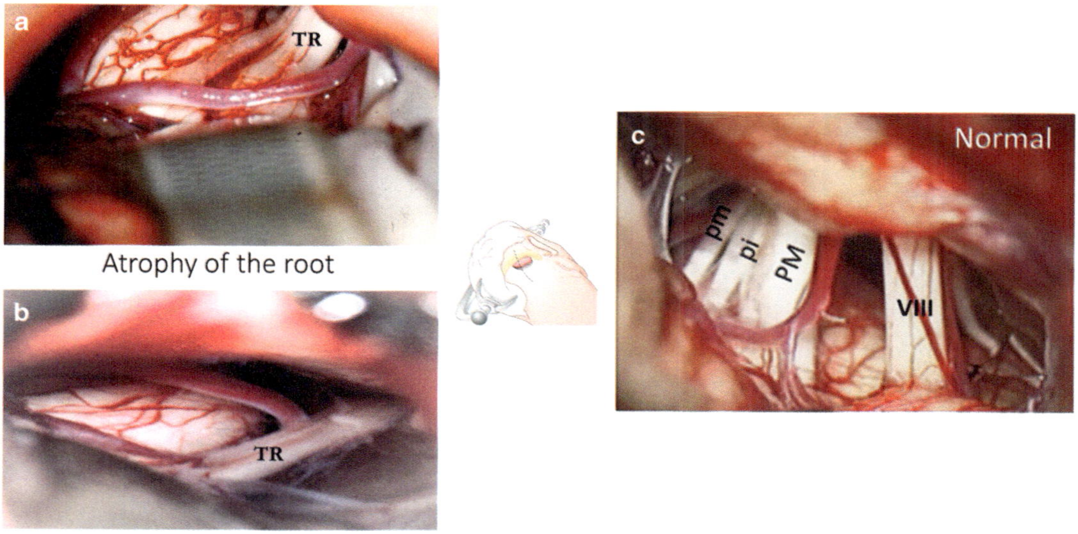


**Fig. 4.14** In many patients suffering from trigeminal neuralgia, especially elder patients, the trigeminal root (TR) is frequently *globally atrophic*, whether root is with or without vascular compression. Illustration with operative photographies, all shown on right side. (**a**) Illustration of a globally atrophic TR, with a greyish aspect at the site of contact with an elongated arterosclerotic superior cerebellar artery lying on the root. (**b**) Illustration of a globally atrophic TR. The contact with an elongated superior cerebellar artery in a supero-medial situation does not seem to be compressive for the root. (**c**) For comparison purpose, illustration of a healthy trigeminal root in the right cerebellopontine angle cistern (*PM* pars major, *pi* pars intermediaris, *pm* pars minor). VIII: cochleo-vestibular cranial nerve

# 5 Trigeminal Neuralgias: Clinical Presentations, Neurological Assessment, and Specialty Investigations

## 5.1 Problems of Characterization

Trigeminal neuralgias correspond to painful manifestations located exclusively in one or more of the three sensory divisions of the trigeminal nerve. Neuralgia is characterized by pain in the form of brief electric shocks, triggered by non-nociceptive stimuli in the cutaneous and mucous territories of the face.

### 5.1.1 Trigeminal Neuralgia May Result from Various Pathologies

Trigeminal neuralgia may result from well-defined pathologies = secondary neuralgias, or develop without apparent pathological cause = primary neuralgias. According to recent classification it is now recommended to term primary neuralgias:

- idiopathic for those where no cause of root alteration can be evidenced (by imaging)
- classical when imaging (preferably high-resolution MRI) can depict a morphological and/or structural alteration of the root, foremost and frequently a vascular compression.

NB: The compressive nature of the depicted vessel(s), and consequently its (their) responsibility in the genesis of the neuralgia, is not easy to ascertain on imaging, so that definition should perhaps stipulate "vessel in relation to the root, likely to be compressive."

### 5.1.2 The Clinical Presentations of Trigeminal Neuralgia

They can be:

- typical, manifested by purely paroxysmal painful discharges
- atypical, when a painful background (most frequently of the burning kind) is associated with paroxysmal pain.

NB: Atypical clinical presentations can be difficult to relate to the form of neuralgia when the continuous background of pain is predominant. It even may happen that the paroxysmal com-


M. Sindou, A. Brinzeu, *Trigeminal Neuralgias: A Neurosurgical Illustrated Guide*, https://doi.org/10.1007/978-3-031-25113-9_5

ponent becomes hidden under the continuous component.

In the mid-twenties, William Sweet gave a purely clinical classification of TN—largely adopted at that time—and termed: typical TN (when pain was purely paroxysmal) and atypical TN (when accompanied by a more or less continuous background of pain (White and Sweet 1969; Gybels and Sweet 1989)). The frequency of atypical neuralgia is variable among series. In a surgical series of around 5000 patients 34.5% of them had atypical presentation (Sindou et al. 2006).

**Key-Point**

Atypical clinical presentations can be difficult to relate to the frame of neuralgia when the continuous background of pain is predominant. It even may happen that the paroxysmal component becomes hidden under the continuous component.

### 5.1.3 The Atypical Trigeminal Neuralgia

The term is not equivalent to atypical facial pain, which is a totally different entity, generally considered of psychological origin. The previously used form: Atypical facial pain is now termed by the ICHD: "Persistent idiopathic facial pain (PIFP)" (IHS 2018). The differential diagnosis between Atypical Trigeminal neuralgia and Atypical facial pain can be very difficult to the point that Sweet qualified the later "La bête noire du neurochirurgien" (in French in his book) (White and Sweet 1969).

Whereas Sweet (Gybels and Sweet 1989) and recently the IHS Committee distinguished Classical TNs in Typical and Atypical on their clinical characteristics, the first being purely paroxysmal, the second "with concomitant continuous pain," Burchiel introduced in 2003 a personal classification system for facial pain (Burchiel 2003). For Burchiel, atypical facial pain was reserved (as in the past) for patients with proven psychogenic pain. Trigeminal neuralgias were divided into Type 1 and Type 2.

Type 1 patients presented predominantly (>50%) with pain that was episodic, lancinating, "electric," triggerable, subject to pain-free intervals, and generally responsive to anticonvulsant therapy, while Type 2 patients presented with more constant (>50%) dull, aching, burning pain, without free intervals, and fundamentally non responsive to anticonvulsant therapy. This classification system was validated showing significant differences in characteristics of the patients in the two groups although in that study the patients had been selected for microvascular decompression (Miller et al. 2009a). Patients with Type 1 were more often associated with arterial compression while venous compression or no compression at all was more frequent in Type 2 patients. Type 1 patients also were less likely to recur after microvascular decompression than Type 2 patients. A flaw of this system is that it has to quantify the degree of atypical pain. It is difficult to ascertain whether someone has 50% or less atypical signs. Further criticism is that in this classification system patients with idiopathic facial pain might be classified as Type 2 trigeminal neuralgia whereas in other classification systems they would not be included in the neuralgia group (Maarbjerg et al. 2015b). However, Burchiel's classification is widely used in the neurosurgical community and particularly so in the series analyzing outcome after surgical treatment.

### 5.1.4 Distinction Between Classical Trigeminal Neuralgia and Painful Trigeminal Neuropathies

This distinction can be a problem. Painful trigeminal neuropathies develop in the territory of one or more divisions of the trigeminal nerve. They are caused by a pathological process or an injury that has created significant neuronal damage. Pain is highly variable in quality and intensity depending on the etiology and the individual. A phenomenon of painful anesthesia and/or dysesthesia may be added. In spite of some difficulties to classify these painful conditions in a few circumstances, the ICHD classification has been tested solid for the distinction between classical TN and painful trigeminal neuropathies (Maarbjerg et al. 2015a).

## 5.2 Mechanisms

Mechanisms of trigeminal neuralgias are still not completely understood. For classical TNs—the most frequently encountered—several theories exist hypothesizing the genesis either peripherally or centrally. For them, the most "attractive" theory is to link the neuralgia to both a peripheral and a central mechanism together.

### 5.2.1 Hypotheses

In classical TNs linked by definition to a NVC, the neuralgia would be generated by the chronic compression and the continuous pulsations caused by the conflicting vessel. The compressive vessel would produce a focal demyelination and would induce ectopic influxes, as well as create short-circuits between fibers (= ephapses) through their damaged sheaths (Gardner 1962). Subsequently the ectopic firing of impulses would lead to an exaggerated sensitivity and hyperactivity of the trigeminal nuclei in brainstem (Møller 1991; Devor et al. 2002a) and in the long run at level of the upper brain structures (DeSouza et al. 2015, 2016; Parise et al. 2014).

### 5.2.2 Structural Abnormalities

Histological studies of root abnormalities in trigeminal neuralgia patients are few due to the difficulty to harvest nerve samples, especially for ethical reasons. Among the most important, are the electron microscopic studies, which showed obvious fiber alterations: denudation of the axons along with ephaptic contact between damaged axons (Kerr and Miller 1966; Kerr 1967a, b; Hilton et al. 1994), in other words focal demyelination (Hilton et al. 1994; Love et al. 1998; Love and Coakham 2001). The most convincing findings are those brought by Rappaport's team from histological studies of samples harvested during microsurgical exploration of the posterior fossa (Rappaport et al. 1997; Devor et al. 2002b). Biopsy samples were taken from 12 patients undergoing microvascular decompression and analyzed with electron microscopy. Massive injury to nerve fibers was found in the areas compressed by the vessel with axonal loss and demyelination, however with few or no inflammatory change, that is, phagocytic cells as is usually found in peripheral nerves. This was accompanied by the persistence of destroyed myelin material in the tissue samples. In these regions while the myelin sheet of axons was present it was altered in several ways, with myelin inclusions inside the axons as well as axonal sprouting when axons were severely damaged. These changes appeared to be related to the degree of compression at surgery.

Results from DTI investigations in Classical TN patients, namely: decrease in Fraction of Anisotropy and increase in Apparent Diffusion Coefficient (Leal et al. 2011b, 2019) reinforce evidence of pathological changes such as axonopathy, axonal loss, demyelination, and residual myelin debris in histological studies of trigeminal fascicles collected from patients with NVC near the TREZ (Hilton et al. 1994; Devor et al. 2002b). The elevation in diffusivity in the affected nerves indicates the presence of obstacles to diffusion, probably because of axonal loss and focal demyelination. Reduced anisotropy could result from damage and removal of highly aligned cellular structures such as axons, or from focal endoneural injury resulting from NVC. These phenomena may explain the theory of focal demyelination of the sensory axons at the site of the NVC (Love et al. 1998), and that ephaptic "short circuits" are responsible for neuralgia, as hypothesized by Gardner (1962). Demyelinated nerve fibers are also known to be sensitive to tiny deformations (Smith and McDonald 1980), so that pulsatile compression by a vessel could, at least in theory, initiate axonal impulses that spread ephaptically within the TREZ

(Love and Coakham 2001; Devor et al. 2002a). Demyelination has also been found in well-documented experimental models of acute (Gledhill et al. 1973) or chronic (Fish and Blakemore 1983) compression of central white matter.

### 5.2.3 Electrophysiological Abnormalities

Peripheral demyelination zones constitute possible sites for the generation of ectopic Action Potentials (APs). In a histological and electrophysiological experimental study in cats and macaques, Burchiel showed that focal demyelination in their trigeminal nerve generate spontaneous ectopic APs and exhibit prolonged high frequency after-discharges induced by short trains of normal stimuli (Burchiel 1980a, b, 1981; Calvin et al. 1982). This is concordant with the observations in patients, of either spontaneous attacks of sustained discharges or discharges after light touch stimulation of trigger zones. The spontaneous ectopic discharges were stopped by the administration of anticonvulsants (diphenylhydantoin). Most importantly spontaneous APs generation was not dependent on the existence of central connections with the trigeminal nuclei, therefore offering support to the peripheral hypothesis of trigeminal neuralgia generation. Those findings have been supported by other electrophysiological studies at the level of the trigeminal ganglion (Rappaport and Devor 1994).

### 5.2.4 Anomalies in Secondary Trigeminal Neuralgias

Tumors of the cerebellopontine angle by compressing the trigeminal nerve may lead to focal demyelination visible on MRI within the root entry zone or its cisternal—transitional zone. In these patients, clinical presentation is often not typical.

Trigeminal neuralgia resulting from multiple sclerosis (MS) is of a frequent occurrence. A hypoesthesia is often associated in particular in the cornea, and clinical presentation is more often atypical, that is, with a background of continuous pain. Focal demyelination is frequently observed at TREZ. Plaques may be also encountered in the trigeminal tracts within the brainstem at their various levels. In these patients location of lesions within the brainstem is an argument suggesting that the peripheral genesis theory does not offer a complete explanation of the disease.

**Key-Point**

We are far from precisely understanding the mechanisms of trigeminal neuralgias.

It is likely distinct mechanisms are responsible for distinct forms of neuralgia.

Both peripheral and central mechanisms can be involved sometimes intricating to various degrees.

### 5.2.5 The Question of Genetic Involvement

There are hypotheses stating that the risk of developing neuralgia is in large part determined genetically; however, these are under a lot of debate (Burchiel 2016). To be noted, there are only rare family observations; Harris counted 30 of 2500 cases studied (Harris 1940).

Up to now, there have been not many and well-characterized risk factors for trigeminal neuralgia. However, one study identified hypertension as a possible factor (Katusic et al. 1991); but this was not subsequently confirmed (Rasmussen 1990; Maarbjerg et al. 2014a, b). Neuralgia is certainly more frequent in women, in whom it starts earlier than in men. Curiously, risk factors linked to sex such as hormone levels have not yet been explored. Another risk factor identified is gain of function mutations found in some other pain syndromes such as erythromelalgia and small fiber neuropathies (Yang et al. 2004; Fertleman et al. 2006; Huang et al. 2014). This has been recently found in one patient with classical trigeminal neuralgia (Tanaka et al. 2016). This however does not appear to be ruled in most patients with classical trigeminal neuralgia. Further research is being performed in a multicentric US Canadian and British study enrolling a group of patients well-described clinically and in whom DNA sequencing will be performed. This may identify association of genes that increase the likelihood of trigeminal neuralgia. It remains to be seen whether this likelihood needs to be associated with vascular conflict for the actual development of the disease or not.

## 5.3 Epidemiology

The incidence of primary trigeminal neuralgias is 4–13 new cases per year per 100,000 population.

The overall prevalence in population-based evaluations is around 0.20–0.5%. The prevalence of TN in people with MS ranges between 1 and 6.3%.

The female predominance is constant in all the series. The prevalence ratio is from 1 to 1.5 to 1 to 1.7.

The majority of cases start after age 50. It is rather a disease of middle age and senescence, with pain occurring three out of four times after the age of 50; late onset after age 70 is not uncommon. https://www.ncbi.nlm.nih.gov/books/NBK554486/

Patients with hypertension present a higher incidence of TN compared to the general population, especially in those harboring a clear-cut vascular compression.

Bilateral forms are rare, 1–2% of cases, and do not progress in parallel.

There are rare family observations; Harris counts 30 out of 2500 cases studied.

The juvenile forms must be regarded as suspicious of secondary neuralgia, in particular in the context of demyelinating or tumor pathologies.

## 5.4 Clinical Presentation in Its Typical Form

Trigeminal neuralgia (TN) is defined by its clinical characteristics of paroxysmal unilateral facial pain in a well-defined territory. Distribution of the pain may be in one or several of the cutaneous and/or mucous territories of the three divisions, with V2 pain being the most frequent territory followed by V3 and V1. It is now well recognized that vascular compression factor is a predominant etiology of primary TN, this condition being termed: classical trigeminal neuralgia.

In its typical form the diagnosis is easy, based on the four following clinical elements (Loeser 1994; IHS 2018).

### 5.4.1 Pain Quality

Pain is intense and paroxysmal characterized by electric-like shocks, sometimes crushing and tearing, more rarely burning. These flashes are brief, in the order of a few seconds; they can be grouped into bursts to form fits of one to two minutes. The frequency of the attacks determines the severity of the condition, from five to ten per day in the mild forms, and repetitive attacks in the most severe ones. The intensity of the pain is described as unbearable. During the attacks, the patient becomes immobilized in a frozen attitude, ceasing all activity; the hemiface is often tense with contractions producing the "tic douloureux." In the course of violent attacks, vasomotor phenomena may occur, such as redness of the teguments, congestion of the eye, or of the nasal mucosa. The fits are followed by a refractory period of one to two minutes. Duration may increase over time with paroxysms becoming prolonged, accompanied by burning sensation and discomfort.

### 5.4.2 Pain Topography

Pain is unilateral, strictly localized to the trigeminal territory, and most often limited to one or two of the trigeminal divisions, at least at the onset of the affection, as shown in Table 5.1. In the majority of cases, pain concerns the maxillary territory (V2). The pain is usually located in the infraorbital area, starting in the upper lip, nasolabial fold, wing of the nose, or upper gum tissue. The mandibular territory (V3) is also frequently involved located in area of the mental nerve, that is, the chin, also the lower lip, and the lower dental territory. The auriculotemporal nerve involvement with temporal pain is rarer, as is the involvement of the lingual nerve with irradiation in the hemi-tongue. Isolated neuralgia of the ophthalmic division (V1) is observed in less than 10% of cases; it generally sites in the supraorbital area.

### 5.4.3 Conditions of Triggering Pains

Provocation of pains by innocuous stimuli is a characteristic of trigeminal neuralgia. The most common is the direct excitation of a skin area, more rarely mucosa. This (these) limited area(s) is (are) most often in the painful area; they are termed "trigger-zones." Light touching, superficial brushing of the teguments, and contact of the tongue on the mucosa are the most effective stimuli. Thermal and noxious stimuli are generally ineffective, as is pressure on the trigger zone. Sometimes patients try to prevent attacks with strong pressure, while avoiding all stimulations such as shaving, washing, brushing teeth, make-up, and so on. The provocation of fits can be also indirect, through speech, mimics, laughing, or eating. This explains the particular attitude of these patients who remain immobile and sometimes reduce their diet. Nocturnal attacks are rare, probably due to the rarity of triggering stimuli at night. Noteworthy painful attacks are followed by a refractory period of a few minutes, which patients use to eat, talk, wash and so on.

**Table 5.1** Distribution of the neuralgia according to the various trigeminal divisions involved[a]

- V1: 7.14%
- V2: 20.23%
- V3: 16.66%
- V1, V2: 13.09%
- V2, V3: 33.33%
- V1, V2, V3: 9.52%
- V1 all: 30%
- V2 all: 76%
- V3 all: 59%

[a]Data from personal series of 579 patients who underwent Micro-Vascular Decompression for Classical Trigeminal Neuralgia (Sindou et al. 2002)

### 5.4.4 Negativity of the Neurological Examination

This is the fourth element, essential for the diagnosis of classical trigeminal neuralgia. The examination is often made difficult by apprehension of the patient for whom even the interview is uncomfortable and can elicit painful attacks. Purpose of the examination is to verify the absence of neurological sign of sensory deficit in the face, in particular in the cornea, and also of motor weakness in the masticatory muscles, as well as in the neighboring cranial nerves. Examination of the corneal reflex is especially important. The observation of the slightest deficit outside of a crisis should suggest a diagnosis of secondary neuralgia, until eliminated otherwise (+++).

### 5.4.5 Evolution

If some forms remain tolerable without intense attacks and stay rather well-controlled by medication, evolution of the classical trigeminal neuralgia is usually toward worsening with shorter and shorter remissions and more frequent discharges in the painful periods. Along its evolution, trigeminal neuralgia tends to take atypical characters and to become permanent. Trigeminal neuralgia does not have the rhythmic, often seasonal development of cluster headache.

### 5.4.6 Trigeminal Pre-neuralgia

To be mentioned, classical trigeminal neuralgia may be preceded by a period of some more or less continuous sensory disturbances from paresthesias to atypical pain. Such manifestations can be termed: pre-trigeminal neuralgia (Fromm et al. 1990).

## 5.5 Other Clinical Presentations

### 5.5.1 Atypical Trigeminal Neuralgia (= Trigeminal Neuralgia with Concomitant Continuous Pain)

Trigeminal neuralgias can take an atypical presentation, characterized by the association to paroxysmal pain of a permanent background of deep aching or burning pain. The paroxysmal component can be on the back row or even be absent, especially if the patient is under anticonvulsant medication. This presentation has been termed by the ICHD: "trigeminal neuralgia with concomitant continuous pain" (IHS 2018).

If the paroxysmal component is missing, it can be difficult to establish relation of the pain with the frame of TN. It is therefore essential to investigate by questioning the existence of paroxysms at the onset of the disease before starting anticonvulsants. In the most "difficult" situations for diagnosis stopping the anticonvulsant drugs may be legitimate; the test usually results in the reappearance of the paroxysmal component.

The trigeminal nature of atypical neuralgia must be clearly identified from the "atypical facial pain" condition, the characteristics of which are presented elsewhere. This distinction is therapeutically crucial. "Atypical facial pain" termed by the IHS "Persistent idiopathic facial pain" is not significantly influenced by the anticonvulsant drugs. Patients with "atypical facial pain" should not be treated surgically.

The incidence of atypical trigeminal neuralgia is variously evaluated according to the series. In our global "surgical" series of more than 6000 of patients operated on over a 25th year period, at the time they were referred for surgery (from 1 to 36 years after onset of the disease, 6.4 years on average), 35% of them presented with an atypical form.

While classification is very intuitive, the proof that the two varieties of presentations fare differently are few and discordant. It has been suggested that along the natural history of all neuralgias one encounters more and more a continuous background of pain (Burchiel 2000); however, this has not been verified in a more recent series of 200 patients under medical treatment alone (Di Stefano et al. 2014). In another similar study on 158 trigeminal neuralgias, Maarbjerg found 49% of patients had a concomitant background of pain with a significant difference in the response to sodium channel blockers (Maarbjerg et al. 2014a, b). Further in a quantitative sensory testing study it was pointed out that patients with a continuous background of pain had sensory loss more often than those that presented with paroxysmal attacks solely (Younis et al. 2016).

Differences in etiology and long-term outcome have not yet been put in evidence. In particular, correlation of neurovascular conflict and typical or atypical presentation could not be made (Maarbjerg et al. 2015b). In some large series of microvascular decompression including patients with TN with atypical elements (while less frequent: 34.5%), the group with atypical TN did not fare worse after neurovascular decompression than patients with typical presentation (Sindou et al. 2008).

### 5.5.2 Trigeminal Neuralgia with Autonomic Involvement

Autonomic symptoms such as nasal congestion, lacrimation, redness of the eye may be present especially in the cases with neuralgia in the ophthalmic division; their presence does not preclude the diagnosis of trigeminal neuralgia. Recommended action is to use a carbamazepine test to distinguish between trigeminal neuralgia and cluster headache.

### 5.5.3 Trigeminal Neuralgia After Long Evolution

These forms are often those the neurosurgeon is confronted with. A long evolution of the neuralgia may induce damage to the nerve therefore contributing to a continuous presence of the pain and reduction of the intermittent attacks. As the neuralgia progresses, it tends to lose its paroxysmal characteristics and to associate a continuous painful background which may predominate in the patient's description. The patient's interview should try to retrospectively find out paroxysms, as well as the provoked character of the pains, at the onset of the condition. This is essential to the diagnosis. It is also possible to observe some degree of hypoesthesia; this must be verified by several times examinations as it could be related to the proximity of the last painful attack. Difficulty of diagnosis may even justify halting the treatment and wait for the apparition of the paroxysmal component that may not manifest under carbamazepine or equivalents.

### 5.5.4 Trigeminal Neuralgia After Trigeminal Surgery

Recurrence is very common after alcoholization or destructive surgery on the peripheral branches of the trigeminal nerve. The lesioning-techniques directed to the trigeminal root or ganglion, whether percutaneous or radio-surgical, often produce more or less significant hypoesthesia in the territory of the targeted fibers, as well as some degree of paresthesias and/or dysesthesias, and sometimes anesthesia dolorosa. Too much destruction of the fibers would create a sort of "trigeminal phantom." All those disturbances fall within the frame of neuropathic pain, always difficult to treat. Fortunately, this type of syndrome rarely appears if surgical lesioning is performed with moderation.

**Key-Point**

*Importance of the pharmacological tests for the differential diagnosis.*

In non-typical presentations, anticonvulsants—on front row: carbamazepine—can be tried; if clearly (at least partly) effective, the diagnosis of neuralgia can be considered.

In atypical clinical presentations characterized by a predominant permanent background of pain, anticonvulsants can be withdrawn to facilitate reappearance of the paroxysmal component, so that to ascertain the diagnosis of neuralgia.

## 5.6 Clinical Assessment

### 5.6.1 Neurological Assessment

Confronted with a facial pain, the first step is to make sure it is trigeminal neuralgia. This is easy if the clinical manifestations are typical, but more difficult if there is atypia since the beginning or if the neuralgia has become atypical while evolving with the age. It is thus essential to question whether the anticonvulsant analgesics (in front row: carbamazepine) have been clearly effective or not, at least at the beginning of the disease. This is the more so important as treatment had to be early stopped for intolerance and not because of its inefficacy. This anticonvulsant—test is for us very indicative to help clarifying the diagnosis of neuralgia.

In some particular neurological situations, complementary investigations can be indicated, as for example laboratory examination of the CSF if the diagnosis of an inflammatory disease is evocated.

Also, neurophysiological explorations may be useful, as for instance the measure of the blink-reflex and the evoked potentials, especially when the diagnosis of Multiple Sclerosis is suspected.

**Key-Point**
Atypical clinical presentation and/or presence of even mild neurological deficit(s) should make the neuralgia suspected to be of secondary origin.

### 5.6.2 Other Specialty Investigations

It is mandatory that all the pathologies potentially responsible for a secondary neuralgia be eliminated, not only by complete neurological examination but also by oriented investigations belonging to the disciplines of odontology, stomatology, otorhinolaryngology, and ophthalmology.

Because some neuralgiform painful manifestations caused by specific pathologies in the face can mimic trigeminal neuralgia, recourse to the other specialties, is wise. Glaucoma, iridocyclitis, sinusitis, and so on may sometimes take the mask of cluster headache, more rarely of trigeminal neuralgia. Disorders of the temporomandibular joint can mimic neuralgia of the V3 division, although they are most often associated with signs of articular dysfunction and temporal myalgias. The pains of tumors of the facial cavities are generally more continuous. The most important difficulties are the pains in relation with the dental pathologies. Frequent are patients complaining about the responsibility of dental cares in their pain. Conversely, it is also frequent that patients ask for teeth cares or even teeth extraction considering they are at the origin of their pain. Thus, the question of the responsibility of the dental surgeon is often implicated, and not infrequently the matter of medicolegal and malpractice complaint.

Nowadays, performing a brain MRI is wise, if not quite necessary, not only to identify a possible cause of secondary neuralgia, but also, in case of primary TN, to depict a NVC or more generally to search for any anatomical factor(s) that could be corrected with "conservative" surgery. Also, MRI, or at least a CT-scan, is important to eliminate any anatomical anomaly which could make a percutaneous intervention, if decided, dangerous as regard to its approach or its lesioning process, as for instance a vascular malformation or a megadolicho-artery bulging into the trigeminal cave.

### 5.6.3 The Way to Assess Pain Intensity in Therapeutic Results

At the time the patients are referred for considering neurosurgery, intensity of pain is generally at 8–10 according to the VAS scale, at least during the pain crises.

On the other hand, the nowadays most admitted scoring system to evaluate outcome after (surgical) treatment is the BNI (Barrow National Institute) scale (Han et al. 1999), as shown in Table 5.2.

**Table 5.2** Scoring system from the Barrow Neurological Institute

| |
|---|
| • *BNI pain intensity score* |
| 1. No pain, no medication |
| 2. Occasional pain, not requiring medication |
| 3. Some pain, adequately controlled with medication |
| 4. Some pain, not adequately controlled with medication |
| 5. Severe pain, no pain relief |
| • *BNI facial numbness score* |
| 1. No facial numbness |
| 2. Mild facial numbness, not bothersome |
| 3. Facial numbness, somewhat bothersome |
| 4. Facial numbness, very bothersome |
| • *BNI total (pain + numbness score)* |
| Excellent (2) |
| Good (3) |
| Fair (4) |
| Poor (≥5) |

# 6 Trigeminal Neuralgias: Neuro-Imaging Assessment

MRI holds a key place for establishing the diagnosis of the neuralgia and identifying an eventual etiology, which will condition the treatment.

## 6.1 Standard Imaging Should Rule Out Secondary Neuralgias

For this, imaging must be able to detect the listed below possible pathologies:

- malformations of the skull base and the occipito-cervical junction, in particular small posterior fossa responsible for so-called crowdy cerebello-pontine angle (CPA), Arnold-Chiari malformation;
- space-occupying lesion of the CPA, arteriovenous malformation, giant aneurysm;
- tumorous process of Meckel cave and/or of parasellar lodge;
- multiple sclerosis, as well as any lesion of the brainstem, whether inflammatory, tumorous, vascular, or ischemic;
- and also, pathologies of the middle cerebral fossa and/or the orbital apex, or of the facial cavities.

As for illustration, such pathologies amounted at 3.6% of the total of our approximative 6000 patients referred over the past 35 years for neurosurgical treatment of their neuralgia.

## 6.2 Detection of the Neurovascular Conflicts

- While standard MRI can detect a possible cause of neuralgia, that is, have it classified as secondary and treated as such, it is not sufficient to study the fine anatomy of the nerves and the vascular structures of the CPA. Detection of the neurovascular conflicts requires high-resolution imaging. According to our experience to detect and depict NVCs, MRI should have the following three special sequences, in combination (Figs. 6.1 and 6.2).

  - The high-resolution 3D-T2 sequence gives fine images with good contrast between the cerebrospinal fluid (in hypersignal) and the vascular and nerve structures (in hypointense signal), achieving a true cisternography of the CPA. This sequence has a different name, depending on the machine used: constructive interference in steady-state (CISS), fast imaging employing steady-state acquisition (FIESTA), driven equilibrium (DRIVE). Limitation of this sequence is the lack of differentiation between vessels and nerves; it must be completed by the following sequences.
  - The 3D-time-of-flight-Angiography (3D-TOF-angiography) sequence visualizes high flux vessels, that is, principally


M. Sindou, A. Brinzeu, *Trigeminal Neuralgias: A Neurosurgical Illustrated Guide*,
https://doi.org/10.1007/978-3-031-25113-9_6

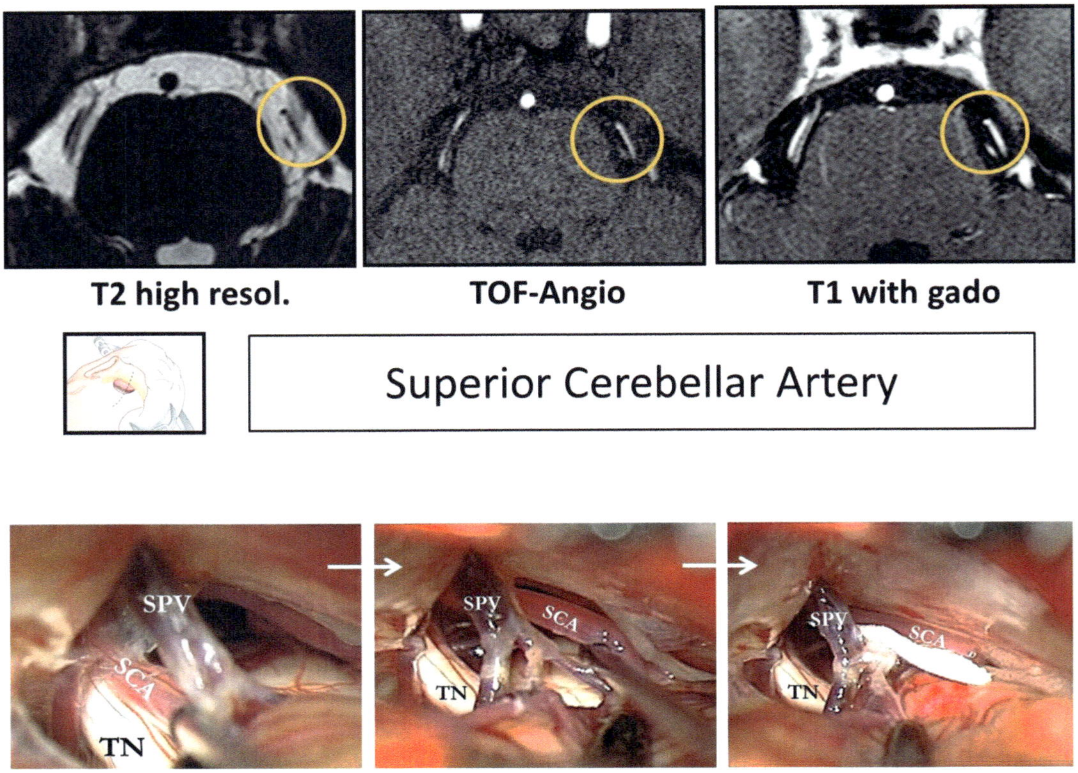


**Fig. 6.1** Imaging diagnosis of an arterial Neuro-Vascular Conflict, from the superior cerebellar artery (SCA) in a patient with left-sided Trigeminal Neuralgia (TN). The MRI 3D-$T_2$ high-resolution sequence shows the root crossed by the conflicting vessel. The 3D-time of flight (TOF)-Angio sequence shows the (arterial) vessel. The 3D-$T_1$ with gadolinium sequence shows the same vessel, and no other vascular structure in the root region (i.e., no additional vein). The microsurgical views illustrate the steps of the trigeminal root (TN) decompression. The SCA has been transposed upward to the tentorium, and its position secured with a piece of semi-rigid Teflon, hold by the superior petrosal vein (SPV) which has been respected. Note that the Teflon plate does not touch the root so that it does not exert any neocompression

the arteries, in hyperintensity, especially if sequence includes a pre-saturation filter.

- The 3D-T1 sequence with gadolinium injection depicts (in hypersignal) all the vascular structures, that is, not only the arteries but also the veins. Thus, by comparing the images of the last two sequences, it is possible to differentiate the veins from the arteries and to precisely identify the type of the vascular compression.

The reliability of high-definition MRI scanning, when it involves the combination of the three sequences, is high. A prospective study comparing imaging data with operative findings in 100 consecutive cases established that the sensitivity of the exploration was 96.7% and specificity 100% (Leal et al. 2010). The protocol allowed to predict the type of the responsible vessel(s) in 88% of the cases, the location along the root and the site around the root in 87.5% and 84.6%, respectively, and the degree of the compression (simple contact/distortion/indentation of the root) by the conflicting vessel in 84.6% of cases ($p < 0.01$).

By principle, the 3-T MRI machine gives better images than the 1.5-T machine. However, in our study the latter gave almost as reliable information, provided the procedure be done carefully. But the 3T-MRI allowed better identification

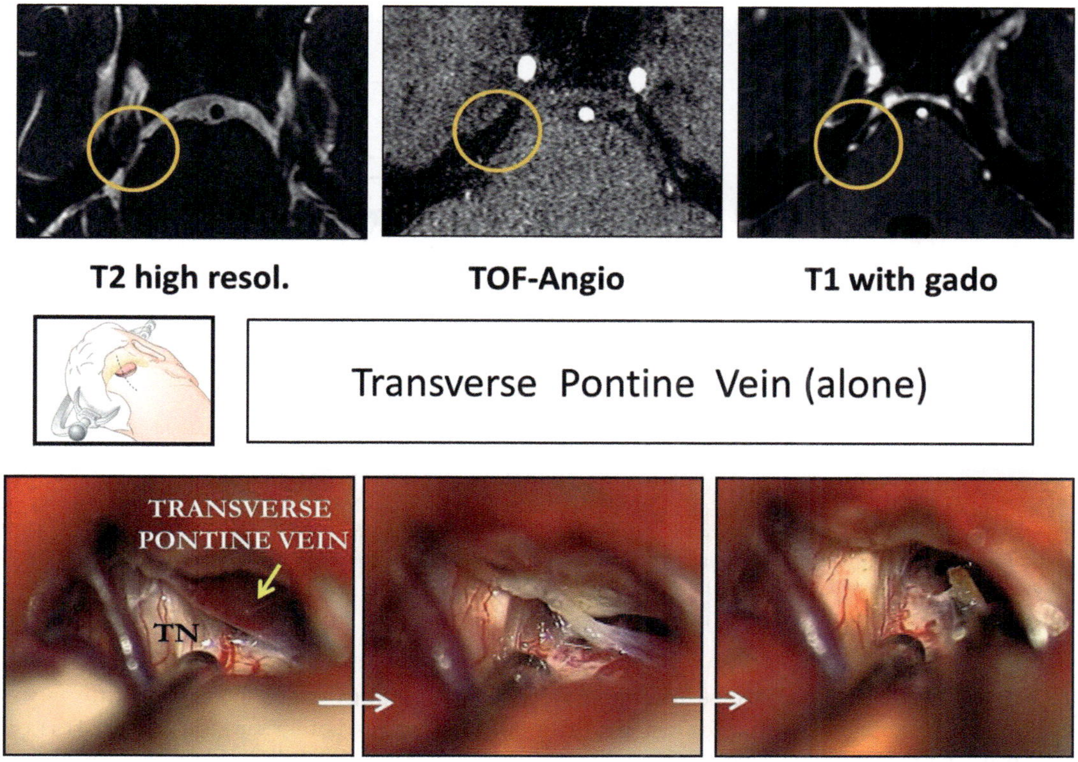


**Fig. 6.2** Imaging diagnosis of a venous Neuro-Vascular Conflict from pure venous compression, namely the inferior transverse vein in a patient with right-sided TN. The MRI 3D high-resolution $T_2$ axial view shows the root crossed by the conflicting vessel. The identifiable conflicting vessel on $T_2$ is not visible in TOF-Angio sequence, but apparent on $T_1$ with gadolinium sequence, which is evocative of a pure venous conflict. Note the small size of the cerebellopontine angle cistern. The microsurgical views illustrate the approach via an infratentorial-supracerebellar route. The transverse vein (arrow) is seen compressive to the inferior aspect of the trigeminal root (TN) at its exit from the porus of Meckel cave. In this case, the coagulation and division of the vein was considered indispensable for the release of the compression

of small caliber vessels, especially the venous ones (Leal et al. 2011a).

## 6.3 Diffusion Tensor Imaging (DTI) MRI

- Further information is possible with Diffusion Tensor Imaging (DTI) MRI, thanks to its capability to evidence alterations in the trigeminal root.

Surely high-resolution MRI—especially if performed with a 3-T machine—may show morphologic changes, namely root deviation, distortion, and engroving (Leal et al. 2011a). Focal atrophy secondary to structural alterations, such as axonal loss and demyelination in the root, can be evidenced by measuring the volume (V) and the cross-sectional area (CSA) at level of the NVC image, and comparing to the ones measured on the unaffected side (Fig. 6.3) (Brinzeu et al. 2018a). However, such morphological changes can be difficult to interpret, so that structural markers of damages can be useful (Leal et al. 2011b, 2019; Parise et al. 2013).

Diffusion-tensor imaging (DTI) enables the analysis of white matter integrity by means of in vivo measurements of molecular diffusivity (Le Bihan 1995). There are numeric indexes to describe anisotropic diffusion and underlying tissue integrity (Pierpaoli et al. 1996). Measuring

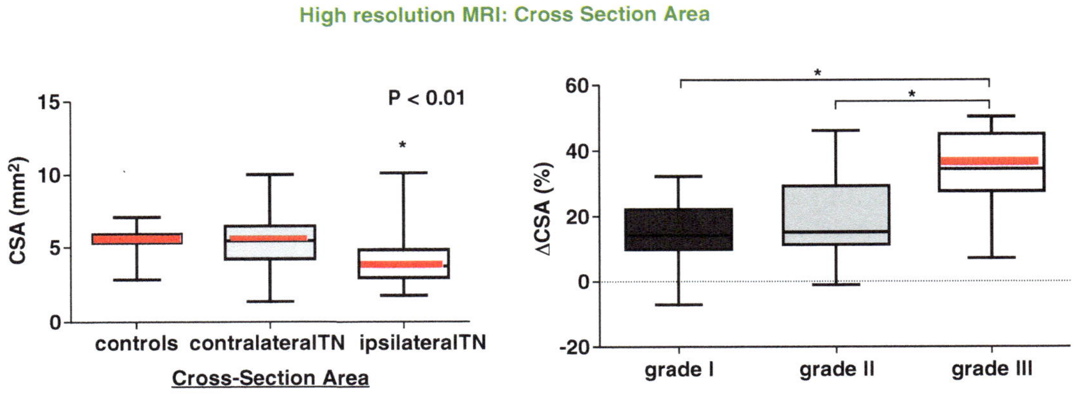


**Fig. 6.3** Study of root Cross Section Area (CSA) with high-resolution MRI (Leal et al. 2014). Left: Graph shows that the mean CSA on the affected side (ipsilateral TN) is significantly lower than the mean CSA on the unaffected side (contralateral TN) and the mean CSA on both sides in control subjects ($p < 0.01$). Right: Correlation between the variation in cross-sectional area (ΔCSA) of the trigeminal root on the affected and unaffected sides (expressed as percentage) and the degree of severity of the compression. Graph shows that the ΔCSA in patients with neurovascular compression (NVC) of Grade III (34.48 ± 11.57%) is superior than in patients with NVC of Grade I (15.58 ± 10.93%) and Grade II (18.76 ± 11.78%) ($^*p < 0.05$)

the Fraction of Anisotropy (FA) is a robust method of assessing the degree of directionality of diffusion (i.e., anisotropic diffusion) that occurs in a particular region (Pierpaoli and Basser 1996). Diffusivity, expressed as the Apparent Diffusion Coefficient (ADC), is a quantitative measure of water motility (independent of orientation) in an individual voxel (Pierpaoli and Basser 1996) and indicates the overall presence of obstacles to diffusion, correlating with not only demyelination but also with neuroinflammatory processes and/or neuroedema (Basser and Pierpaoli 2011). This method can be applied to the study of abnormalities in white matter tracts, independent of their cause, to ascertain structural alterations.

At present these sophisticated methods, time-consuming to set-up and interpret, are mostly carried out for research. However, they could be used in difficult cases for classifying trigeminal neuralgias and therefore deciding treatment.

Used for assessing patients, DTI revealed a loss of anisotropy and an increase in diffusivity in affected nerves before surgery (Fig. 6.4) (Leal et al. 2011b). These diffusion alterations correlated well with atrophic changes in patients with TN caused by NVC. After removal of the compression, the loss of FA remained but ADC normalized in the affected nerves, suggesting improvement in diffusion of the trigeminal root (Leal et al. 2019).

**Key-Point**

*The diagnosis of classical trigeminal neuralgia requires demonstration of morphologic changes in the TGN from vascular compression.*

This can be difficult on preoperative MRI when the vessel suspected to be conflicting is in simple contact with the root (Grade I of compression).

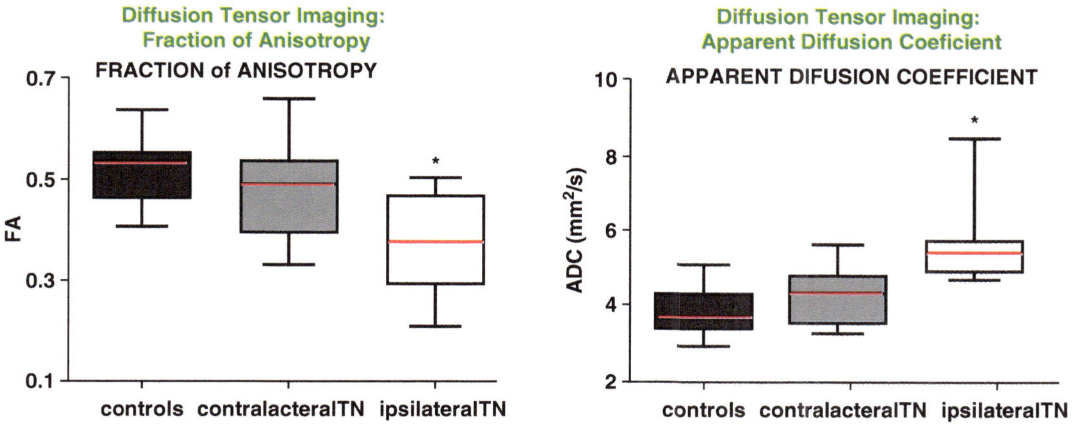


**Fig. 6.4** Study with diffusion tensor imaging: fraction of anisotropy and apparent diffusion coefficient (Leal et al. 2011b). Left: Graph shows that the mean fraction of anisotropy (FA) on the affected side (ipsilateral TN) is significantly lower than the mean FA on the unaffected side (contralateral TN) and the mean FA on both sides in control subjects ($p < 0.05$). Right: Graph shows that the mean apparent diffusion coefficient (ADC) on the affected side (ipsilateral TN) is significantly higher than the mean ADC on the unaffected side (contralateral TN) and the mean ADC on both sides in control subjects ($^*p < 0.05$)

# 7 Differential Diagnoses of Trigeminal Neuralgias

The main differential diagnoses are the trigeminal pains linked to an identifiable pathology or an injury to the trigeminal system or its territory. They belong to two different entities. The first one corresponds to the "secondary trigeminal neuralgias," the second to the "painful trigeminal neuropathies." Other diagnoses not directly related to pathologies of the trigeminal nerve mimic trigeminal neuralgia, quite frequently the trigeminal autonomic cephalalgias in their various forms.

## 7.1 The Secondary Trigeminal Neuralgias

The secondary TNs belong to the nosologic group of trigeminal neuralgias, but they are linked to identifiable diseases attaining the afferent primary fibers to the gasserian ganglion, the root, or the brainstem. The pain can be purely paroxysmal or associated with a more or less continuous background of pain. Examination often shows sensory changes. MRI is the most appropriate mean to identify the responsible pathology. Clinical neurophysiology and biology may also help.

Among many, main causes can be attributed to the following pathologies.

Space-occupying processes in posterior fossa or skull base region represent the first cause of secondary trigeminal neuralgias. Among those, tumors of the cerebello-pontine angle (CPA) or the Meckel cave in contact with the trigeminal root are the most frequent, as for example meningiomas (Fig. 7.1) or epidermoid/dermoid cysts (Fig. 7.2). Fewer are the tumors of the TGN itself, principally the schwannomas; they can be located in the trigeminal cave, the CPA, or both. All these tumoral processes evolve with increasing deficits.

When the diagnosis of nature cannot be ascertained on sole imaging, one can recourse to percutaneous biopsy through the foramen ovale to determine appropriate treatment (Messerer et al. 2012; Sindou et al. 2012).

Also, arterio-venous malformations (a few of which are located within the trigeminal root itself), arterio-venous dural fistulas, giant aneurysms may be at the origin of secondary TNs.

Cranial abnormalities can be responsible or be favorizing factors for neuralgias; among these, skull base platybasia or malformations of the cranio-cervical junction such as Chiari malformation.

Infectious pathologies, although infrequent, may be encountered, as for example Lyme disease (Fig. 7.3).

Multiple sclerosis (MS) is undoubtfully a frequent etiology of secondary trigeminal neuralgia (Fig. 7.4). MS accounts for 2–4% of the TN pop-


M. Sindou, A. Brinzeu, *Trigeminal Neuralgias: A Neurosurgical Illustrated Guide*,
https://doi.org/10.1007/978-3-031-25113-9_7

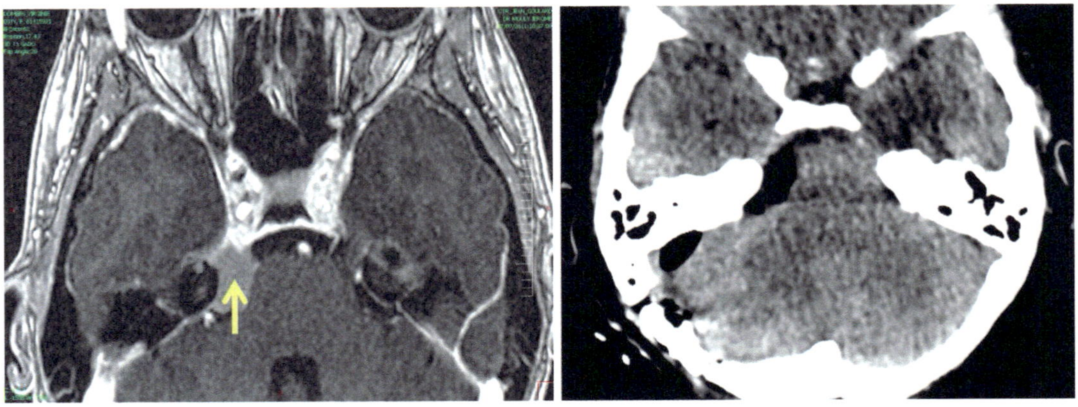

**Fig. 7.1** Meningioma. Atypical trigeminal neuralgia on right side in $V_2$–$V_3$ territories in a 38-year-old female. MRI-$T_1$ + gadolinium sequence shows petrous apex and trigeminal cave meningioma (arrow). Gross total removal of the tumor through a retrosigmoid approach (as shown in post-op CT) obtained favorable outcome on both pain and sensory function of the trigeminal nerve

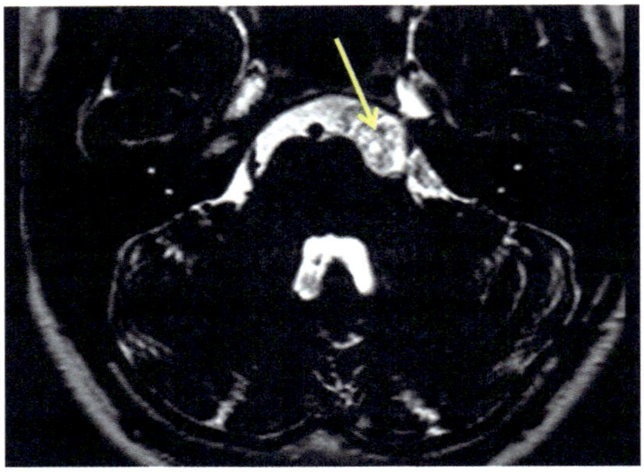

**Fig. 7.2** Epidermoid cyst. Typical trigeminal neuralgia on left side in $V_2$–$V_3$ territories in a 32-year-old male. MRI-$T_2$ sequence shows an epidermoid cyst at upper part of the left cerebello-pontine angle cistern (arrow). Neuralgia was relieved after total resection of the tumor including the cyst membranes stuck to the trigeminal nerve

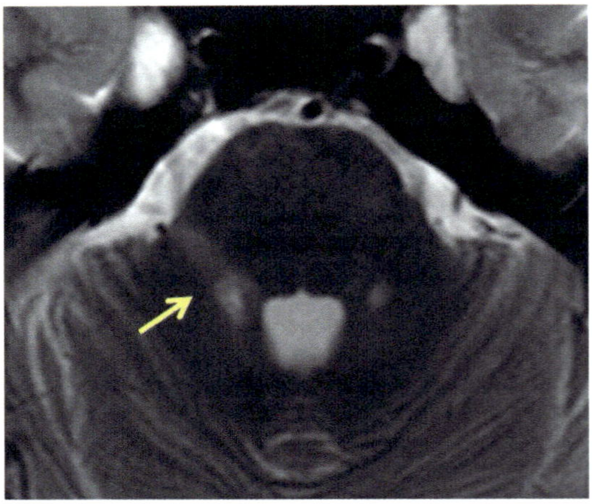

**Fig. 7.3** Lyme disease. Typical trigeminal neuralgia on right side in $V_2$–$V_3$ territories in a 55-year-old male. MRI-$T_2$ sequence shows abnormal signal in pons corresponding to the intra-axial trigeminal pathways (arrow). Etiology was considered sequella of Lyme disease. Neuralgia was relieved by thermorhizotomy, but with numbness in $V_2$–$V_3$ trigeminal divisions

ulation. TN occurs during the course of the disease in 2–5%, according to series. Importantly, TN may constitute the first revealing symptom of the disease (MS).

The MS plaques are most often in the pons, on the trigeminal pathways to the brainstem nuclei, more rarely in the TREZ. According to the ICHD Cephalalgias 2018, the MS TN can be classified as central neuropathic pain (IHS 2018).

NB: Complete neurological examination, high-resolution MRI (and/or CT scan), and electrophysiological explorations are mandatory to identify or exclude the various pathologies that might create secondary TNs. This is the more so as important as their treatment should be as etiopathogenic as possible.

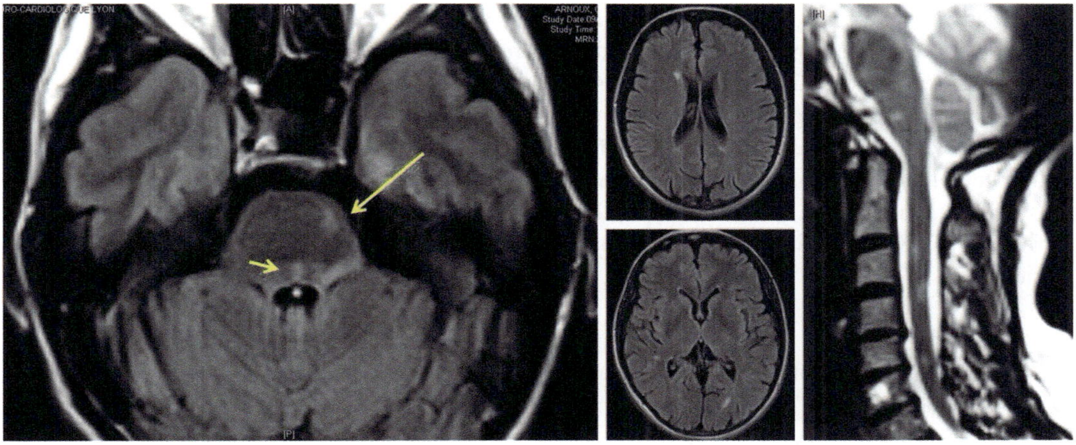

**Fig. 7.4** Multiple sclerosis. Atypical trigeminal neuralgia on left side in $V_2$–$V_3$ territories in a 35 year old female affected with a slowly evolving multiple sclerosis. MRI shows disseminated plaques especially located in brainstem within left trigeminal trigeminal pathways (arrows). Plaques are also visible in white matter of brain and spinal cord. Neuralgia was relieved by percutaneous thermorhizotomy, with numbness in left $V_2$–$V_3$ division territories

## 7.2 The Painful Trigeminal Neuropathies

Painful trigeminal neuropathies may develop in the territory of one or more divisions of the trigeminal nerve, caused by a pathological process or an injury that has created significant neuronal damage.

Pain is highly variable in quality and intensity depending on the etiology and the individual. A phenomenon of painful anesthesia and/or dysesthesias may be added. A burning continuous background often associated with paresthesias is the dominant component of the pain. Allodynia and hyperalgesia are common, which participate—according to the IASP taxonomy—to attach this pain to the frame of neuropathic pain. Sensory deficit can be detected, as well as reduction of the corneal reflex when the ophthalmic division is involved.

Such painful neuropathies are frequently encountered, as sequela of herpes zoster attacks, or after injuries which can be from traumatic origin, or observed after dental, buccal, ENT, maxillofacial, and craniofacial surgeries. In all those surgeries the peripheral branches of the TGN are structures at risk. After intracranial neurosurgical procedures, anesthesia dolorosa may appear as the consequence of aggressive tumors resection, especially those invading the skull base or occupying the cerebellopontine angle region.

Neurosurgeons are also well aware that any of the lesioning-procedures to treat primary TN can leave as a sequela some degree of trigeminal neuropathy, whatever the lesioning-agent may be.

## 7.3 The Trigeminal Autonomic Cephalalgias (TACs)

### 7.3.1 Cluster Headache

In its typical form everything opposes cluster headache to trigeminal neuralgia. The age of onset is younger and the predominance of men is clear. The pain is throbbing, burning, and heartbreaking. Topography is that of the external carotid artery with frequently a retro-orbital maximum and a posterior irradiation in "branch of glasses" with an associated occipital pain. The attack lasts from one to several hours without remission. The evolution is quite characteristic with painful periods of several weeks, the patient suffering every day for a few hours, with a remarkably fixed daily rhythm.

The mechanism of cluster headache is still incompletely understood and puzzling. However, functional imaging studies suggest the existence of an activation of the posterior hypothalamic region with involvement of the trigemino-parasympathetic reflex, the clinical signs of sympathetic dysfunction being secondary to them.

Nevertheless, the distinction can be difficult with some other trigeminal autonomic cephalalgias (TACs), the criteria for which have been revised in 2018 by the international Headache Society (IHS) (2018).

### 7.3.2 Other Types of TACs

Several other syndromes have been described besides the classic cluster headache, that may give rise to diagnostic discussion with trigeminal neuralgias.

"Cluster-tic" combines the two types of attacks independently or in succession, neuralgia preceding cluster headache. Therapeutic tests with carbamazepine and injectable triptans are useful. If trigeminal neuralgia is the predominant disease, the pain will disappear with carbamazepine, while if there is a combination, the two medications will be necessary for obtaining the pain relief of both components.

"Paroxysmal hemicranias" consist in painful attacks—similar to the pain of cluster headache syndrome—but shorter in duration (2–30 min) and several times a day. The condition affects mostly the female gender and responds well to indomethacin. This syndrome may become more or less permanent, and thus takes the form of "Hemicrania continua," with the same characteristics. This syndrome similarly responds to indomethacin.

The syndrome of "short-lasting unilateral neuralgiform headache attacks with conjunctival injection and tearing (SUNCT)" is characterized by very short, orbital and unilateral (one to a few minutes), and numerous (3–200/day) attacks, accompanied by very intense tearing and redness of the eye.

Close to the previous one is the syndrome of "short-lasting unilateral neuralgiform headache with cranial autonomic features"; the difference consist in the location of the pain elsewhere than in the orbital territory.

For these two syndromes it is necessary to ask for an MRI centered on the sellar region, as sometimes one can find a pituitary adenoma or other types of tumors or lesions. More often these syndromes are of idiopathic nature. Pain does not respond well to Indomethacin; Lamotrigine or Topiramate can be tried.

## 7.4 Neuralgias Outside the Trigeminal Territory

The most frequent neuralgic pains affecting the cephalic extremity are the Occipital neuralgias; in a large majority of the patients, differential diagnosis is easy as the respective territories are quite different. Perhaps the most difficult differential diagnosis with trigeminal neuralgia is the vago-glossopharyngeal neuralgia; this is the more so true as the territories of the Vth nerve and of the IXth–Xth nerve complex have important overlaps, and that both neuralgias can be intricated.

### 7.4.1 Vago-Glossopharyngeal Neuralgia

The neuralgia of the Glossopharyngeal cranial nerve (the IXth CN), which it seems preferable to term Vago-Glossopharyngeal Neuralgia (VGPN) because of the frequent additional involvement of the sensory territory of the vagus nerve (with its auricular and pharyngeal branches) (the Xth CN) (Gybels and Sweet 1989) is not easy to differentiate from some forms of trigeminal neuralgia (Chen and Sindou 2015).

This VGPN compared to trigeminal neuralgia is rare since its incidence is estimated at only 1% of the latter. The pain, most often paroxysms characterized by electrical shooting-like attacks, begins in the back of the throat, at the base of the tongue and/or the tonsil, and radiates to beneath the angle of the jaw or in the depth of the ear. Attacks are most often violent, strictly one-sided and always deep. The pain is caused usually by swallowing, sometimes by talking, yawning, coughing, sneezing. The trigger zone is the pharyngeal mucosa, the tonsil, and the depth of the external auditory canal. The attacks, which can last from seconds to minutes are followed at least in the early forms by a "refractory period" during which the trigger zone is unexcitable, and that the patient takes advantage for eating.

In its classical form, clinical examination does not detect any neurological deficits and investigations remain negative with the mention of possible NVC. At present, high-resolution MRI can depict with good reliability the responsible neuro-vascular conflict, so that MVD can be safely performed (Fig. 7.5).

Syncopal attacks may be associated to the pain and a cause of misdiagnosis. It has also been described forms with acute digestive manifestations, with abdominal pain, vomiting, and even diarrhea; these symptoms can be explained by involvement of the vagus nerve (Antherieu et al. 2016).

Recently, a form of involvement of the Xth cranial nerve, particularly on its contingent corresponding to the laryngeal nerve, leading to laryngeal hemispasm, mostly by vascular compression, has been described. This dramatic-looking syndrome has been given the evocative acronym of HELP (Hemi-Laryngo-Pharyngeal Spasm) (Honey et al. 2017).

### 7.4.2 Neuralgia of the Intermedius Nerve

This neuralgia is extremely rare. Territory is mainly the concha of ear, sometimes accompanied by lacrimation, salivation, and disturbance of taste. Differential diagnosis is very difficult with the purely otalgic form of the vago-glossopharyngeal neuralgia.

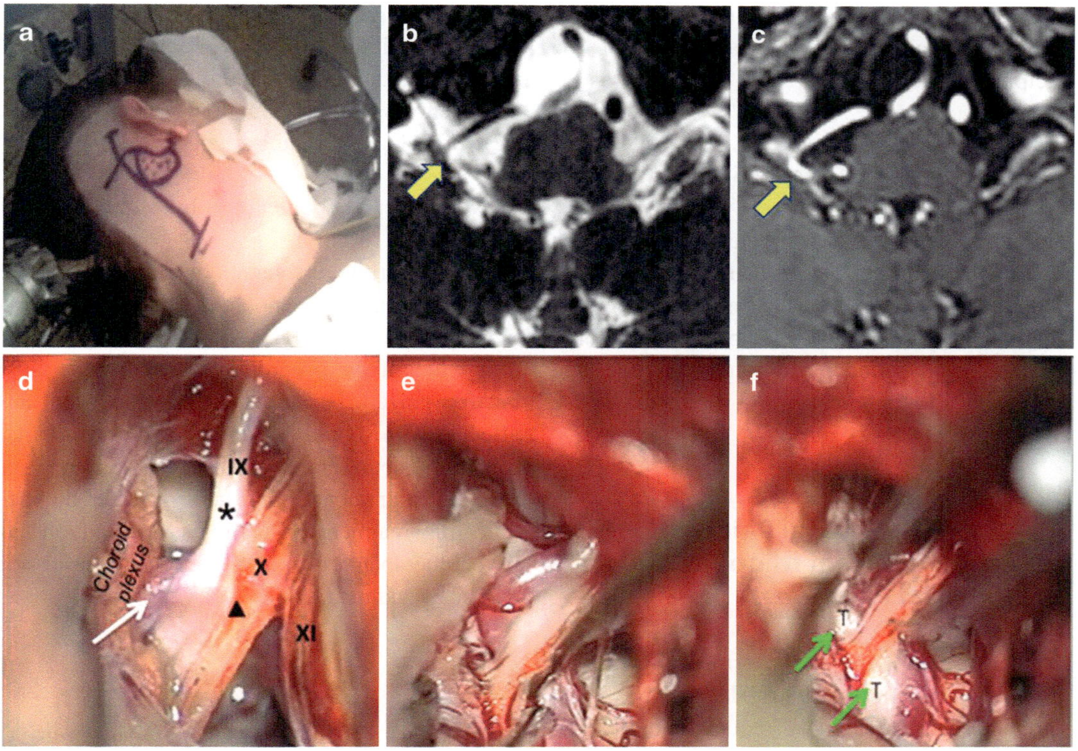


**Fig. 7.5** Vago-glossopharyngeal neuralgia on right side due to Neuro-Vascular Conflict (NVC) from posterior-inferior cerebellar artery (PICA) treated by micro-vascular decompression (MVD). Landmarks of the keyhole approach (retromastoid, retrocondylar, and retrosigmoid) for vagal and glossopharyngeal MVD. (**a**) High-resolution MRI with $T_2$ (**b**) and $T_1$ + gadolinium (**c**) sequences show the NVC (arrows). Infrafloccular microsurgical approach on the right side. The offending PICA is ventral to the Root Entry Zone (REZ) of the ninth (asterisk) and the tenth (triangle) nerves. Note the atrophic and greyish aspect of the ninth and tenth rootlets testifying of local demyelination. (**d**) The compressive PICA (arrow) is detached after dissection and freeing of the rootlets from arachnoid adhesions. (**e**) The Teflon felt bundle (T, green arrows) is placed so that the artery is maintained apart from REZ of ninth and tenth rootlets (**f**)

### 7.4.3 Neuralgia of the Superior Laryngeal Nerve

This neuralgia is also very rare. Its seat is the lateral wall of the throat, the submandibular region under the ear canal; it is triggered by swallowing, screaming, and turning the head. It is difficult to diagnose with the pharyngeal form of the glossopharyngeal neuralgia.

### 7.4.4 Occipital Neuralgia

Occipital neuralgia is frequent and characteristic. It corresponds to the territory of the great (or small) occipital nerve or the third occipital nerve. It is triggered by the pressure at the emergence of these nerves in the muscles of the neck and/or by rotation—flexion of the neck. It is often accompanied by paresthesias and allodynia of the occipital territory.

### 7.4.5 The Neck-Tongue Syndrome

This rare syndrome is characterized by sudden pain in the occipital region or the upper part of the neck, with an abnormal sensation in the tongue, on the same side. This pain is commonly triggered by the sudden rotation of the head, and corresponds to the territories of the lingual nerve and the second cervical root.

## 7.5 Atypical Facial Pain (= Persistent Idiopathic Facial Pain)

Atypical facial pain—now termed by international classification of the IHS as "persistent idiopathic facial pain"—is frequent and misleading. The pain is dull, aching, and of nagging quality.

The permanence of the pain, the area often located deeply in the nasolabial fold, sometimes at the frontal or maxillary sinus or in a dental region ("sine materia" toothache), as well as the negativity of the clinical assessment, make it very different entity from TN. When comparing trigeminal neuralgia to persistent idiopathic facial pain, criteria testing led to a sensitivity of 95.1% and a specificity of 83.8% (Maarbjerg et al. 2014a, b, 2015a). However, the distinction between neuralgia with or without a continuous background of pain has not been however tested in its impact on outcome.

The previously used form: Atypical facial pain is now termed by the ICHD: "Persistent idiopathic facial pain (PIFP)." Diagnostic criteria are the following:

(A) Facial and/or oral pain fulfilling criteria B and C
(B) Recurring daily for >2 h/day, for >3 months
(C) Pain with both of the following characteristics
   1. poorly localized, and not following the distribution of a peripheral nerve
   2. dull, aching, or nagging quality
(D) Neurological examination: normal
(E) Dental cause been excluded

Not better accounted for by another ICHD diagnosis.

This syndrome is retained by elimination as "a facial pain which does not have the characteristics of other cranial neuralgias and cannot be attributed to any identifiable disorder." This syndrome must be recognized because the patients who are affected with should not undergo surgery. Unlike trigeminal neuralgia, atypical facial pain does not respond to anticonvulsant therapy. It has no specific drug treatment. Psychologist consultation and psychotherapeutic support are most useful for diagnosis and management.

**Key-Point**

The most difficult and misleading differential diagnosis is the distinction between atypical trigeminal neuralgia and atypical facial pain, the so-called persistent idiopathic facial pain according to the recent terminology, this latter not being in any way a surgical indication.

# Pharmacological Treatment of Trigeminal Neuralgias

8

The unbelievable number of treatments tried for trigeminal neuralgia since its first descriptions in the seventeenth century are a testimony to the undue suffering incurred by the affliction: everything including poisons (arsenic, hemlock), opiates, galvanotherapy, and so on. Unfortunately the only positive results of this corresponded in fact to spontaneous remission. Progressively physio pathological hypotheses were introduced leading to that of a paroxysmal activity in the trigeminal nuclei formulated by Trousseau as early as 1853. This paved the way to the first validated pharmacological treatment with the introduction of diphenylhydantoin by Bergouignan based on the rationale of utilizing an antiepileptic for the treatment of trigeminal neuralgia (Bergouignan and D'Aulnay 1951; Bergouignan 1958, 1970). Subsequently carbamazepine was developed specifically for the treatment of trigeminal neuralgia by W Schindler in 1953 (Schindler 1954) and its use popularized by Blom in the early sixties (Blom 1962). This was followed by the development of oxcarbazepine a decade later with the purpose of reducing the side effects of carbamazepine in particular in its antiepileptic use which had, immediately after its release, become very popular.

Later, other drugs were introduced in attempts to compensate the disadvantages of carbamazepine and oxcarbazepine. None were specifically developed for trigeminal neuralgia and all have lesser efficacy in large series than these two, however still finding a role in replacing the carbamazepine class when side-effects are too important. Trigeminal neuralgia being a rare disease, there is little financial incentive to design new molecules for its treatment; however, some advanced studies are ongoing in particular with vixotrigine (Zakrzewska et al. 2018; Kotecha et al. 2020).

Pharmacological treatment of trigeminal neuralgia is therefore based on the use of antiepileptics with a few other potential contributions. The European Academy of Neurology summarized all treatments with any proven efficacy and gives clear indications for their use (Bendtsen et al. 2019, 2020). Two main drugs of similar efficacy are the mainstay of the pharmacological treatment: carbamazepine and oxcarbazepine. All other drugs have lower efficacy and are not particularly adapted for trigeminal neuralgia. Other antiepileptic drugs include lamotrigine and the now classical anti neuropathic pain: gabapentin and pregabalin. Other drugs that have been studied at least in part and have come clinical evidence are baclofen and botulinum toxin A.

Carbamazepine and oxcarbazepine have been directly compered in a clinical study (Di Stefano et al. 2014) clearly concluding in the similarity between the two. Initial treatment with carbamazepine yielded 98% pain sedation while oxcarbazepine yielded 94% pain sedation both at the higher spectrum of the dosage. In the subsequent months following initiation of treatment, 27% of


M. Sindou, A. Brinzeu, *Trigeminal Neuralgias: A Neurosurgical Illustrated Guide*,
https://doi.org/10.1007/978-3-031-25113-9_8

carbamazepine users and 18% of oxcarbazepine discontinued following joint decision with their physicians because of side effects of the medication (i.e., not because of loss of efficacy). The side-effect profile is not identical between the two molecules and therefore they can be switched with good efficacy at least initially after the switch. Loss of efficacy over time is observed by the increase in number and intensity of paroxysms or by the development of continuous background pain (Di Stefano et al. 2020). This is however observed in less than 10% of patients over periods of at least 5 years (Di Stefano et al. 2021). Alternative or adjuvant molecules can be tried in general with lesser efficacy and significant risks of side-effects (Di Stefano et al. 2018).

The overwhelming efficacy of carbamazepine and oxcarbamzepine for the initial treatment of TN has led to the proposition of their use as a test and secondary criterion for the diagnosis for trigeminal neuralgia. For one patients should be encouraged in the initial phase of treatment to up-titrate doses to a level that leads to sedation of the pain. This often comes with the price of side effects at least in the form of drowsiness. If positive patients can modulate their treatment quite well with both carbamazepine and oxcarbazepine juggling between the forms with immediate release which are extremely useful for halting a salvo of paroxysmal episodes and slow release for a background treatment (with lower levels of drowsiness).

From the surgeon's point of view, who sees the patients later in the evolution of their disease, it is important to seek out the initial effect of these two drugs and probe for the effect on pain. Patients who have discontinued the medication have a tendency to dislike the medication (mostly because of the side effects), and this emotional reaction hides the actual effect on pain. It is confirmatory of trigeminal neuralgia and encouraging concerning the results of surgery to know that the initial effect of carbamazepine was positive.

From the medical clinician's point of view, it is also important to remember that the other medication (not carbamazepine or oxcarbazepine) for trigeminal neuralgia has lower efficacy overall and is less adapted. It can be tried single standing or as an adjuvant but when carbamazepine or oxcarbamzepine fail, surgery should be considered, and outside contraindications, it is probably the best option. In these types of cases seeking surgical opinion allows the patients to better understand their disease and choose the preferred treatment and some if not many will prefer surgery to the fog of long-term use of high dose antiepileptics (Poole et al. 2022).

## 8.1 Carbamazepine (Tegretol®)

Carbamazepine use for trigeminal neuralgia is now notoriously effective. One would expect—if the other diagnostic criteria are fulfilled—to achieve pain sedation with carbamazepine at least initially. If there is no effect of carbamazepine at high doses, the diagnosis of TN should be put under serious scrutiny and the entire differential performed once again. Carbamazepine has no clear effect on cluster headaches or idiopathic headaches. On the other hand, it can be active on secondary trigeminal neuralgia, in particular those of multilocular sclerosis.

The dosage varies depending on the patient between 600 and 3600 mg (which surpasses the manufacturer and regulator's recommended doses). The dose is determined by trial and error after a gradual introduction which makes it possible to reduce the inaugural side-effects: drowsiness, drunkenness, digestive intolerance. This is particularly true in the elderly where the risk of falls and ataxia are high.

We therefore start with 100 or 200 mg daily, increasing by 100 mg every other day. A dose of 600–800 mg in three divided doses provides relief for most patients, but sometimes higher doses of 1200 or even 1600 mg may have to be used. Plasma concentrations are between 6 and 12 mg/l.

The use of slow release forms is useful for chronic treatment but in the initial phase of treatment we prefer the use of rapid release forms.

The effectiveness of the product is appreciable from the first days of treatment, truly constituting a diagnostic test. Overall from the first 8 days, 60% of patients see their pain disappear, 20%

improve, and 20% resist and with up-titration of doses, one should expect 98% pain sedation in the initial phase.

The constraint of carbamazepine is represented by its side-effects: nausea, drunkenness, drowsiness, fatigue, diplopia, ataxia, nystagmus, sometimes dysarthria, sometimes cognitive disorders. These are not complications per se and constitute a direct side-effect of the use of the molecule. They are also the main limiting factor for long-term effective use.

The list of complications of carbamazepine is long but they are rarer than the side effects. These should be known and sought by the practitioner. Severe complications such as hyponatremia, agranulocytosis, systemic lupus erythematosus, and skin "rash" are rare but dangerous. Allergic-type complications can obviously also occur as well as blood disorders: megaloblastic anemia, aplasia, or agranulocytosis can occur early, requiring monitoring of the blood count after 1 month, then at least every 6 months. Skin intolerances are rare but sometimes serious, requiring treatment to be discontinued. It is often morbilliform and urticarial rash appearing around the seventh day of treatment, sometimes hypersensitivity syndrome with skin signs, hyperthermia, lymphadenopathy, lymphocytosis, eosinophilia, requiring emergency stop. Liver damage is mainly biological, cytolytic type.

In the subsequent months following introduction of the treatment a significant proportion of patients discontinue use because of side effects and sometimes but more rarely complications. Side-effects lead to 27% of patients discontinuing use. Overall, in the first year approximately one-third of patients drop out of the treatment plan. For these patients either oxcarbazepine or another antiepileptic can be an option. The expectation is that oxcarbazepine will yield the same efficacy and may not have the same side-effects—this has been clinically verified. Other antiepileptics are clearly of lesser efficacy and sometimes a shot in the dark as of such should not be tried if the surgical option is real.

Long-term use of carbamazepine has been studied with a loss of efficacy in about 10% of patients over time that is not due to direct side-effects of complications but to the increase of the frequency of pain attacks and their intensity. This is also true for the long-term use of oxcarbazepine. Switching between the two is still an option but there is also the option of an additional treatment such as lamotrigine, gabapentinoids, or baclofen if the patient tolerates such additions. Again, the surgical option should be taken into account—if it is possible—because of the multitude and importance of cumulative side effect and complications as well as drug interactions.

All these constraints do not, however, call into question the remarkable effectiveness of carbamazepine, which remains the first treatment option along oxcarbazepine.

## 8.2 Oxcarbazepine (Trileptal®)

The complications of carbamazepine in the treatment of epilepsy have motivated the research behind oxcarbazepine developed 20 years after carbamazepine but oddly introduced in clinical practice in the 1990. Nowadays at least in the US it is prescribed more often than carbamazepine (by about 30%). In the field of trigeminal neuralgia the efficacy of oxcarbazepine is very similar to that of carbamazepine. Side-effects are also similar although the drop-out rate is somewhat less important in the first year of treatment being 18% compared to 27%.

From the point of view of complications Oxcarbazepine does not require routine hepatic or hematologic monitoring. Routine plasma measurements are also not necessary as is recommended with carbamazepine when drowsiness, dysarthria or ataxia, or nystagmus is observed. However, oxcarbazepine induces hyponatremia far more often than carbamazepine. Overall the profile of side effects and complications is similar but not identical and allows switching between the molecules.

Oxcarbazepine is started with a dose of 600 mg/day in two divided doses and can be increased to 1200 or even 2400 mg in particularly refractory neuralgia.

In the long term the two molecules are very similar and as of such no preference can be stated.

However, in the short run, carbamazepine seems more versatile and adaptable to the patients' needs who can take half and quarter doses with quick results when pain attacks occur. Adaptability by the patient and rapid onset results—as well as habbit—are reasons we prefer carbamazepine to oxcarbazepine. There is no evidence they differ in the long run and switching in case of problems with one of them should be the rule (except for hyponatremia perhaps). They are not used in association.

## 8.3 Other Antiepileptics

**Recognized by Current Recommendations**

*Lamotrigine* (Lamictal®) is a sodium channel blocker and glutamate antagonist. It can be used between 200 and 600 mg in neuralgia resistant to carbamazepine. Its main risk is skin allergy: one case of Stevens-Johnson-Lyell syndrome/in 1000 cases treated. Its introduction should be gradual, at 50 mg/day with an increase of 50 mg/week. Its usefulness is especially for trigeminal autonomic pain of the SUNCT type. It has a limited number of clinical studies concerning its use in the treatment of trigeminal neuralgia. Its main role is as an addon to carbamazepine or oxcarbazepine in an ongoing treatment that loses efficacy. In this matter it has been studied in a clinical randomized controlled trial (Zakrzewska et al. 1997). The doses used were 400 mg/day. Its use as a standalone therapy is not clinically validated and it is also impeded by the necessity to slowly titrate doses. It might be considered in patients that have serious contraindications to surgery.

*Gabapentinoids* (gabapentin and pregabalin) are currently in wide use for neuropathic pain. Their role in trigeminal neuralgia is limited but they might be considered for long standing neuralgias with an important continuous background of pain. One rule of the thumb is that doses are necessarily high (1800 mg for gabapentin and 900 mg per day for pregabalin). A preference for pregabalin can be expressed in concordance to the linear relation between dose and plasma concentration. In patients with resistance or complications to carbamazepine and contraindications to surgery this might be the best standalone options. In patients with continuous neuropathic pain in the trigeminal territory they also may be considered in particular in the settings of old trigeminal neuralgias or secondary neuralgias.

**Rarely Used Drugs**

*Diphenylhydantoin* (Di-Hydan®) (300 mg/day) is practically abandoned because of its side-effects: ataxia, nystagmus, cerebellar syndrome, hypertrophic gingivitis, etc. It might be an option if nothing else is available.

*Clonazepam* (Rivotril®) at a dose of 2–6 mg/day has been used for the treatment of refractory trigeminal neuralgia with rapidly repetitive pain attacks with significant patient suffering. It causes significant somnolence but cannot be halted rapidly. It cannot be used for long-term treatment.

*Topiramate* (Epitomax®) can be used between 150 and 300 mg/day in the event of carbamazepine escape. Side effects are rare, cognitive, and behavioral (depression, psychosis); frequent weight loss and paresthesia are observed.

*Levetiracetam* (Keppra®) at high doses of 3–4 g/day can be tried on refractory forms.

## 8.4 Non-antiepileptic Drugs

The use of non-antiepileptic drugs may be considered, however their efficacy compared to antiepileptics is inconclusive and current recommendations only cite their use as addons. Here can be mentioned:

Baclofen can be added to the antiepileptics as an oral adjuvant slightly increasing the efficacy with however the price of side effects. No serious clinical studies can be cited but it remains a discussed option.

Botulin toxin A has been tried with injections performed around the trigger zone. In initial studies a 20% cure rate was cited but no long-term studies have been performed and newer studies in the field are lacking. Again this is an option that might be considered in selected cases that do not benefit from other treatments.

**Key-Points**

Medical treatment is the first line treatment and the most used treatment for trigeminal neuralgia. First and foremost, this is represented by specific antiepileptics such as *carbamazepine and oxcarbazepine* that have virtually identical efficacy and similar side effects and complications. These two are very much effective at sufficient doses. The main limiting factors in the short run are the side effects in particular those of drowsiness. These account for about a quarter of patients that discontinue use. Switching between them is an option. Long-term loss of efficacy exists, and it involves one-tenth of patients. Add-on treatments can be considered, and they are represented mainly by lamotrigine, gabapentionids, and baclofen. Alternative treatments exist but with low efficacy and should be considered only in cases where surgery is not desirable. Gabapentinoids and lamotrigine are the main standalone alternatives.

In cases when carbamazepine and oxcarbazepine fail for whatever reason the consideration of alternatives should immediately include surgery as well, since the efficacy of alternative pharmacological treatments is low.

Studies have shown that patients that have the opportunity to consult surgeons early in the course of their TN, and thus know and have the possibility to choose between treatments, exhibit better satisfaction and long-term results.

# 9 Micro-Vascular Decompression (MVD) and Other Open Microsurgical Procedures for Trigeminal Neuralgias

The Micro-Vascular Decompression (MVD) method—now considered the gold-standard for treating classical trigeminal neuralgia—only slowly emerged along the last five decades among the numerous other techniques of the neurosurgical arsenal (which will be briefly recalled at beginning of this section). At present this conservative technique has the favor because it is established on solid pathophysiological bases; MVD does like most of the techniques which predominate in surgery, "at end anatomy prevails."

## 9.1 Brief on the Evolution of the Surgical Treatments

*Improving techniques to become more effective and safer took a long period of time along decades, both for open surgery and the percutaneous lesioning-techniques.*

The first surgical intervention proposed for trigeminal neuralgia was the Gasserian ganglionectomy. Conceived by Wears in 1885 and pioneered in practice soon after by Rose (Rose 1890), the procedure was then performed by Hartley (Hartley 1893), Horsley (Horsley 1891a, b) and Cushing (Cushing 1900). But it was quickly abandoned due to the frequent occurrence of keratites and anesthesia dolora. In 1901 Frazier, at the instigation of Spiller, developed the extradural sub-temporal Retrogasserian neurotomy (Spiller and Frazier 1901). Then in 1920 Dandy introduced the Juxtapontine radicotomy via sub-occipital laterocerebellar route (Dandy 1925). Limited to the pars major, the section, especially if reduced to its inferolateral two-thirds, was able to obtain analgesia without complete anesthesia of the face, in particular of the cornea. In 1938 Sjoqvist performed the Trigeminal tractotomy by cutting the descending spinal trigeminal tract at level of the medulla, this tract being the vector of the fibers for the thermoalgesic sensation of the face (Sjoqvist 1938; Olivecrona 1942; Kunc 1959). This intervention was then refined and popularized by Kunc (Kunc 1964, 1977; Kunc et al. 1978).

In 1952 Taarnhoj, assuming that trigeminal neuralgia could be due to constriction of the Gasser ganglion by fibrosclerosis of the dura-mater of the trigeminal cave, proposed the Decompression of the ganglion by opening its dural roof (Taarnhøj 1952, 1982). This technique, which had the theoretical interest of being conservative, was later abandoned due to the frequent recurrences after surgery. Shortly after, Shelden in 1955, interpreting the immediate good effect of the Taarnhoj's method as due to an operative trauma to the ganglion and neighboring nerve fibers, proposed the Hammering of the ganglion through direct approach (Shelden et al. 1955). This gave rise to the more recent method of balloon compression by Mullan (Mullan and Lichtor 1983).


M. Sindou, A. Brinzeu, *Trigeminal Neuralgias: A Neurosurgical Illustrated Guide*,
https://doi.org/10.1007/978-3-031-25113-9_9

In parallel, to mitigate the risks of the interventions by direct approach, percutaneous techniques were developed on the principle of the "old" method of Alcoholization of the Gasserian ganglion, proposed as early as 1906 by Taptas (1911) and performed via lateral approach by Harris (1912a, b, 1940) then via the transforamen ovale approach by Hartel (1912). Instead of alcohol, Jaeger in 1957 proposed the Injection of hot water at the site of the ganglion (Jaeger 1959), and Jefferson in 1963 the Injection of phenol (at the concentration of 1/20th in glycerin) (Jefferson 1963). In 1941 Kirschner introduced the Electrocoagulation of the gasserian ganglion as the lesion-maker; surgery was performed under general anesthesia and using a stereotaxic percutaneous approach to the ganglion with penetration of the electrode through the foramen ovale (Kirschner 1933). The technique was then successively improved by Thiry who used a current of lower intensity in order to avoid the total loss of the tactile sensitivity (Thiry and Hotermans 1974), then by Schürmann who replaced general anesthesia by neuroleptanalgesia to control the effects of the coagulation in the patient awake (Schürmann et al. 1972).

In the early seventies, Sweet refined and popularized the technique under the name of Controlled differential thermocoagulation of the trigeminal ganglion and rootlets (Sweet and Wepsic 1974). A radio-frequency generator was used as the heat source, a thermistor to measure the temperature at the tip of the electrode, and short sequences of general anesthesia or neuroleptanalgesia—only during the painful steps of the intervention—to allow the patient's cooperation. The method is able to obtain analgesia without complete anesthesia and in the sole painful area, thanks to the somatotopy of the fibers at the targeted level.

Still within the framework of percutaneous techniques performed under fluoroscopic control, Hakanson introduced in 1981 the Neurolysis of the Gasser ganglion by injection of glycerol into the trigeminal cistern of the Meckel cave via the foramen ovale (Håkanson 1978), and Mullan in 1979 the Compression of the Gasser ganglion using the inflatable balloon of a Fogarty probe as the lesion-maker (Mullan and Lichtor 1983).

Besides, in the fifties, Leksell applied the technique of Stereotaxic gamma-knife radiosurgery to trigeminal neuralgia (Leksell 1971). But this method only lost its anecdotal character with the advent of high-resolution MRI, which made precise targeting of radiation possible.

Along with these lesioning methods, the conservative method of Microsurgical vascular decompression developed in successive stages. The method is based on the observation made by Dandy, of the frequent observation of vascular conflicts in patients operated on in the cerebellopontine angle for trigeminal neuralgia to perform a juxtapontine radicotomy (Dandy 1932). However, vascular decompression was not performed until 1956, when Gardner reported treatment by simple decompression of the trigeminal root (Gardner 1962). The method was then soon adopted and refined with the microsurgical techniques by Jannetta, who firstly used the subtemporal extradural transtentorial route (Jannetta and Rand 1966; Jannetta 1967), then the retromastoid approach (Jannetta 1977), the later after Hardy from Montreal University advised this route as the most appropriate for performing MVDs (Provost and Hardy 1970). Thanks to Jannetta, the method was popularized and became widely accepted as the first surgical option for treating conservatively the nowadays so-called classical trigeminal neuralgia (Cruccu et al. 2016).

## 9.2 Anatomical-Pathological Findings in Patients with Neuro-Vascular Conflicts

### 9.2.1 Incidence of the Neuro-Vascular Conflicts

According to literature review a neurovascular conflict (NVC) is found in 90.5% of the patients with classical trigeminal neuralgia (76.3–100% depending on the series). In our surgeries performed in Lyon University Hospital a NVC was identified in 97% of the patients operated on for decompression (Sindou et al. 2002). An artery was the compressive vessel in the vast majority (90.70%). In the other 6.30%, the compressing vessel was a vein. In most cases the artery was the SCA (88%) (Fig. 9.1), whereas the AICA was found in 25.1% (Fig. 9.2), and a VBA in 5.2% (Fig. 9.3). Totality was more than 100% due to frequent implication of several vessels in the same patient. A venous compression, in association with an artery or alone (Fig. 9.4), was encountered in 38.7% (Dumot and Sindou 2015). Multiple conflicts, arterial (Fig. 9.5), or mixed arterial and venous (Fig. 9.6) were seen in one-third of the patients.

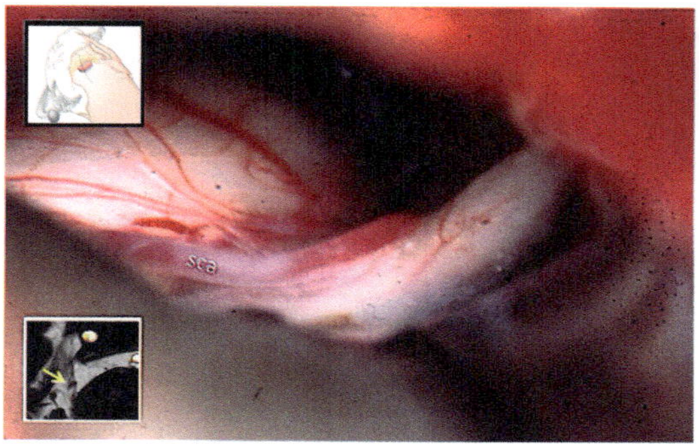


**Fig. 9.1** Patient with classical typical trigeminal neuralgia on right side. *Superior cerebellar artery* (sca) being the cross-compressing vessel as seen on MRI; degree of compression estimated at II out of III, that is, exerting traction on the trigeminal root by pushing it down

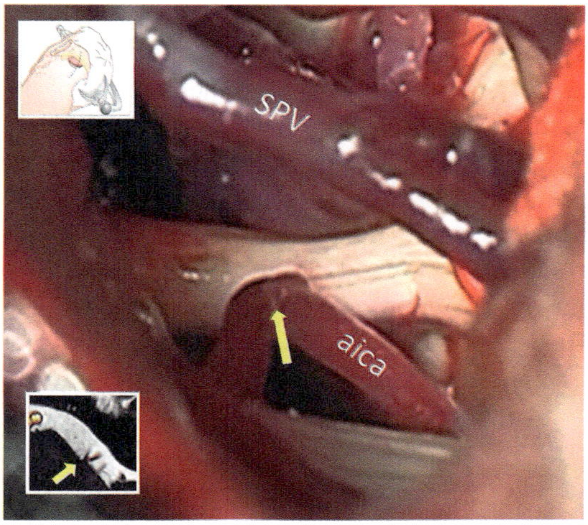


**Fig. 9.2** Patient with classical typical trigeminal neuralgia on left side. *Anterior inferior cerebellar artery* (AICA) as the conflicting vessel at the ventral part of TREZ as seen on MRI; degree of compression estimated at I out of III, that is, only contact with the root (but after wide opening of the arachnoid of the cerebello-pontine angle). Note Superior petrosal vein (SPV) preserved

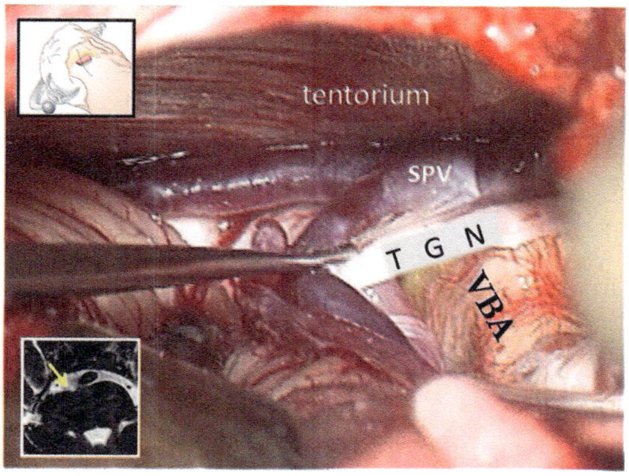


**Fig. 9.3** Patient with classical atypical trigeminal neuralgia on right side. *Megadolicho-Vertebro-Basilar artery* (VBA) as the compressive vessel, severely stretching the trigeminal nerve root (TGN) and compressing brainstem as seen on MRI. Superior petrosal veins (SPV) preserved

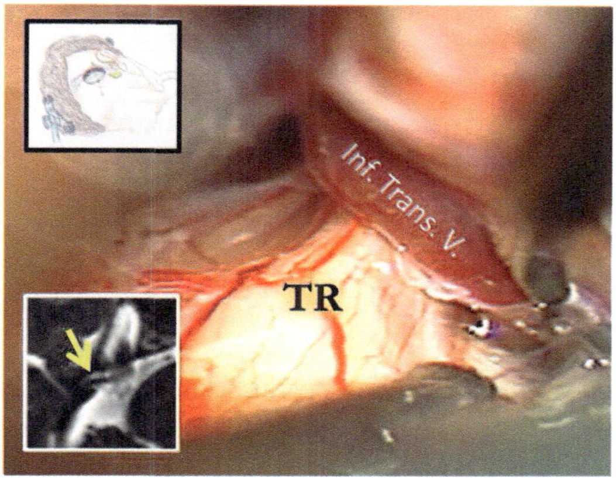


**Fig. 9.4** Patient with classical typical trigeminal neuralgia on right side. The *inferior transverse vein, belonging to the deep superior petrosal venous system*, as the neurovascular conflict; degree of compression estimated at III out of III, that is, strangulation of the trigeminal root (TR) at exit from the porus of Meckel cave, as seen on MRI

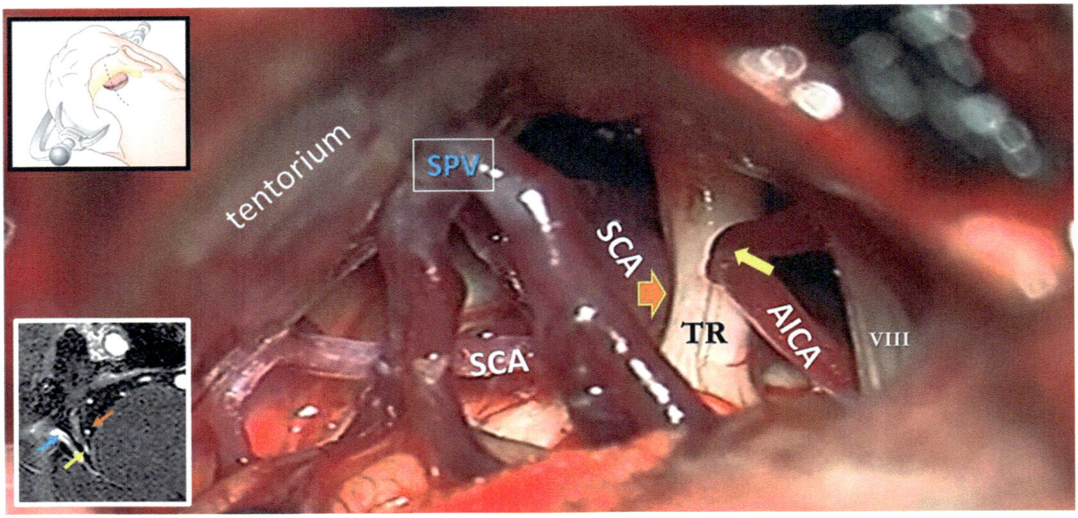


**Fig. 9.5** *Multiple arterial conflicts on MRI and at surgery*, from: the superior cerebellar artery (SCA), estimated grade III, at trigeminal root entry zone (brown arrow); and the anterior inferior cerebellar artery (AICA), of grade I out of III, at mid-cisternal portion of the trigeminal root (TR) (yellow arrow). *SPV* superficial Superior petrosal venous system (blue). VIII: Cochleo-vestibular cranial nerve exposed

### 9.2.2 Situation of the NVC Along the Trigeminal Root

In most publications the situation of the NVC along the trigeminal root was reported to predominate in the Trigeminal Root Entry Zone (TREZ), a region considered more excitable because of the central myelin nature of its neural tissue (see section on Anatomy of the TGN, this book). However, our observation was that conflicts were at the TREZ in only 50%; in the other half they were either mid-cisternal, in 40%, or at porus trigeminus, in 10% (Fig. 9.7) (Sindou et al. 2002, 2007; Dumot and Sindou 2015). At the porus the most frequently encountered vessel was a transverse pontine vein.

### 9.2.3 Location of the NVCs Around the Trigeminal Root

Location of the NVCs around the trigeminal root did not solicit much attention in literature. In our series most of the patients: 318 (89.3%) had the compression from above, of which 220 (61.7%) from a superomedial direction and 98 (27.5%) from a superolateral direction. An inferior compression was present in 38 patients (10.7%) (Fig. 9.8). Those data were correlated to the distribution of pain (Sindou and Brinzeu 2020). Odds ratios were computed for each location of compression and painful territory involved. Distribution of the pain was significantly different according to the location of the conflict ($p = 0.0005$, Fisher Exact test). Patients with superomedial compression had an odds ratio of 2.7 [95% confidence interval (CI) 1.66–4.41] of manifesting with V1 pain. Conversely V3 pain was less likely to occur with superomedial compression than the other types of pain (odds ratio 0.53, 95% CI 0.34–0.83). Inferior compression on the other hand was more likely to manifest with V3 pain with an odds ratio of 2.56 (95% CI 1.21–5.45). Overall V2 pain had an odds ratio close to 1 regardless of the type of compression. These findings suggest an association between the location of the NVC with its resulting insult and the distribution of pain supporting a somatotopic view of the organization of the trigeminal root and a role of the conflict in the clinical manifestation of trigeminal neuralgia.

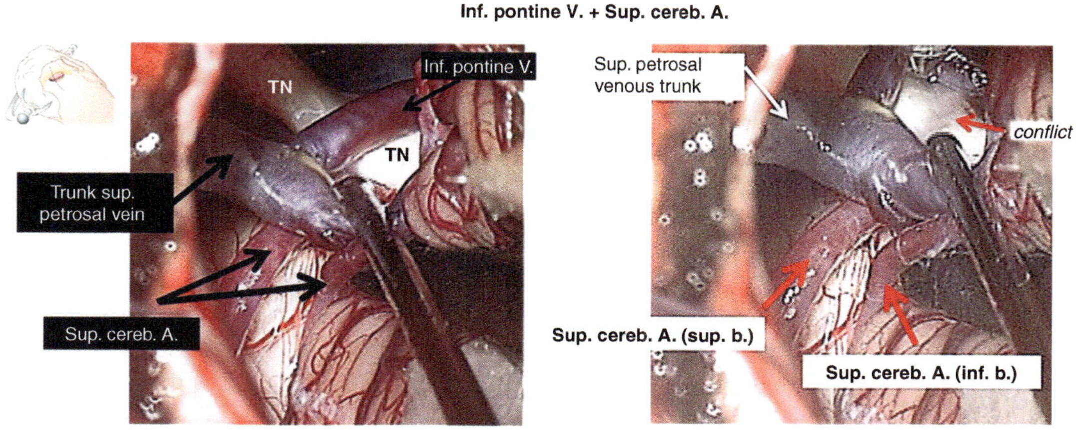


**Fig. 9.6** Multiple (mixed) arterial and venous conflicts. Exposure, through an infratentorial–supracerebellar approach on right side and inside the cerebello-mesencephalic fissure, of the superior petrosal venous trunk which drains the superior petrosal vein and its pontine affluent to the superior petrosal sinus. The trigeminal nerve root (TN) is squeezed between the inferior pontine vein, dorsally, and the superior cerebellar artery with its two division branches, ventrally, the later pushing down the root to the pontine vein; See on the right image the print of the pontine vein on the root, marked by a focal greyish discoloration at the conflict site, of grade III out of III of compression (red arrow); Decompression was performed by liberating the root from the venous compression and by pushing upward the superior cerebellar artery with a plate of Teflon to maintain it apart (not shown in the image)

### 9.2.4 Degrees of Compression of the NVCs

Compression by vessels can be of more or less important degrees. Those have been categorized by Sindou (Sindou et al. 2007) as merely a contact with the root, or displacing it, or even deforming it with groove and focal demyelination. They were termed compression of grade *I* (Fig. 9.9), *II* (Fig. 9.10), and *III* (Figs. 9.11 and 9.12), respectively. See Table 9.1. In grade III, an aspect of focal demyelination can be seen under the operating microscope manifested by a greyish zone at the site of the compression (Fig. 9.13).

In our series CVNs were of grade I in 19%, II in 38%, and III in 43% (Sindou et al. 2007; Leal et al. 2010).

The degree of compression was found to play a highly significant role for prognosis ($p = 0.0001$), as shown from the Kaplan-Meir statistical study on outcome (Fig. 9.14). Probability of long-term pain relief at 15 years of FU was of 85% and 73% for high grades of compression, III and II respectively, versus of 65% only for grade I (i.e., simple contact of the vessel with the root) (Sindou et al. 2007, 2008).

### 9.2.5 Other Anomalies of (or in) the Posterior Fossa

Other anomalies of (or in) the posterior fossa have been described in patients with classical TN neuralgia, which may play a role in the genesis of the neuralgia, such as the small size of the posterior cranial fossa the nerve being compressed within a virtual cerebello-pontine angle cistern (Parise et al. 2010, 2013). Also, surgical observation frequently noticed (in 12.6%) the trigeminal root angulated on crossing over the upper petrous ridge (Brinzeu et al. 2018b). This was especially found in patients with a particularly atrophic cer-

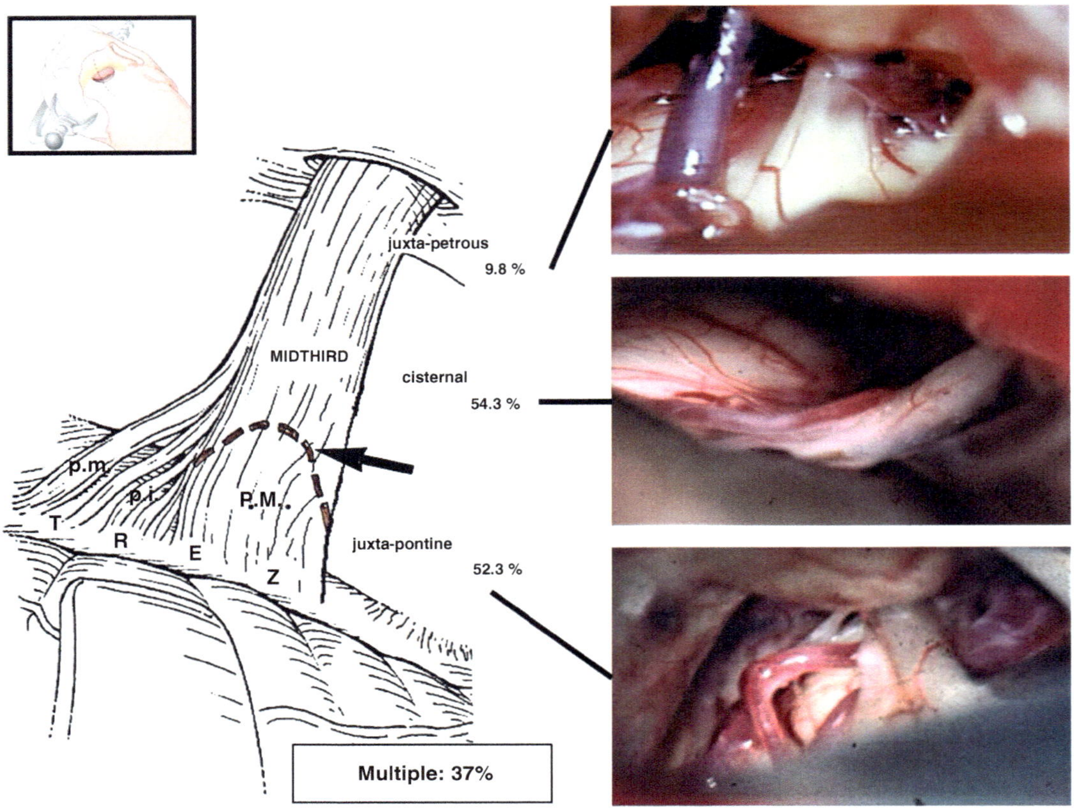


**Fig. 9.7** Situation of the Neuro-Vascular Conflicts along the root. Repartition of the NVCs in the patients with trigeminal nerve explored for MVD (393 patients explored) according to respective situations at juxtapontine trigeminal root entry zone (TREZ), at mid-third of the root (= cisternal), and at exit of root from porus of Meckel cave (= juxta-petrous). In 37% of the patients NVCs were several in the same individual (Sindou et al. 2002). Examples of operative views of NVCs (all presented on right side for didactic reason): Juxtapontine: right NVC from the superior cerebellar artery (SCA) in a superomedial location at TREZ, of grade II of compression; Cisternal: right NVC superiorly to midportion of the root from SCA, pushing root down, of grade II of compression; Juxtapetrous: right NVC inferiorly to root at its exit from porus of Meckel cave due to an inferior transverse vein, of grade III of compression with a marked greyish zone of focal demyelination

ebellum, as at the extreme in the sagging phenomenon. In other studies, anomalies of the root itself were described (Sindou et al. 2002, 2007), such as severe global atrophy of the nerve (42%) or local thickening of the arachnoid surrounding the nerve (18.2%). When encountered these anatomical anomalies which likely contribute to the neuralgia, if not taken into account, could well explain some failures of the decompressive surgery.

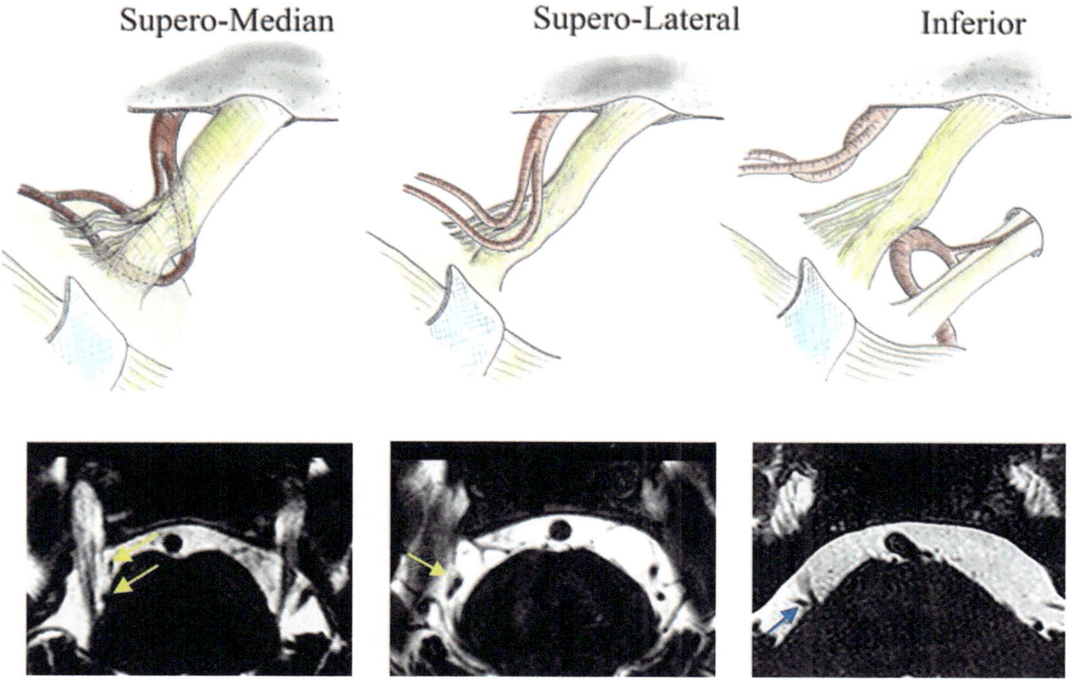


**Fig. 9.8** Location of the Neuro-Vascular Conflicts around the root. Repartition of the NVCs, in the patients with trigeminal nerve explored for MVD (356 patients explored and having a clearcut arterial conflict) according to their respective locations around the root (Sindou et al. 2002). Examples of NVCs on MRI with $T_2$-sequence (all presented on right side for didactic reason). Most of the patients 318 (89.3%) had the conflict coming from above, of whom 220 (61%) with the compression from supero-medial direction and 98 (27.5%) from supero-lateral direction; an inferior compression was present in 38 patients (10.7%)

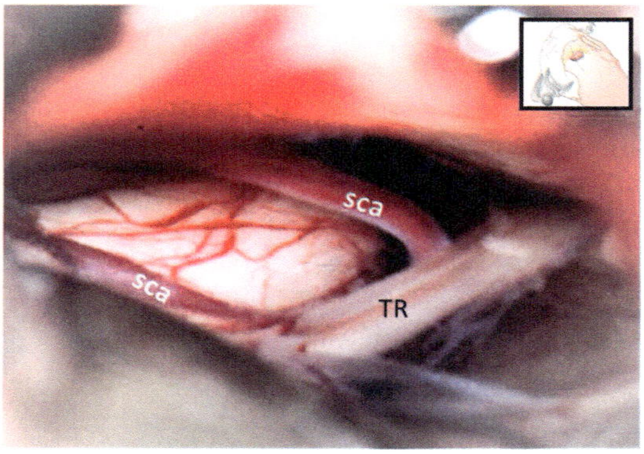


**Fig. 9.9** Grade I: Mere contact to the root. Neuro-Vascular Conflict from superior cerebellar artery (sca) in cistern, of grade I. Note the global atrophy of the root (TR). Patient with right-sided neuralgia

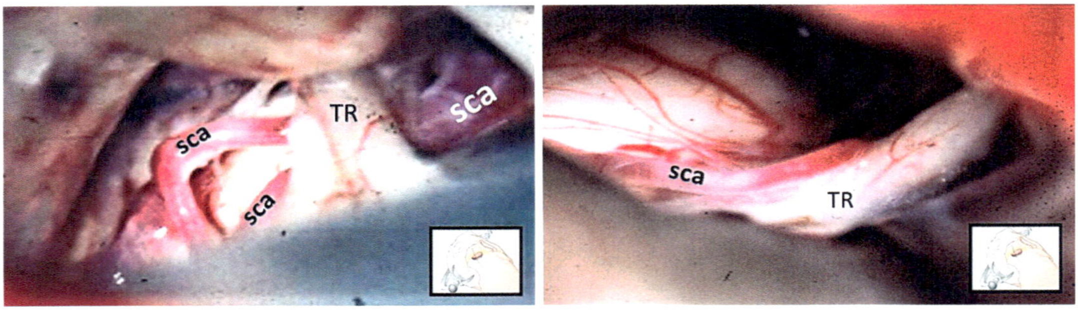


**Fig. 9.10** Grade II: Displacement and/or Distortion of the root. Left: Neuro-Vascular Conflict from superior cerebellar artery (sca) and its two division branches in superomedial location, at TREZ, of grade II. Patient with right-sided neuralgia. Right: Neuro-Vascular Conflict from SCA in superolateral location pushing down the root at its midportion, of grade II. Patient with right-sided neuralgia

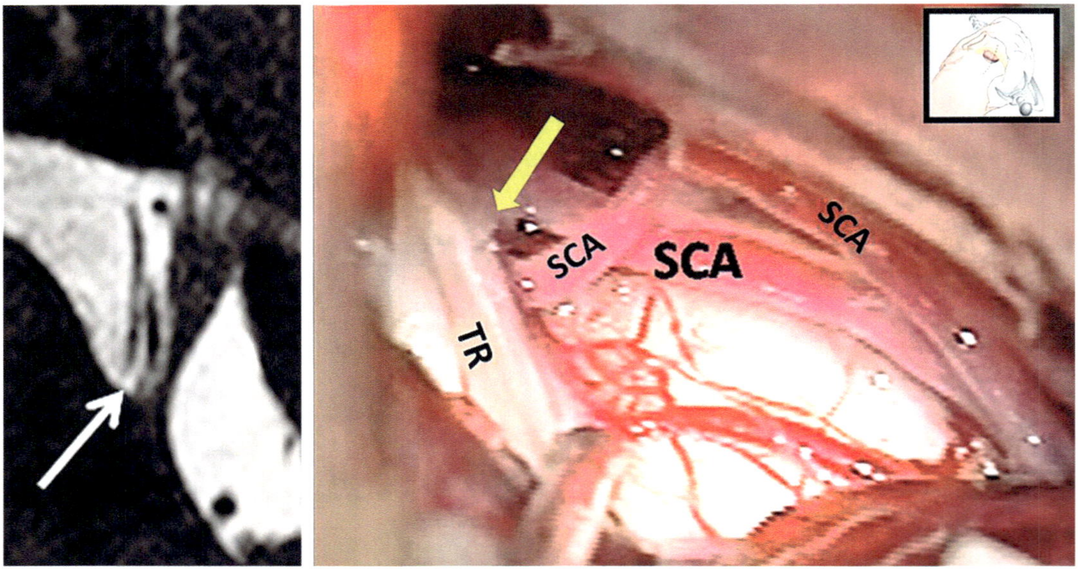


**Fig. 9.11** Grade III: Indentation/Focal Atrophy of the root. Neuro-Vascular Conflict from superior cerebellar artery (SCA) and its two division branches engrooving the TREZ and midportion of the root (TR), of grade III. Patient with left-sided neuralgia. Note good predictability from MRI

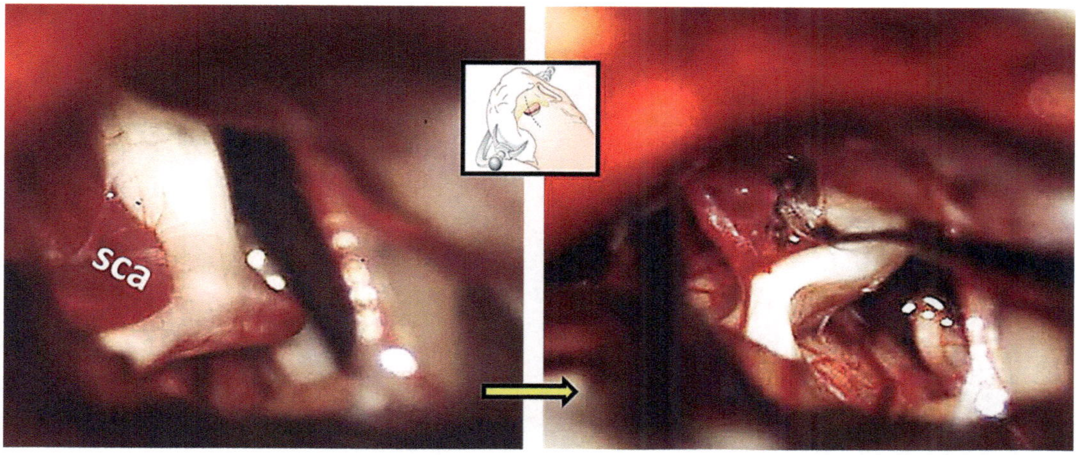


**Fig. 9.12** Grade III extreme: Transfixion of the root. Neuro-Vascular Conflict due to loop of elongated superior cerebellar artery (sca) transpiercing the root, of grade III. 45-year-old female patient with right-sided neuralgia

**Table 9.1** Grades of severity of the root compression by the conflicting vessel, at surgery and on preoperative imaging

| Surgical and imaging descriptions of the different grades of compression | |
|---|---|
| Surgical description[a] | Imaging description[b] |
| **0** Neurovascular relation without contact | **0** Neurovascular relation without contact |
| **I** Simple contact without visible alteration of the root | **I** Contact: absence of interposed CSF layer |
| **II** Displacement/distortion of the root | **II** Deviation of the root |
| **III** Indentation of the root/engrooving/focal demyelination | **III** Indentation of the root |
| *In this grading system, veins are graded according to the same scale as arteries* | |

[a]Based on Sindou et al. (2007)
[b]Based on Leal et al. (2010)

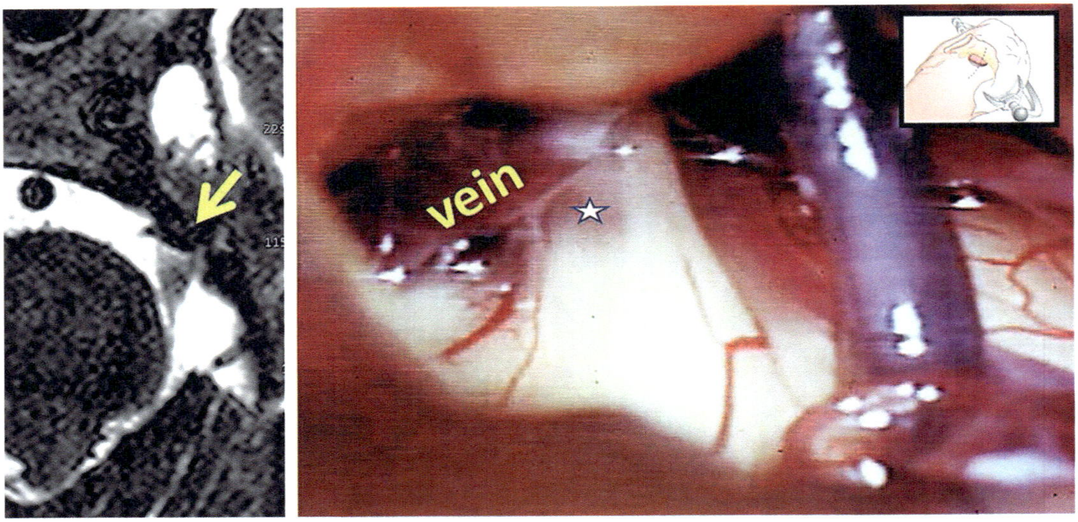


**Fig. 9.13** Grade III with focal demyelination of root due to pure venous compression. Severe cross-compression of root by Inferior Transverse vein, detectable on T2-MRI. Note the marked focal demyelination at inferior aspect of the root, linked to the venous compression (white star). 42-year-old female patient with left-sided typical neuralgia

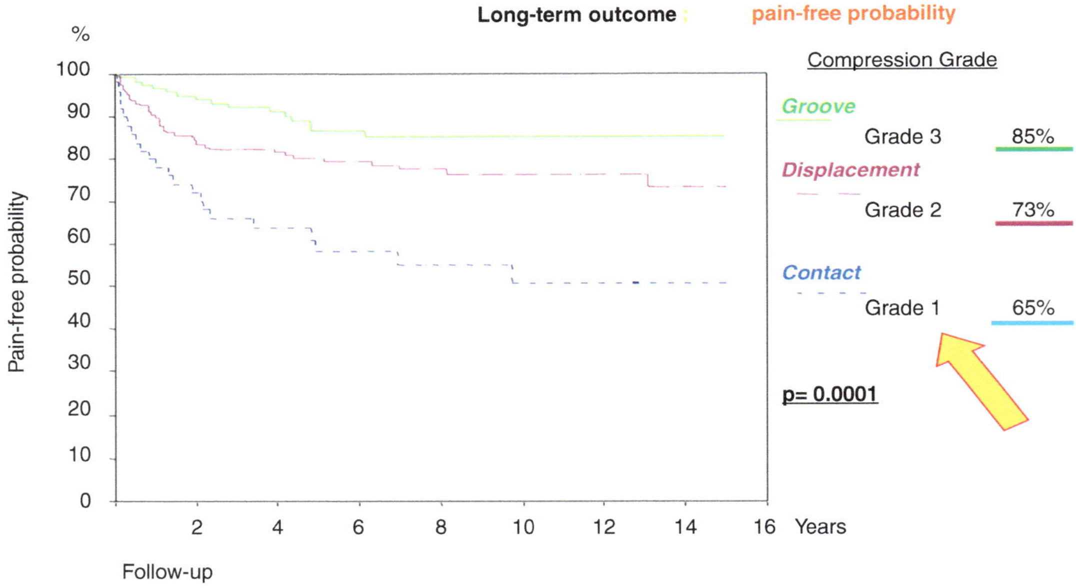


**Fig. 9.14** Long-term Outcome probability according to the degree of compression of the Neuro-Vascular Conflict. Kaplan–Meier statistical analysis showing probability of a lesser percentage of pain relief in the group of patients in whom degree of compression was found grade I (i.e., simple contact) at surgery (Sindou et al. 2007)

## 9.3 Mechanisms of Pain in the Roots Compressed by the NVC

In classical TNs, linked by definition to a Neuro-Vascular Conflict (NVC), the neuralgia would be generated by the chronic compression and the continuous pulsations of a neighboring vessel. The vascular agent causes, at a minimum a simple contact with pulsations on the root (Grade I), or to greater degrees, its displacement or distortion (Grade II), or even more an indentation responsible for local atrophy and demyelination (Grade III). The chronic compression by producing a focal demyelination would induce ectopic influxes, thereafter conveyed via short-circuits between fibers (= ephapses) through their damaged sheaths (Gardner 1962). Subsequently, the firing of the centers under the ectopic influxes would generate hyperactivity of the trigeminal nuclei in brainstem (Rappaport and Devor 1994; Devor et al. 2002a), and perhaps also on long run at level of the upper brain structures (Parise et al. 2014). These chronic lesions, at the source of neuronal hyperactivity, would explain the epileptiform nature of such neuralgias and the pharmacological effectiveness of the anticonvulsants.

Recourse to the Micro-Vascular Decompression procedure was based on those anatomical observations and pathophysiological considerations, and at present the decision taken on the demonstration by imaging of the responsible compressive vessels.

## 9.4 Main Technical Risks of the MVD Procedure for Trigeminal Neuralgia

The occurrence of a number of complications can be minimized by obeying some technical principles in performing the procedure.

### 9.4.1 Risk of Hearing Loss on the Approach: How to Avoid

The safer way to avoid hearing loss when approaching the trigeminal root is to take the infratentorial-supracerebellar route. It has been clearly evidenced with intra-operative BAEP recordings that lateral-to-medial retraction of the cerebellar hemisphere entails a high risk of excessive stretching of the cochlear (and vestibular) nerves (Fig. 9.15), as well

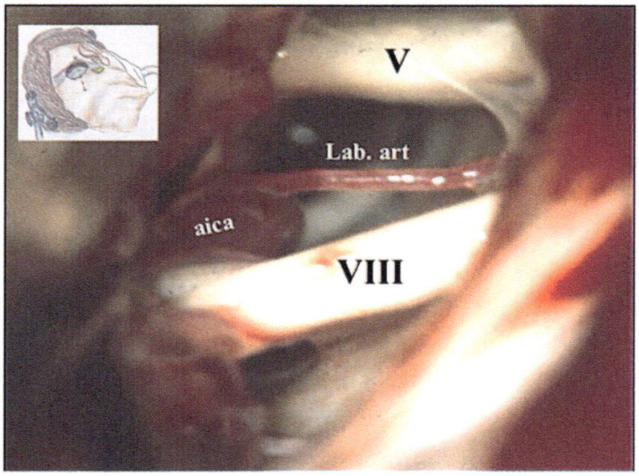


Hearing function at risk by Stretching of the VIIIth Nerve due to lateral-to-medial retraction of cerebellum

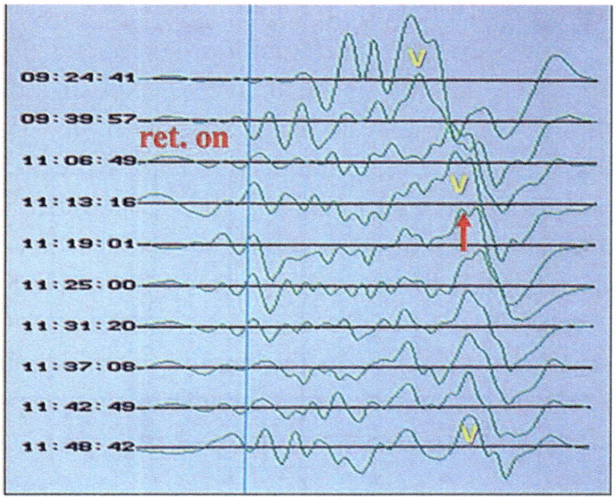


Increase in latency of peak V after retractor on

**Fig. 9.15** The most frequent neurological risk of the Micro-Vascular Decompression procedure is the occurrence of hearing and/or vestibular disturbances. Main mechanism is *stretching of the cochleo-vestibular nerve* (VIII) which especially may happen in the maneuver of lateral to medial cerebellar retraction, as illustrated in the operative photography. Consequence is an increase in latency of peaks III and V as shown in the recordings of the intraoperative Brainstem Auditory Evoked Potentials (BAEPs). An increased in latency of peak V of 1 ms constitutes the early warning signal for the surgeon (Sindou et al. 1992; Polo et al. 2004)

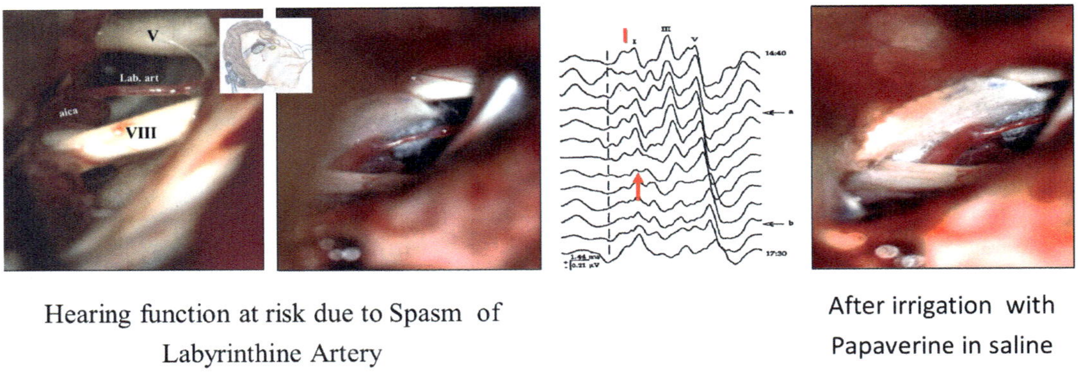


**Fig. 9.16** Hearing function can be at risk in the eventuality of *vasospasm of the labyrinthine artery* (lab.art.) or of the Anterior Inferior Cerebellar Artery (AICA) under their manipulation, as illustrated in the center operative photography. A warning signal of cochlea ischemia is reduction in amplitude of peak I, as shown on the BAEPs recording. The spasm can be reversed within a few seconds by irrigation of papaverine in solution (only a few droplets, because of the acid PH of Papaverine) as evidenced in the right operative photography (Sindou et al. 1992; Polo et al. 2004)

as of manipulations of the labyrinthine artery (Sindou et al. 1992; Polo et al. 2004) (Fig. 9.16). A limited approach through a keyhole craniectomy, prevents not only from excessive CSF depletion and also avulsion of the bridging petrosal veins, but also from wide exposure of the facial-cochleo-vestibular nerve complex. Craniotomy and dural opening should be turned just below the transverse sinus (Fig. 9.17) and subarachnoid trajectory under the cerebellar tentorium (Fig. 9.18).

However, the infratentorial-supracerebellar approach has the disadvantage of exposing the thin trochlear nerve to direct surgical injury. For this reason, it is recommended to expose the SCA and its branches by incising the peripeduncular arachnoid, not at the level of the trochlear nerve itself but as below as possible in the mesencephalo-cerebellar fissure. By doing so, a “curtain” of arachnoid posterior to the nerve will assure its protection from trauma by the instruments, especially brutal aspiration by the sucker.

### 9.4.2 Risks from Venous Sacrifices: How to Avoid Venous Infarction

Veins constitute a frequent and dangerous obstacle to access the trigeminal nerve through the classic infratentorial-supracerebellar route. In this approach the superior petrosal venous system (SPVS) is a structure at risk (Dumot and Sindou 2018), so that the neurosurgeon is confronted to the difficult dilemma of sacrificing or not one or several of its constituting veins (Fig. 9.19). Some surgeons prefer to sacrifice the superficial SPVS almost systematically in totality or at least partially to improve access, rather than taking the risk of disinsertion of the trunk of the superior petrosal vein from the Superior Petrosal Sinus, which can be at the origin of dramatic bleeding. Others advocate attempting to respect the venous system as much as possible (Dumot and Sindou 2018).

A literature search from 36 articles reporting venous complications after microvascular decompression led to establish at 1.6% the rate of confirmed venous infarcts (Sindou and Dumot 2020). In our 688 cases own series reviewed, 0.32% had cerebellar infarct that necessitated surgical decompression, and 0.58% medically managed cerebellar swelling (Sindou and Dumot 2020). Other complications such as peduncular hallucinosis or hearing or gait disturbances have been reported as linked to sacrifice of the sSPVs (Sindou and Dumot 2020). Complications from venous sacrifices are probably under-reported because most are transient or not always easy to

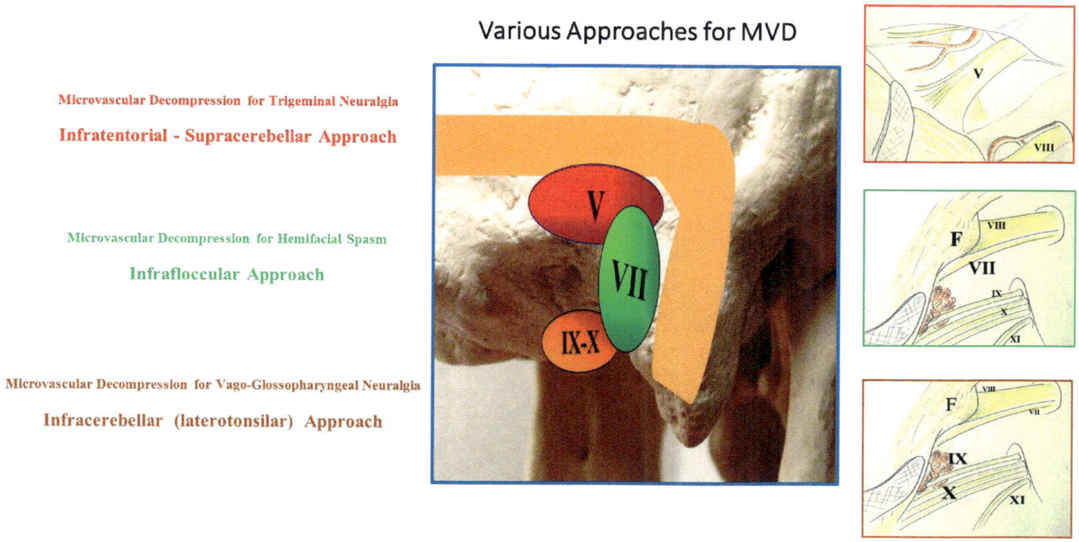


**Fig. 9.17** Recommended approaches for Micro-Vascular Decompression of the various cranial nerves of the cerebello-pontine angle have been designed to avoid stretching of the cochleo-vestibular nerve, and so decrease occurrence of corresponding disturbances. Recommendations have been established on the basis of Brainstem Auditory Evoked Potentials recordings (Sindou et al. 1992)

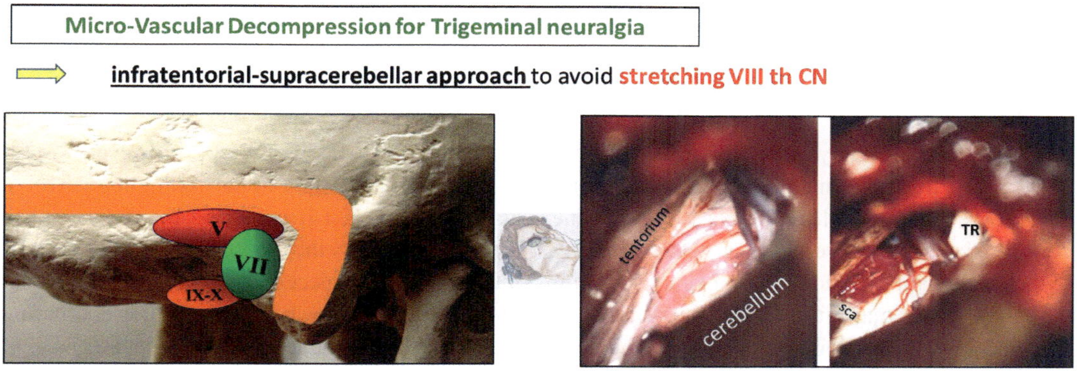


**Fig. 9.18** Preferential access to trigeminal root (TR) is through infratentorial—supracerebellar approach. Operative views illustrate decompression from a conflict by the superior cerebellar artery (sca), using the transposition method (i.e., without any material in contact with the root). Of note: Superior petrosal venous system preserved

relate to a venous origin. Further, on images differentiation between contusion caused by excessive cerebellar retraction and venous infarct is sometimes puzzling, the more so because of possible co-responsibility (Sindou and Dumot 2020). Prediction of harmful consequences of sacrificing veins is far from reliable, therefore attempting to respect veins is advised. To do so on approaching, the trigeminal root should be reached passing through the windows in between the SPV affluents, taking care not to avulse them, as shown in Fig. 4.7.

Study of a personal series including 326 consecutive patients who underwent MVD for primary trigeminal neuralgia showed a relatively high incidence (38%) of venous Neuro-Vascular Conflicts (NVC) or a close relationship of a vein with the root (Sindou et al. 2002). Venous com-

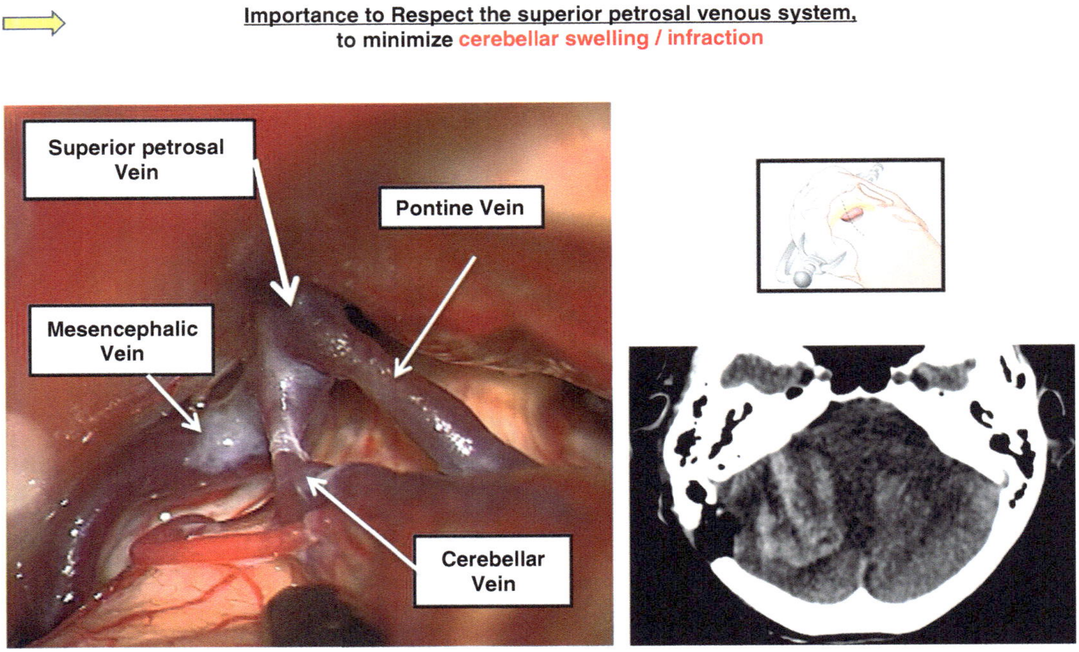


**Fig. 9.19** Importance to respect the superior petrosal venous system. The CT-scan shows a postoperative venous infarction of the right cerebellar hemisphere linked to the sacrifice of the superior petrosal vein, performed to access the trigeminal root; The operative view of the superior petrosal venous system and its affluents (here notably developed) illustrates how it would be dangerous to sacrifice this draining system

pressions were not only at TREZ (in 16.9%) but also at the mid-cisternal portion (39.7%), and also at the porus of Meckel cave (33.1%). The compressive veins were either a vein belonging to the superficial superior petrosal venous system (sSPVS), in the majority the pontine affluent of the superior petrosal vein, or a vein from the deep superior petrosal venous system (dSPVS), almost always a transverse cross-compressing vein adjacent to the porus. Conservation of the vessel is admissible only if its mobilization away can be successfully obtained; this implies complete freeing of the trigeminal root from all arachnoid adhesions. Otherwise, coagulation and division have to be performed.

### 9.4.3 Risks Linked to the Decompression: How to Avoid Neo-Compression

Simple decompression without any material inserted, as well as absence of root manipulations, would be idealistic (Fig. 9.20). However, to prevent for re-malposition of the conflicting vessel—as a matter of fact it would be imprudent not to maintain durably the conflicting vessel apart—introduction of a piece of material, including synthetic prosthesis, may be useful. A study comparing the prosthesis (in the study: Teflon material) touching the root (= Interposition) and not-touching the root (= Transposition) supports performing the procedure without the implant in contact with the root ($p = 0.05$) (Sindou et al. 2008) (Fig. 9.21). This is easier with the superior cerebellar artery because of its laxity and rare perforating branches, more difficult with the anterior-inferior cerebellar artery as it generally has important perforators to the brainstem and also the labyrinthine artery arising from its cisternal portion.

Of theoretical interest, the significantly better long-term cure rate when the implant is not in contact with the root favors the "pure" decompressive effect of the MVD procedure, rather than a conduction block-like mechanism, as objected in some critical publications (Adams 1989).

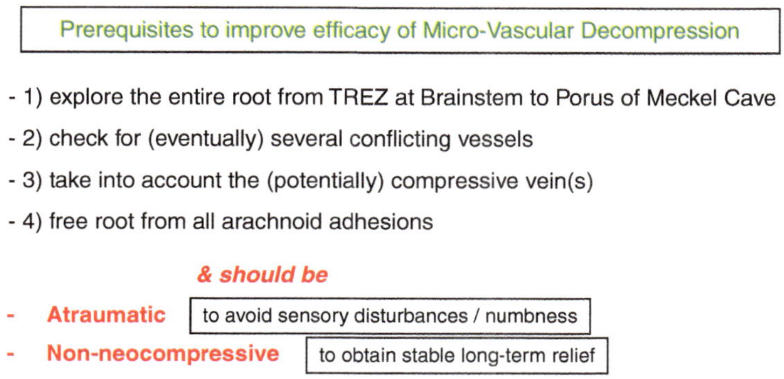


**Fig. 9.20** Prerequisites to improve efficacy of Micro-Vascular Decompression

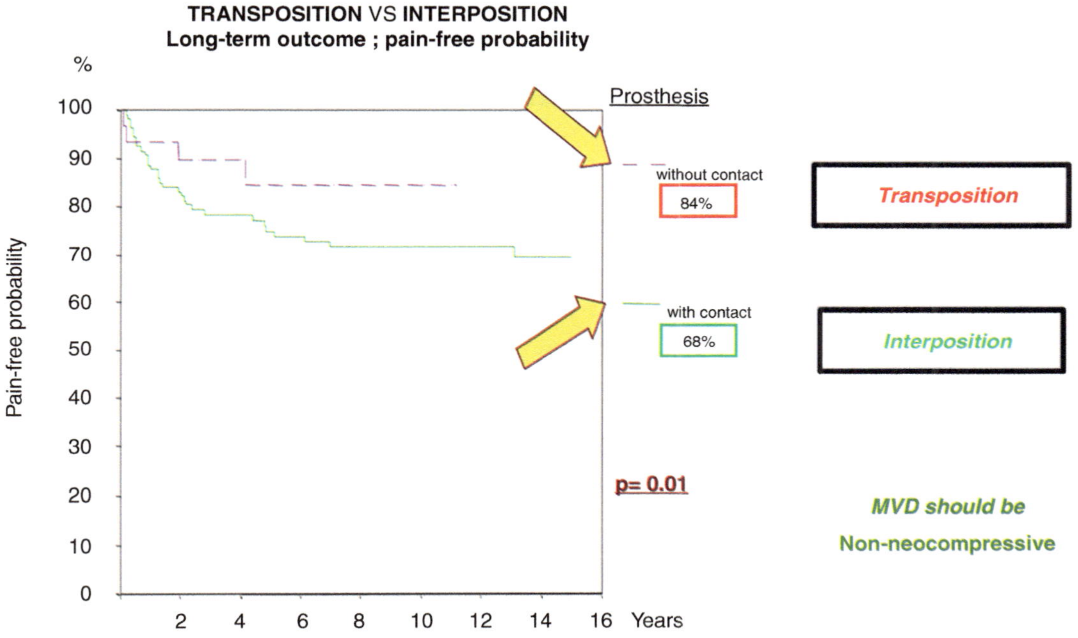


**Fig. 9.21** Micro-Vascular Decompression (MVD) should be non-neocompressive. Goal of MVD is to maintain the conflicting vessel apart of the compressed trigeminal root. This can be achieved by *transposition* of the vessel or by *interposition* of material inserted in between the root and the vessel. Kaplan-Meier statistical analysis shows higher probability of better long-term outcome when the transposition method can be performed ($p = 0.01$) (Sindou et al. 2008)

## 9.5 Surgical Steps

- Under general anesthesia with endotracheal ventilation, the patient is installed in the contralateral decubitus position, with the head moderately elevated, slightly flexed and rotated 15° toward the contralateral side, and secured with a three-pin holder (Fig. 9.22). The ipsilateral shoulder is taped and pulled caudally and posteriorly. Hair is shaved in the retromastoid region. The mastoid process and superior nuchal line which are the landmarks for the retromastoid craniectomy are identified by palpation with the index finger. A skin incision 5 cm in length is made obliquely, 1 cm medial to the bisector of the angle formed by the nuchal line and the posterior margin of the mastoid process. The underlying subcuta-

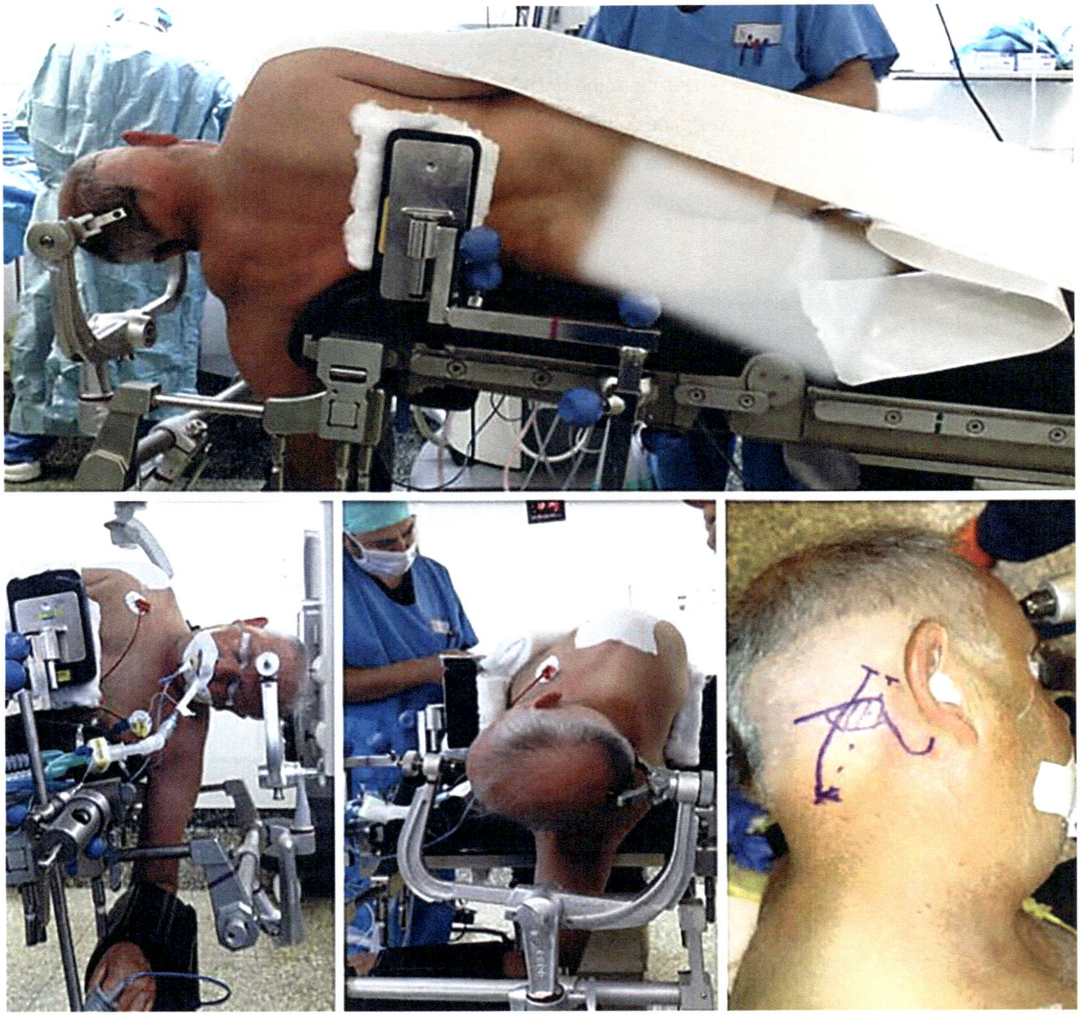

**Fig. 9.22** Installation. Microvascular decompression in a patient with a right classical trigeminal neuralgia due to neurovascular conflict. Patient installed in lateral decubitus with (moderate) traction on shoulder. Operating table with (only slight) inclination to decrease cephalic venous pressure and avoid excessive CSF leakage. Note the 15° contralateral rotation of head and the landmarks of the craniectomy (hatched area) below the occipital crest/transverse sinus and posterior to base of the mastoid process/sigmoid sinus. Cutaneous incision is 1 cm medial to the bisector of the angle formed by the nuchal line and the posterior edge of the mastoid process

neous tissue and muscles are divided using electrocautery. If the occipital artery is encountered, it is divided between two silk ligatures. The posterior aspect of the mastoid process is cleared of soft tissue. The mastoid emissary vein within the bone is obliterated with Surgicel first then with wax.

- Only a few specific instruments are necessary (Figs. 9.23 and 9.24).
- The retromastoid craniotomy is performed by turning a burr hole just posterior to the base of the mastoid process and just below the nuchal line, then by enlarging the hole with a Kerisson rongeur, so that, first, the transverse sinus, and, second, the posterior border of the sigmoid sinus, are exposed (Fig. 9.25). The burr hole must not be made too laterally toward the mastoid process as this would endanger the

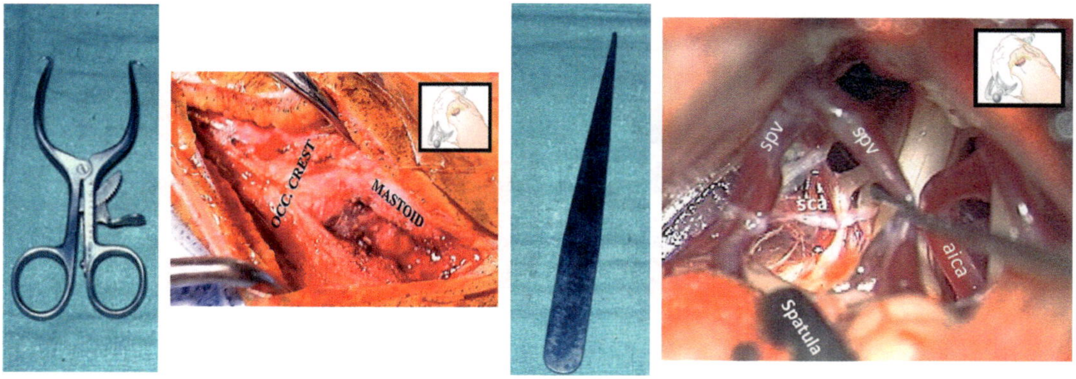


**Fig. 9.23** Instruments for approach. Self retractor to expose occipital crest and mastoid process (left images); Spatula of the Sugita-Fukushima type, with narrow extremity on the cerebellar hemisphere, for opening the mesencephalic and the pontine cerebellar fissures (right images)

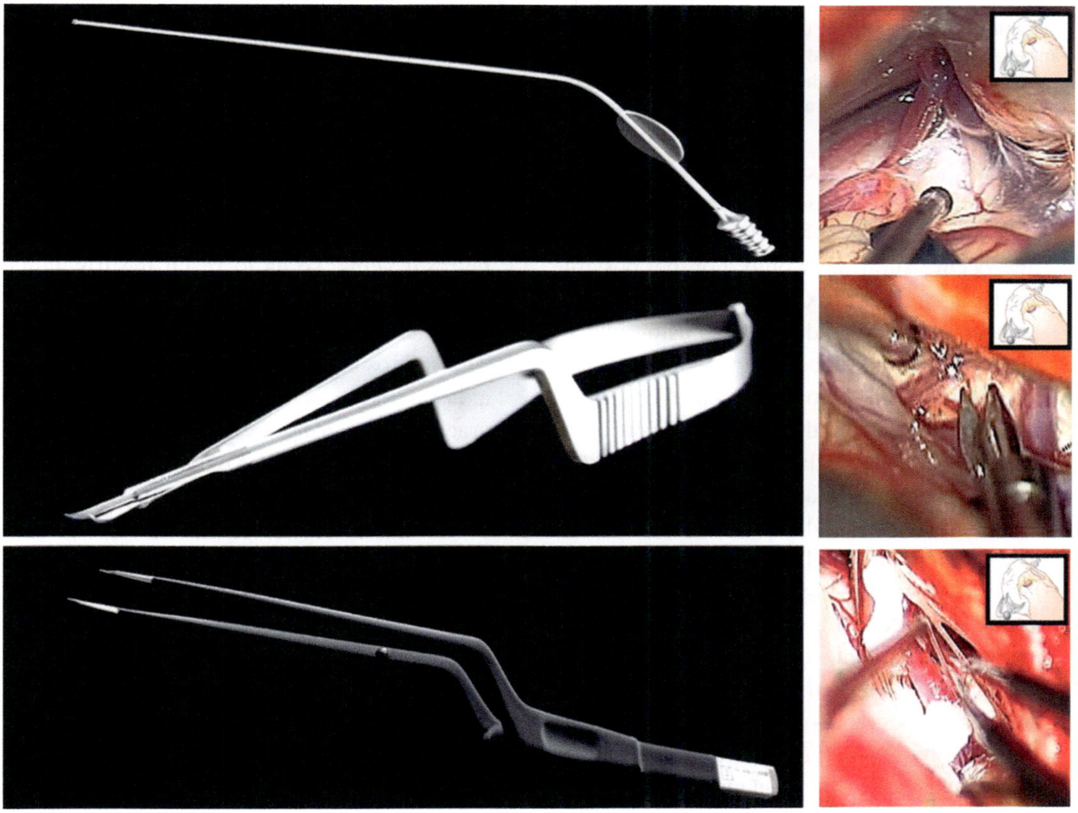

**Fig. 9.24** Microsurgical Instruments. From top to bottom: Suction tube with ball-point tip, which may serve for CSF aspiration, and also as freehand keyhole retractor and dissector probe; Microscissors with fine and curved tips for sharp dissection; Bipolar forceps with extrafine arciform tips to ease delicate dissection and well-limited coagulation

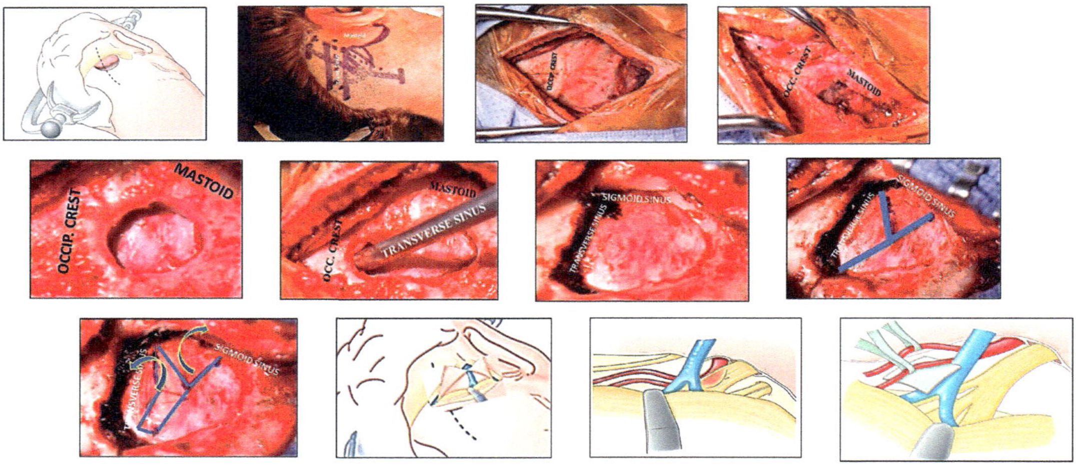


**Fig. 9.25** Steps of the craniotomy for Micro-Vascular Decompression of the trigeminal nerve (on right side for illustration). Upper row: Cutaneous landmarks of the transverse sinus (= occipital crest) and of the sigmoid sinus (= posterior edge of the mastoid process). Middle row: Craniectomy (2–3 cm in diameter) with exposure of the transverse sinus (safely cleavable from bone) using kerisson rongeur; landmarks of the incisions for the dural flaps: one reflected on the transverse sinus, the other on the sigmoid sinus (be aware of fragility of its wall). Lower row: Infratentorial–supracerebellar route to the trigeminal root to perform the decompression

sigmoid sinus, the external wall of which is most often reduced to a thin endothelial layer adhesive to the bone. If effraction and bleeding occur, suturing would not be possible owing to its friable texture; packing to achieve hemostasis could lead to its occlusion; patching with a small piece of aponeurosis generally allows the sinus to stay patent. Conversely, bone resection over the transverse portion of the lateral sinus is relatively safe as its external wall is stronger and less adhesive to the bone than the sigmoid one.

- The craniectomy is elliptic in shape, 2 cm in large × 1.5 cm in height on average, but with variations according to cases and their anatomical singularities, as MVD should be by nature a "tailored operation." If mastoid cells are opened as is common, they are occluded by affixing a piece of subcutaneous tissue (e.g., fat plus aponeurosis). Plugging wax into the cells would lead to (often delayed) serous otitis. Then the dura is opened by making two small flaps, a superior one retracted along the transverse sinus and a lateral one along the sigmoid sinus. A self-retaining retractor—of the Yasargil type—mounted with a thin blade (Sugita-Fukushima type) is placed on the superior cerebellar surface, no more anteriorly than the level of the superior petrosal veins, so as to reach the trigeminal root via an infratentorial-supracerebellar approach.
- The microscope is positioned with its visual axis parallel to the superior petrosal sinus. The arachnoid covering the dorsolateral aspect of the cerebral peduncle is opened parallel to the tentorial incisura and 1–2 mm below the trochlear nerve. This is done with a microsucker in one hand to attract and immobilize the arachnoid and sharp microscissors in the other. Care must be taken not to injure the thin and fragile trochlear nerve, especially with excessive suction (Fig. 9.26).
- The superior petrosal trunk and its three main tributaries: the (dorsal) mesencephalic, the (superior) cerebellar, and the (lateral) pontine veins, are then dissected free from the surrounding arachnoid. This allows downward retraction of the cerebellum without tearing the superior venous trunk and stretching the cochlear-vestibular nerve complex. Avulsion of the superior petrosal trunk from the supe-

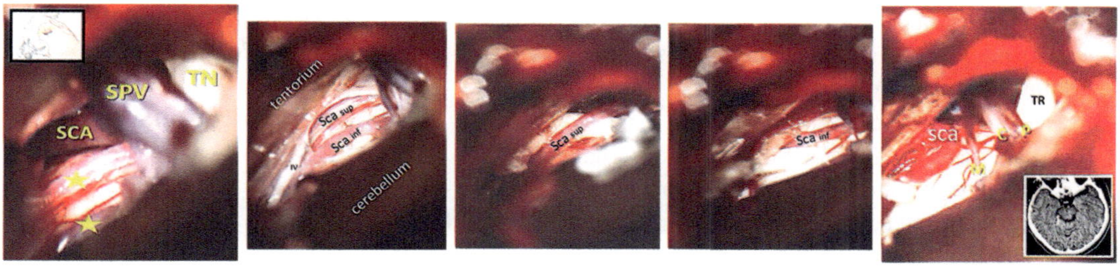


**Fig. 9.26** Steps of the infratentorial–supracerebellar approach for Micro-Vascular Decompression of the trigeminal nerve (on right side for illustration). From left to right: Exposure of the trigeminal nerve (TN) through infratentorial–supracerebellar route. Note that the superior petrosal venous system (SPV) hides the neurovascular conflict between the TN and the two branches (asterisk) of the superior cerebellar artery (SCA). Incision of the arachnoid, just inferiorly to the trochlear nerve (IV), with exposure of the superior and inferior branches of the SCA. A sling made of teased Teflon fibers (2 mm in width, 3 cm in length) is passed around each of the SCA branches. The SCA branches are detached from the trigeminal root (TR) by pulling on slings. At final, decompression has been performed by transposition of the Sca away from the TR. Note that the three affluents (mesencephalic, cerebellar, pontine) of the SPV were respected; Post-op CT shows the Teflon slings maintaining SCA in place

rior petrosal sinus would lead to profuse bleeding. The arachnoid is then opened laterally and inferiorly toward the VIIth and VIIIth cranial nerves; limited dissection of the arachnoid around these nerves will reduce the likelihood of hearing complications. The retractor tip is then placed to expose the cerebellomesencephalic and cerebellopontine fissures, so that the entire root can be examined through the various triangles defined by the petrosal veins, from pons to Meckel's cave, and all possible NVCs identified. The root is then dissected free by dividing the pia-arachnoid filaments (= chordae). Not infrequently the arachnoid is thickened and strongly adhesive to the trigeminal rootlets; dissection shall be as atraumatic as possible.

- The vessels most often responsible for the NVC are the neighboring cerebellar arteries (89.7%), mostly the SCA, more rarely the AICA, only in a few cases the VBA. Vessels can also be veins of the superior petrous system, either in association with arterial conflict (29.1%) or as a pure venous compressive factor (8.9%). Compressions are classically at the trigeminal root entry zone. In fact, they can sit at any level of the root, not only at level of the entry zone (in 52.3% of the cases) but also of the cisternal portion of the root (in 54.3%), and not infrequently at exit of the root from the porus of the Meckel cave (in 9.8%) (Dumot and Sindou 2015).
- Use of endoscopy for MVD of the trigeminal root does not seem to bring significant help, contrarily to MVD for the facial and cochleovestibular nerves. Important is to design a tailored keyhole approach, not too narrow and adapted to what is predicted from the preoperative MRI exploration.
- The principle of the microsurgical vascular decompression (MVD) procedure, which is conservative by nature, consists in freeing the root from the vascular compression by careful separation of the nerve and vessel, and to keep the latter at distance, using the "Interposition" or, preferably, the "Transposition" method.
- Arteries may be endangered by their stretching or kinking, especially during transposition. Avulsion of perforators might occur if care is not taken to avoid excessive traction on trunk or branches. Manipulation of vessels often generates "mechanical" vasospastic reactions with potentially severe ischemic consequences, as it happened in two of our patients (0.1%). Therefore, throughout the vascular manipulations, gentle irrigation with saline, and if vasospastic reaction occurs application of (only a few because of its very

acid PH) droplets of papaverine solution (1 ml in 10 ml saline), are important measures to maintain arterial flow.

- Avulsion of the petrosal veins might lead to profuse hemorrhage soiling the cisternal spaces. In the eventuality of bleeding, preservation of vein patency should be attempted by affixing small pieces of Surgicel to the tear. Compact packing that would compress and/or occlude the vein(s) must be avoided; this could create congestive oedema or hemorrhagic infarction of cerebellum and brainstem.
- After decompression completed, venous hemostasis is confirmed by requesting the anesthesiologist to perform sustained digital compression at the neck of both jugular veins or, if this is not possible, by carrying out a Valsalva maneuver with the ventilation machine. Arterial hemostasis is ensured again by irrigating the vessels with (a few) droplets of papaverine in saline, in order to reverse all possible spasm due to surgical manipulations.
- The dura-mater is closed with single stitches. In order to achieve watertight closure, if necessary, a piece of aponeurosis, harvested from the subcutaneous fascia (or the fascialata at thigh if the latter is not practicable), is affixed externally to the dura. As a matter of fact, "Keyhole" approaches render hermetic closure of the dura (under tension) difficult. We do not recommend the use of fibrin glue because of its rapid resorption, which leads to delayed CSF leak.

  Additional fatty tissue is affixed onto the mastoid cells when opened during craniectomy. Advice is not to pack wax into the opened cells, as it may migrate into the middle ear and cause chronic serous otitis with otalgia, or be responsible of granulomas and secondary infection. Bone chips are put back over the craniectomy defect preferably if mastoid cells were not opened. Finally, the muscular, subcutaneous, and cutaneous layers are closed with interrupted sutures. Finally, a compressive dressing is applied to avoid pseudomeningocele and decrease the risk of CSF fistula or of rhinorrhea through the Eustachian tube if mastoid cells were opened.

## 9.6 Surgical Technique of MVD According to Vessels

### 9.6.1 The Superior Cerebellar Artery (SCA)

SCA is the most commonly conflicting vessel. Its normal situation corresponds to a course from anterior and lateral to posterior and medial around the brainstem, with a bifurcation at a certain distance superiorly to the TREZ, before distributing to the medial and lateral superior cerebellar surfaces and the dorsolateral aspect of the peduncle. When responsible, SCA is elongated and has one of the two types of relationship to the root: either anteromedially to the TREZ or superolaterally lying on the rootlets in their cisternal portion. Since its collaterals are generally long, transposition of SCA is most often relatively easy to perform (Fig. 9.27 left).

The SCA and its (two) division branches are detached from the nerve and transposed upward just beneath the tentorium. For doing so, slings—made of Teflon felt shredded fibers—3 cm in length and 2 mm in width, are passed around each of the arteries to pull and detach them, as much as possible without touching the nerve. Transposition is maintained by wedging the slings in between the superior aspect of the cerebellum and the inferior surface of the tentorium. Then, to avoid secondary mal-repositioning of the arteries, a small square piece of semi-rigid prosthesis (made of Dacron or Teflon) is placed on the superior petrosal vein as a console to hold the transposed arteries, which also prevents the prosthesis for touching the root.

### 9.6.2 The Anterior Inferior Cerebellar Artery (AICA)

When AICA is the offending vessel, compression is generally exerted by an upward loop onto the inferior aspect of the pars major at its brainstem entry (Fig. 9.27 right).

Transposition of AICA is usually difficult because it frequently has short perforators to the brainstem, and gives origin to the labyrinthine artery.

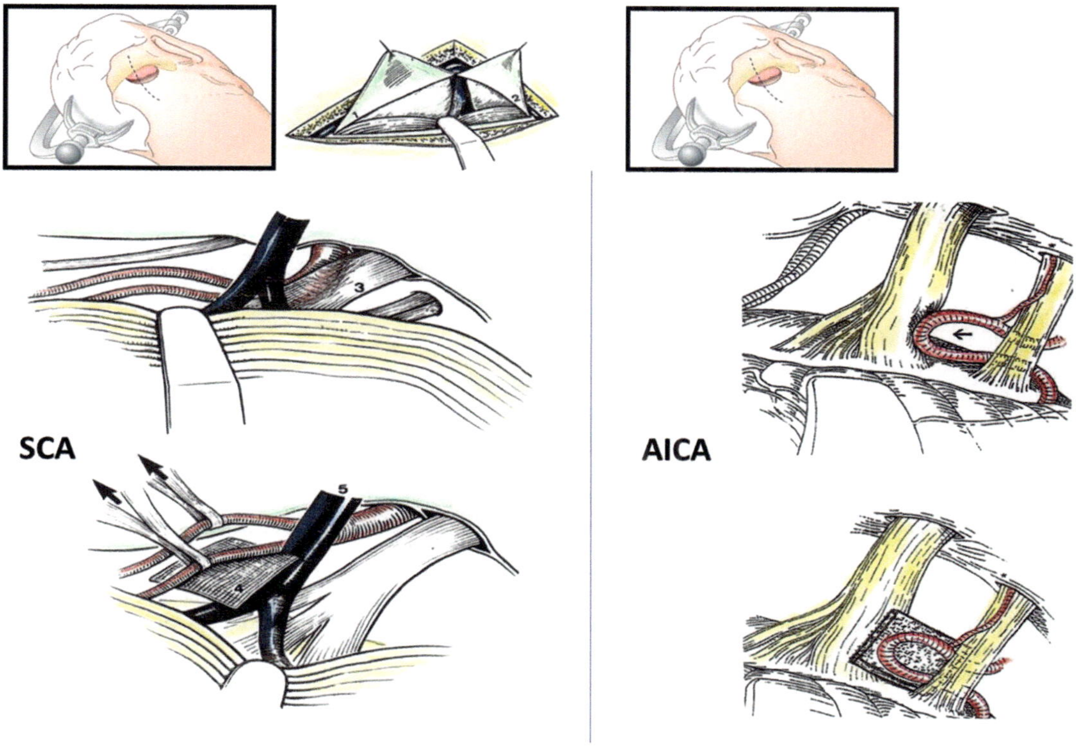


**Fig. 9.27** Non-Neocompressive technique for decompression of the superior (SCA) and the anterior-inferior (AICA) cerebellar arteries. Left: decompression of SCA (for right-sided neuralgia): Upper row: 1 = dural flap retracted upward onto the transverse sinus, 2 = dural flap retracted laterally onto the posterior edge of the sigmoid sinus; infratentorial—supracerebellar approach; Middle row: 3 = trigeminal root compressed by the SCA from above; Lower row: transposition of the SCA and its two branches, using slings of Teflon fibers, secured with a plate of semi-rigid Teflon (4) not touching the root. Note respect of the superior petrosal vein (5). Right: Decompression of AICA (for right-sided neuralgia): Upper row: trigeminal root entry zone compressed inferiorly by AICA; Lower row: decompression by using interposition of semi-rigid Teflon plate with the so-called bridging technique

In most cases the loop cannot simply be pulled away, and a small ball-shaped cushion of Teflon felt fibers, or a small piece of semirigid Dacron or Teflon prosthesis according the bridging method, has to be interposed between the root and loop.

### 9.6.3 The Vertebrobasilar Artery (VBA)

For conflicts due to a Megadolicho-VBA the preferable method is transposition of the compressive vessel. This can be ideally achieved by using sling(s) made with strong prosthetic material, as from Goretex, fixed to neighboring dura. However, especially if VBA is huge, atheromatous and/or calcified, effective decompression may be impossible. In such an eventuality a partial sensory rhizotomy at the juxtapontine portion of the root can be performed (Fig. 9.28).

**Key-Point**
Transposition of the conflicting vessel, without any material touching the root, affords better long-term relief of the neuralgia than the Interposition technique.

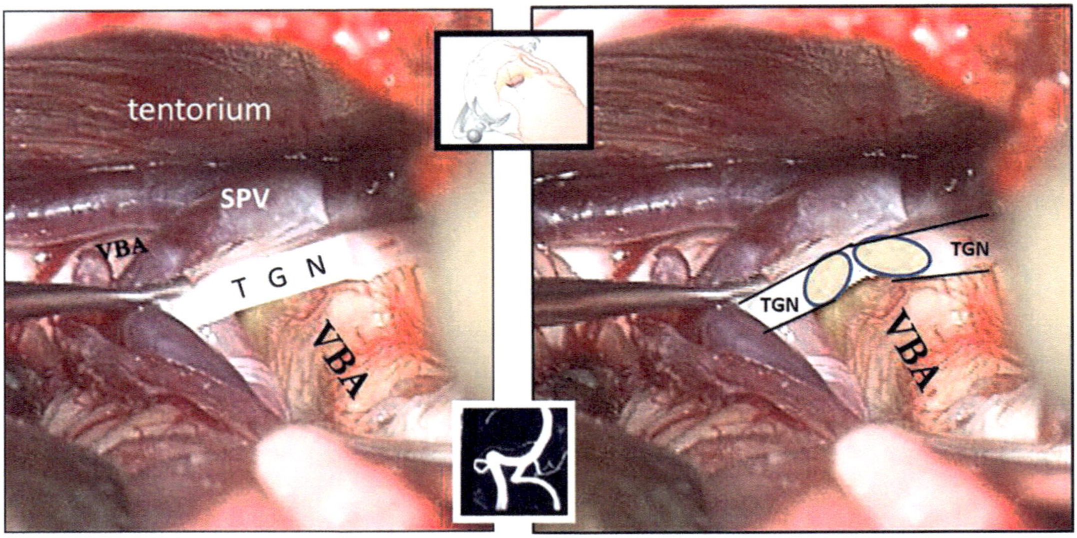


**Fig. 9.28** Trigeminal nerve (TGN) compression by Megadolicho-VertebroBasilar artery (VBA) (on right side on illustration). Left: TGN stretched from below by huge atheromatous VBA; Right: because decompression revealed impossible, a *partial sensory rhizotomy* of the TGN was performed, namely of the infero-lateral two-thirds of the root. *SPV* Superior Petrosal Venous system

### 9.6.4 Material for Decompression

Regarding the material used for decompression, especially for Neuro-Vascular Conflicts of arterial origin, there is no consensus among the various teams dealing with this surgery.

- Opening of the arachnoid to provide more space in the cerebellopontine angle cistern for the neurovascular structures, with simple separation of the conflicting vessel(s), although the most elegant, revealed to be insufficient in the majority of cases.

- Implants can be used, either for the simple Interposition between the vessel and the nerve or to maintain the conflicting vessel apart (Transposition technique). Prevention of arteries to become conflicting again is important as arteries are "shape-memory" structures that tend to return to their previous offending position.
- Pieces of autologous muscle or aponeurosis, that were frequently utilized, are considered by most as generating secondary fibrosis and adherences. Fat would be better tolerated but is scarcely used.
- There has been a long list of implanted material trials.
- Absorbable gelatin (Gelfoam*, Pfizer), knitted cellulose (Surgicel *, Johnson and Johnson), and fibrin glue as well, resorb within only a few days;
- Ivalon sponge (Unipoint Industries, Hight Point, NC), largely used in the US, has been found by some to be aggressive and neo-compressive for the neighboring neural structures;
- PTFE-Teflon in its various presentations: shredded or knitted is at present the most used material; Polyester Dacron is more rarely utilized. Respective illustrations are presented in the neighboring figure (Fig. 9.29).

In spite of the absence of experimental studies in MVD indication, Shredded Teflon® Felt (PTFE felt, C.R. Bard Co, Bard Implants Division, Billerica, MA) has become the preferred product for MVD. To be recalled, from a previous publication (Sindou and Mercier 2018), TEFLON-

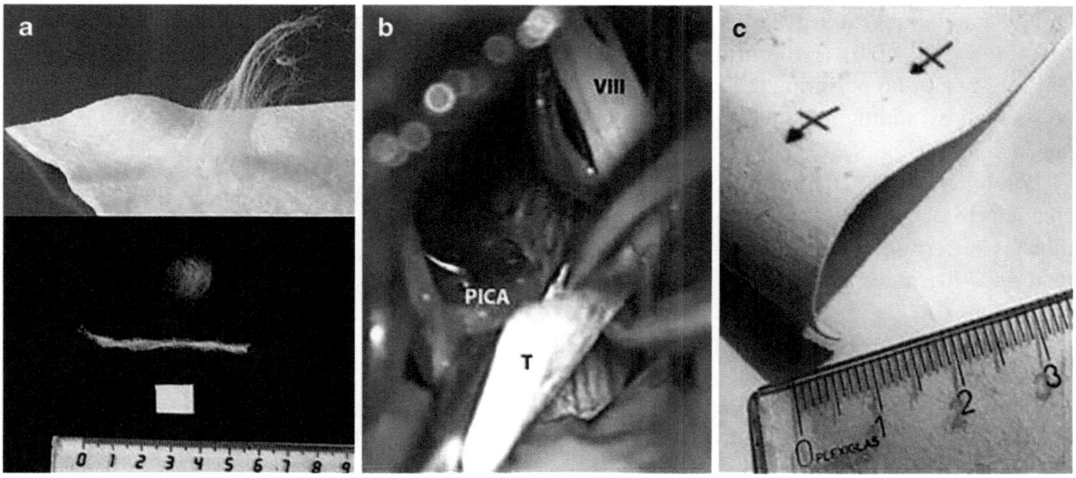


**Fig. 9.29** Material for Micro-Vascular Decompression. Left (**a**) Shredded PTFE Teflon®felt prepared by teasing constituting fibers (upper view), to make balls or ribbons (lower view). Simple pieces (15 × 8 mm in this illustration) are not recommended because of their propensity for (harmful) adhesiveness to neurovascular structures; Center (**b**) *Example of Bridging technique on the Facial nerve for treating Hemifacial Spasm, with semi-rigid material.* EdwardsOutflow Tract knitted PTFE Teflon® is semi-rigid material. Picture shows insertion in between the PICA to maintain it away and the facial REZ as well as the VIIIth complex. The plaque (10 × 15 mm) is placed on the ventrolateral aspect of brainstem (pons) ventrally and the flocculus dorsally, so that it has a "bridging effect" over the facial and VIIIth cranial nerves; Right (**c**) Sauvage®knitted Polyester Dacron® is a more supple material than the two others

PTFE® means PolyTetraFluorEthylene. Introduced for use in the treatment of paralyzed vocal cords, TEFLON-PTFE® is a biologic implant on the market for the past 40 years. Teflon® for MVD is the same product as the one used for cardiovascular patching. According to literature, Teflon® Felt appears to be a good inert material (Li and Sun 2016). However, a few publications have reported inflammatory reactions or granulomas (Cho et al. 1994; Megerian et al. 1995; Fujimaki et al. 1996; Rath et al. 1996; Liao et al. 1997; Premsagar et al. 1997; Kureshi and Wilkins 1998; Bobek and Sagher 1999; Chen et al. 2000; Matsushima et al. 2000; Vitali et al. 2007). Teflon® Felt utilized in the form of a compact piece may generate strong adhesions to the adjacent neurovascular structures due to its filamentous nature. This has been reported in the literature on the occasion of redone surgery, and is also our observation. The most current way of using Teflon® felt is to tease its fibers from the felt; this can be done with a pair of forceps or by pulling on the fibers between the gloved thumb and index fingers, which is not easy. Then the fibers, after being moistened with saline solution, can be shaped into different tailored forms according to different situations: rolled into a ball or in an oval or peanut shape, more or less compact and of various sizes. Fibers can be agglomerated into ribbon-shaped bundles (of ±2 mm in width and 2–4 cm in length). These ribbon-shaped slings are passed around the vessel loop(s) for their transposition; they are used to exert a pulling effect and to maintain the vessel away so that it has no contact with the decompressed root.

In addition to the shredded Teflon® felt material, that we are preferentially using, two other products, of the knitted type, can be utilized as plates (plaques) for interposition:

- the "Edwards Outflow Tract Knitted PTFE" when a relatively rigid plate is needed
- the "Sauvage knitted Polyester DACRON®" when a more supple sheet is preferable.

Both products are manufactured by BARD Peripheral Vascular Inc. 1625 West 3rd street, Tempe, AZ 85281, USA (www.bardpv.com).

For maintaining transposition apart, the sling technique (Fig. 9.30) or the bridging technique (Fig. 9.31) can be performed. Transposition can be secured by adding a plaque to hold the transposed vessels (Fig. 9.32).

Foreign material may generate granulomas, characterized by giant cell inflammatory reactions. Concerning Teflon—the mostly utilized material—literature compilation reports occurrence rates of 1.7–3.0% of the MVD procedures using it. Granulomas were estimated responsible for 13–50% of all the recurrent neuralgias after MVD which utilized Teflon material inserted. Our experience is that granulomas, and also aggressive adhesiveness of the material manifested by a real incorporation of the Teflon fibers to the root tissue (as observed in trigeminal nerve re-explorations), only occur in the cases in whom the material was in contact with the root itself. Those observations are solid arguments to advocate Transposition as much as possible, and to reserve Interposition when transposition without touching the root is not possible (Sindou et al. 2007).

**Key-Point**

Ideally the material used to maintain the conflicting vessel away from the root should not be in contact with the trigeminal nerve parenchyma.

## 9.6.5 Venous Neuro-Vascular Conflicts (NVCs)

Study of our personal series showed an incidence of 38% of possible implication of veins in the genesis of the neuralgia (Dumot and Sindou 2015). Compression may be pure venous, amounting at 8.9% (Fig. 9.33), or in association with an artery, at 29.1% (Fig. 9.34). This high level of percentages should be nuanced as it is

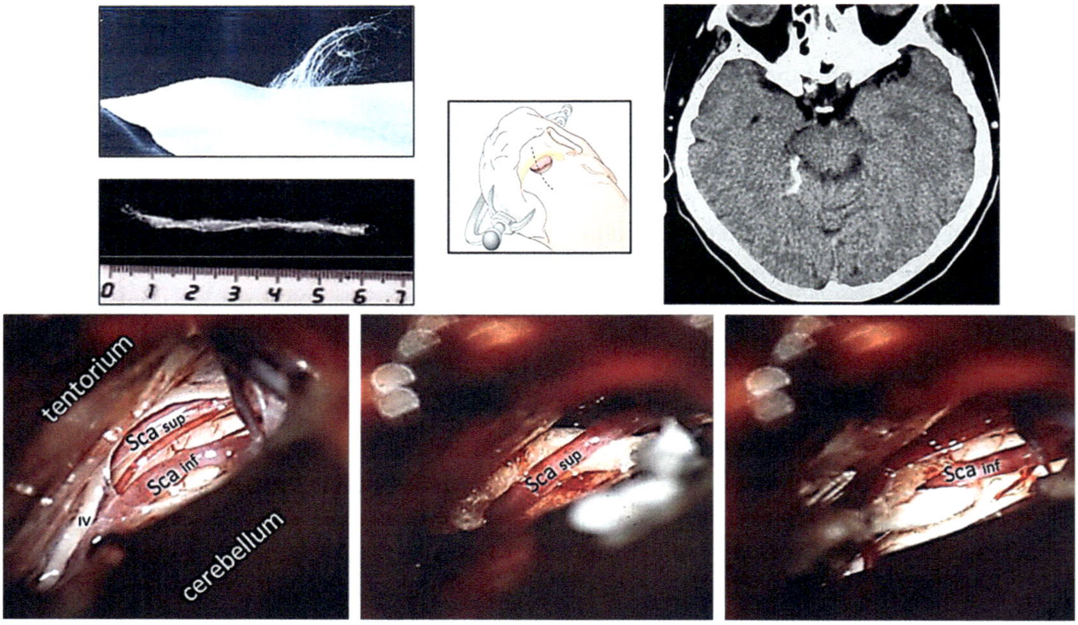


**Fig. 9.30** Transposition technique for Micro-Vascular Decompression of the trigeminal nerve (right side on illustration). Transposition of the two division branches of the superior cerebellar artery (Sca sup. and Sca inf.), using slings (ribbon-shaped) made of Teflon fibers, harvested by teasing from shredded PTFE Teflon felt. Operative steps seen through infratentorial—supracerebellar route. Post-op. CT-scan shows the Teflon slings below tentorium maintaining arteries in place

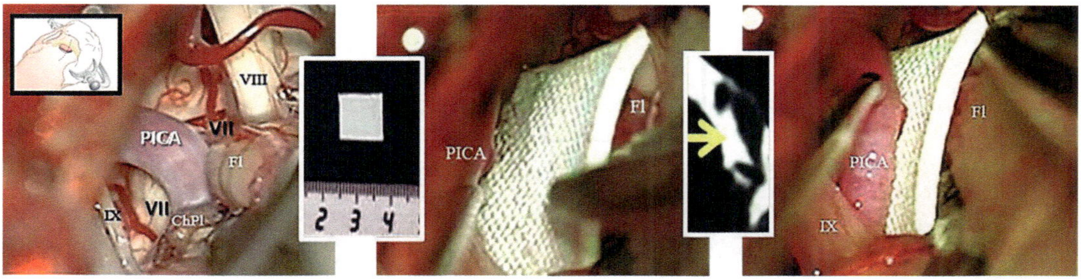


**Fig. 9.31** Bridging technique for Micro-Vascular Decompression. Operative example of "bridging technique" in a patient with primary hemifacial spasm on left side, due to compression of the facial nerve (VII) by posterior inferior cerebellar artery (PICA). Decompression was performed using a semi-rigid plaque made of knitted PTFE Teflon. The plaque was inserted between PICA and VIIth and placed on the ventral surface of the brainstem anteriorly and the flocculus (Fl) posteriorly, so that the material has a "bridging effect" over the facial and the cochleo-vestibular (VIII) cranial nerves, without any contact with them. See Choroid plexus (Ch.Pl.) emerging from Luschka foramen and glossopharyngeal nerve (IX)

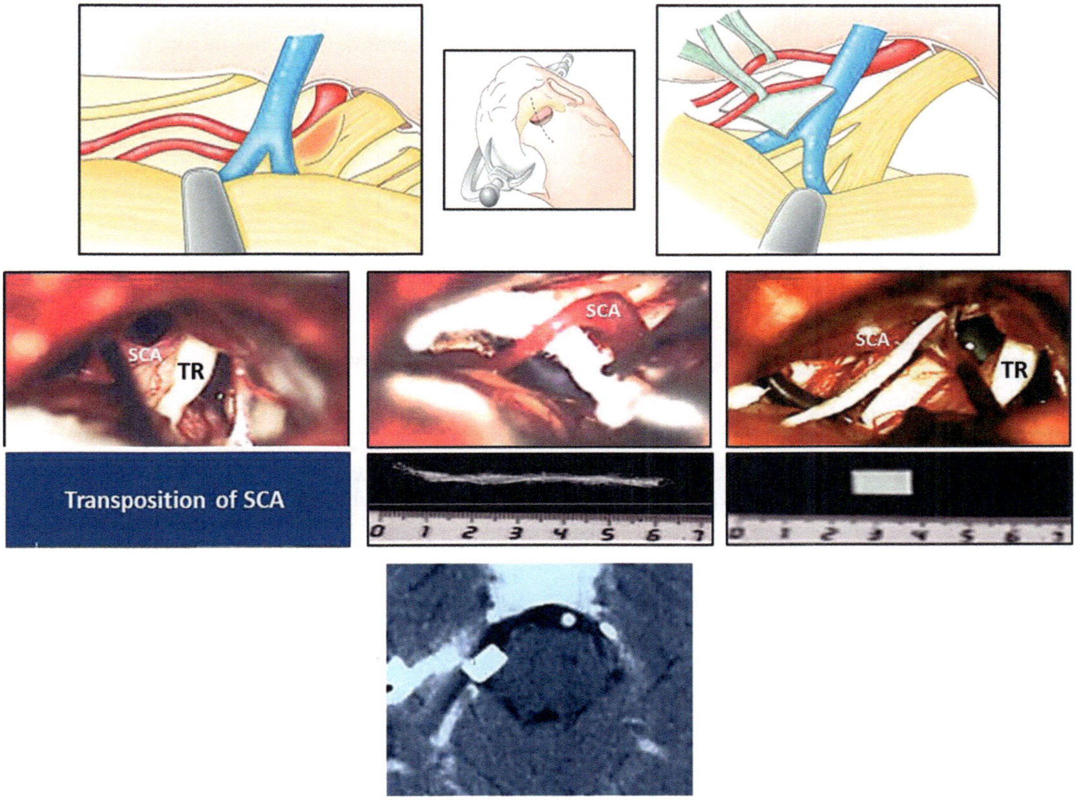


**Fig. 9.32** Secured Transposition for Micro-Vascular Decompression (MVD) . Transposition technique using both: sling(s) and plaque, to secure transposition. Example of MVD in a patient with classical trigeminal neuralgia on right side, due to neurovascular conflict from superior cerebellar artery (SCA). Sling, made of Teflon fibers harvested from shredded PTFE Teflon felt, is passed around SCA as a first step. Then transposition is secured by inserting a plaque (made of semi-rigid knitted PTFE Teflon) between artery and superior petrosal vein, in order not to be in contact with the decompressed trigeminal root (TR). Post-op CT-scan shows both pieces of "foreign" material in place

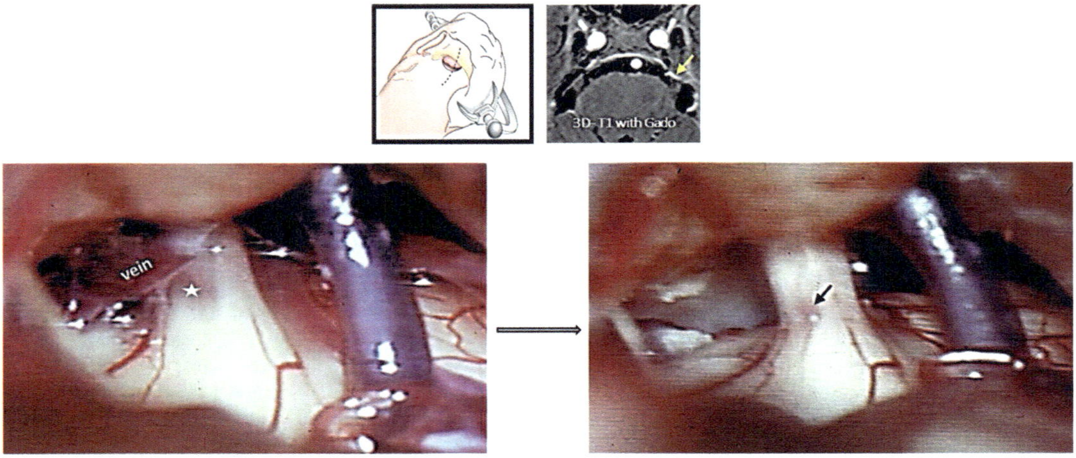


**Fig. 9.33** Venous decompression for deep transverse inferior vein. Left classical trigeminal neuralgia due to pure venous neurovascular conflict, as seen on the axial section of T1 + Gadolinium MRI sequence. The conflicting vessel is an inferior transverse pontine vein, belonging to the deep superior petrosal venous system (left operative view). The venous compression created a focal demyelination, manifested by a greyish aspect in the root (star). Decompression was achieved by coagulation and suppression of the compressive vein, as seen on the right operative image where the demyelination zone is visible (arrow)

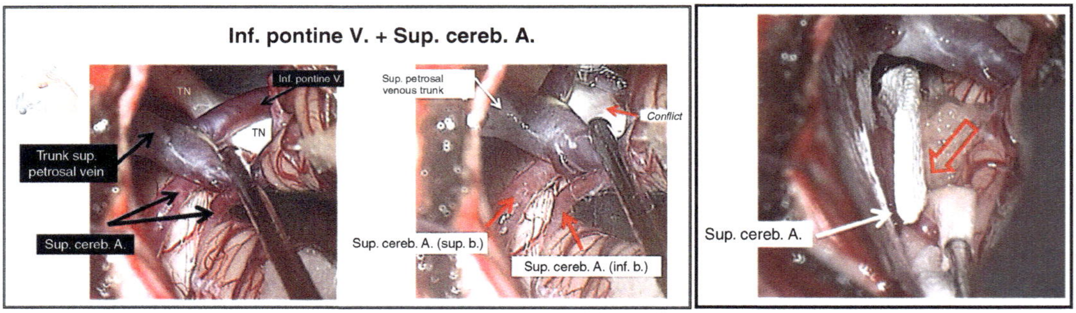


**Fig. 9.34** Operative steps for Mixed (venous and arterial) Neuro-Vascular Conflict. Left: Exposure of the neurovascular structures implicated in the conflict, right-sided. The trigeminal nerve root (TN) is squeezed between the inferior pontine vein, dorsally, and the superior cerebellar artery (SCA) with its two branches, ventrally, the later pushing down the root to the pontine vein. Center: After dissection and freeing of the root from the vein the site of the conflict is visible, with a groove and a greyish aspect testifying of local demyelination at the site of the venous compression (red arrow). Right: Decompression of the TN by transposition of the SCA and its two branches using a semi-rigid plaque of Teflon to maintain them away

often difficult to be certain of their responsibility, except when the vein markedly engrooves the root. The suspected compressive veins were either veins belonging to the superficial superior petrosal venous system (sSPVS), in a majority the pontine affluent of the superior petrosal vein, or a vein from the deep superior petrosal venous system (dSPVS), almost always a transverse cross-compressing vein adjacent to the porus of Meckel cave.

Conservation of the vessel is admissible only if its mobilization away can be successfully obtained; this implies complete freeing of the trigeminal root from all arachnoid adhesions. Otherwise, coagulation and division have to be performed. Decompression could be performed without sacrificing the vein in 63.2% of our venous conflicts (Dumot et al. 2017).

According to our observations, we differentiated two main types of venous NVCs (Dumot and Sindou 2015). In the first type, which corresponds to mixed venous and arterial conflicts, an elongated artery pushes the root against a nearby vein, the vein marking a print into the displaced root (Fig. 9.34). In such conditions, transposing the artery is often sufficient for an effective decompression. In the second type, which corresponds to pure venous cross-compressions, like those frequently seen at the exit of the root from the porus of Meckel's cave, mostly due to the inferior transverse vein of the dSPVS, generally the vein exerts a real cross-compression, as shown in Fig. 9.33. In such an eventuality, coagulation with division of the vein is most often the solution.

When a vein is coursing parallel to the nerve, it is difficult to be certain of its pathological role. The vein may be kept intact, pushed away and maintained apart, as prediction of the tolerance of sacrificing veins is far from to be reliable.

## 9.7 Outcome After MVD

### 9.7.1 Pain Relief

Outcome has been analyzed by their respective authors in a large number of individual series and in a few meta-analyses. Table 9.2 summarizes some important reported series (Table 9.2). The quality of pain relief and its long-term persistence are not always easy to compare from one series to another due to their disparities and the technical peculiarities of the procedures used not reproduced exactly.

In our various articles along time (Sindou et al. 2002, 2006, 2007, 2008; Dumot et al. 2017) the neuralgia was estimated relieved if the patient had no pain or only sporadic pain episodes that did not require treatment, that is, BNI I or II, respectively. In our 356 patients studied with a Kaplan-Meir statistical analysis, probability of

**Table 9.2** Outcome after Micro-Vascular Decompression (Literature review)

| | | | | MVD | | | | |
|---|---|---|---|---|---|---|---|---|
| Nb. patients | Follow-up (mean in year) | Relief of the Neuralgia Initial (%) | Relief of the Neuralgia Late (%) | Side-effects Hypo-esthesia (+/++) | Side-effects Vth nerve motor weakness | Complications Dysesthesia | Complications CN palsy | Complications Permanent Severe Morbidy |
| 246 | 5.1 | - | 83 | | | | | |
| 178 | 5.2 | 94 | 84 | | | | | 1.10% |
| 109 | 4.8 | - | 76 | | | | | |
| 133 | 5 | - | 84 | | | | | 0.70% |
| 1155 | 6 | 98 | 70 | (++) 16.5% | 0% | 1.60% | 3% | 0.30% |
| 135 | 1.4 | - | 83 | | | | 3% | |
| 281 | 10 | 92 | 86 | | | | | |
| 146 | 5.7 | 96 | 89 | | | 1.40% | | 1.30% |
| 146 | 3.2 | 85 | 89 | | | | | |
| 225 | 10 | 76 | 63 | | | 1.40% | 5.30% | 0.80% |
| 1188 | 5 | 98 | 80 | | | | | |
| 114 | 2 | - | 82 | | | | | |
| 156 | 10 | 93 | 74 | | | | | |
| 220 | 5.3 | 89 | 84 | | | | 2% | |
| 362 | 8 | 86 | 80 | (+) 10% (++) 4% | | | 1.90% | 0.30% |
| 119 | 3.3 | 91 | 81 | | | | | |
| 266 | 7 | 98 | 71 | | | | | |
| 156 | 9.7 | 88 | 82 | | | | | |
| 154 | 5.6 | 84 | 72 | | | | | |
| 226 | 6 | 85 | 83 | | | | | |

Publications retained correspond to series with more than 100 operated cases, a follow-up of at least 1 year, and precise information on initial pain relief and outcome at last follow-up; in those, side effects and/or complications were more or less detailed

Summary of results for the main MVD series published (Bederson and Wilson 1989; Klun 1992; Cutbush and Atkinson 1994; Illingworth 1995; Barker et al. 1996; Rath et al. 1996; Kondo 1997; Lee et al. 1997; Broggi et al. 2000; Tronnier et al. 2001; Tyler-Kabara et al. 2002; Chen and Lee 2003; Olson et al. 2005; Zakrzewska et al. 2005; Sindou 2006; Bond et al. 2010; Sarsam et al. 2010; Oesman and Mooij 2011; Sandel and Eide 2013; Zhang et al. 2013) cure was 81.2% at 1 year and 73.4% at 15 years (Fig. 9.35). The long-term outcome was similar whether the clinical presentation was typical or atypical (Sindou et al. 2006) (Fig. 9.36); however, the background of pain needed a certain delay to disappear. Important, outcome was found dependent on the grade of the conflict. Grade I compression patients fared worst with a 65% of probability to benefit pain relief at 15 years, whereas grade II and Grade III showed a probability of cure at 15 years of 75% and 85%, respectively (Sindou et al. 2007) (Fig. 9.37).

A recent personal review covering 17 large series of the literature and totaling 5124 patients showed approximately similar results among the various reported articles (Sindou and Brinzeu 2018). Immediate pain relief was obtained in 80–98% of the patients (91.8% on average), with persistence of complete relief in 62–89% (76.6% on average) at end of follow-up (which ranged from 5 to 11 years depending on the series, 7 years on average).

In the largest published series, the one of Jannetta, studied by Barker and which included 1185 patients followed up to 20 years (median 6.2 years), 82% had an excellent immediate relief and 70% kept this relief after 10 years of FU (Barker et al. 1997).

In a recent review of the European Academy of Neurology of 21 published series regrouping 5149 patients with an average FU varying from 3 to 10.9 years, the reported initial pain relief, the FU pain-free, and the recurrence rates of the MVD group ranged from 80–98.2%, 62–89%, and 4–38%, respectively, with an average initial pain relief, FU pain-free, and recurrence rates

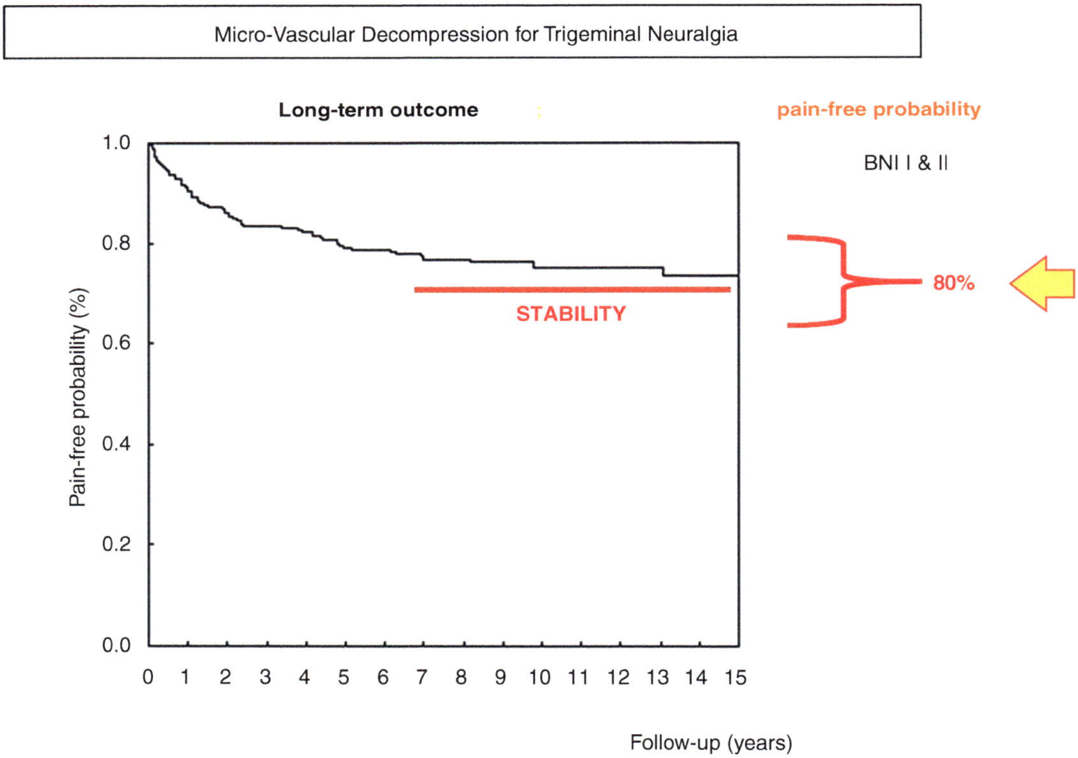


**Fig. 9.35** Long-term (15 years) probability for patients affected with classical trigeminal neuralgia treated with microvascular decompression (MVD) of being pain-free (BNI I or II): 80%. Data from a personal series of 1800 patients treated with MVD. Study with Kaplan-Meier statistical analysis. Note the relative stability of the curve after 2 years of follow-up (Sindou et al. 2007)

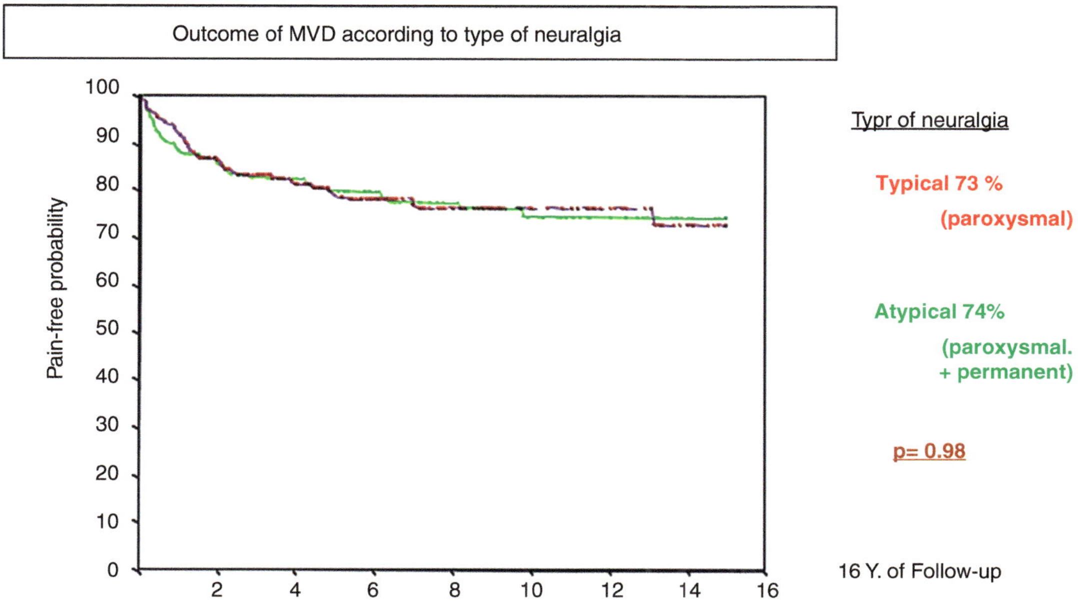


**Fig. 9.36** Long-term (15 years) probability for MVD to obtain pain relief (BNI I or II) in classical trigeminal neuralgia *according to clinical presentation*: typical (i.e., with pure paroxysmal crises) or atypical (i.e., paroxysms associated with a background of continuous pain). Comparative study shows same effectiveness in both presentations ($p = 0.98$). However, in the group of patients with atypical presentation, disappearance of the continuous pain component often needs a delay of several months to a few years to occur (Sindou et al. 2007)

calculated as 93,7%, 84%, and 21.2%, respectively (Bendtsen et al. 2019).

In 2007 we conducted a study on the factors which could influence the prognosis of MVD (Sindou et al. 2007). The analyzed factors were categorized as follows.

1. The factors related to the neuralgia: side, topography, and extent, did not exert an adverse influence. Neuralgia with atypical manifestations had the same satisfactory outcome as typical neuralgia, provided permanent background of pain not secondary to previous lesioning-procedures (Sindou et al. 2006).
2. Regarding the anatomical factors, the type of the compressive vessel: arterial or venous (provided being cross-compressive for the later), as well as its location along or around the root, were not significant for the outcome. In contrast, the severity of the compression did play a significant role, with more severe compression being associated with a better outcome ($p = 0.0001$) (Sindou et al. 2007). The presence of a severe focal arachnoiditis had a significant pejorative role on the long-term prognosis ($p = 0.002$) (Dumot et al. 2017; Mazzucchi et al. 2019) (Fig. 9.38). On the contrary, the existence of a global atrophy of the root did not reveal to be a pejorative factor, at least on the paroxystic component of the neuralgia when atypical ($p = 0.36$) (Sindou et al. 2007) (Fig. 9.39).
3. The factors related to the patient: gender, age at surgery (Fig. 9.40), past history of systemic hypertension, and—although surprisingly—the duration of the neuralgia prior to surgery, did not play a role in prognosis.

However, our findings do not converge with some other literature reports on the following factors. Factors found with a higher risk of recurrence in the literature were early onset of the disease, female gender, preoperative duration of the neuralgia, and venous conflicts.

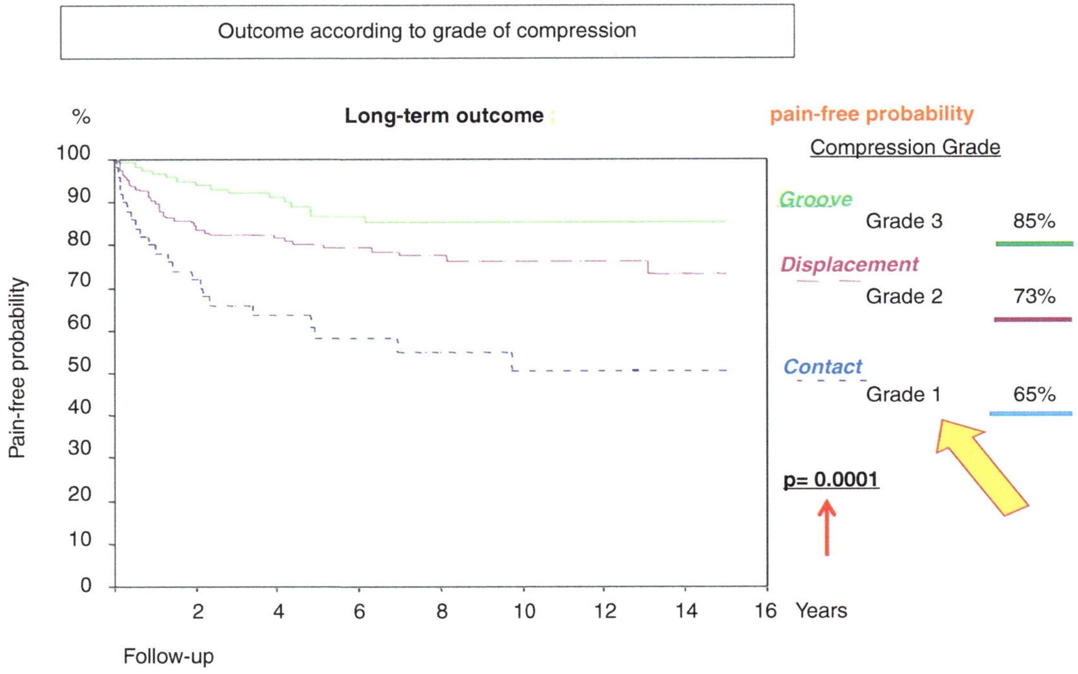


**Fig. 9.37** Long-term (15 years) probability of MVD efficacy (BNI I or II) *according to the grade of compression of the conflicting vessel* as estimated at surgery ($p = 0.0001$) Probability of obtaining relief was only 65% for the group of patients having grade I of compression (i.e., simple contact). This raises the hypothesis of other (or additional) factor in the genesis of the neuralgia (Sindou et al. 2007)

### 9.7.2 The Puzzling Case of the Venous Compressions

The role of venous neurovascular conflicts (NVCs) as a cause of trigeminal neuralgias is controversial as to ascertain responsibility of veins is most often difficult.

Our experience is that implication of veins may be frequently suspected to be responsible of nerve root conflicts. This happened in 38% of all classical neuralgias in our overall series of 326 studied cases, and as the main responsible vessel in 17.5% (Dumot and Sindou 2015). Implication can be either as an element of a mixed arterial/venous conflict, in 29% of the cases, or constituting a pure venous compression, in 9%.

In mixed NVCs, the artery generally pushes the root onto the vein with a demyelination on the venous side, as shown in Fig. 9.34. In pure venous NVCs, the vein—often an inferior transverse vein nearby the porus trigeminus—is found exerting a cross-compression onto the root, as shown in Fig. 9.33.

Retaining a vein as a plausible compressive vessel must be very critical. According to our view, main criteria is vein exerting a real cross-compression, especially if the vessel prints a mark of demyelination manifested by a focal greyish discoloration of the root. Responsibility of veins coursing parallel to the root should be retained only very prudently.

Results on the neuralgia after MVD in the cases in whom implication of a venous compression has been retained have been evaluated in our series through Kaplan-Meir statistical analyses (Dumot et al. 2017). These are detailed in the following illustrative figures: probability to be pain-free at 10 years after decompression of venous

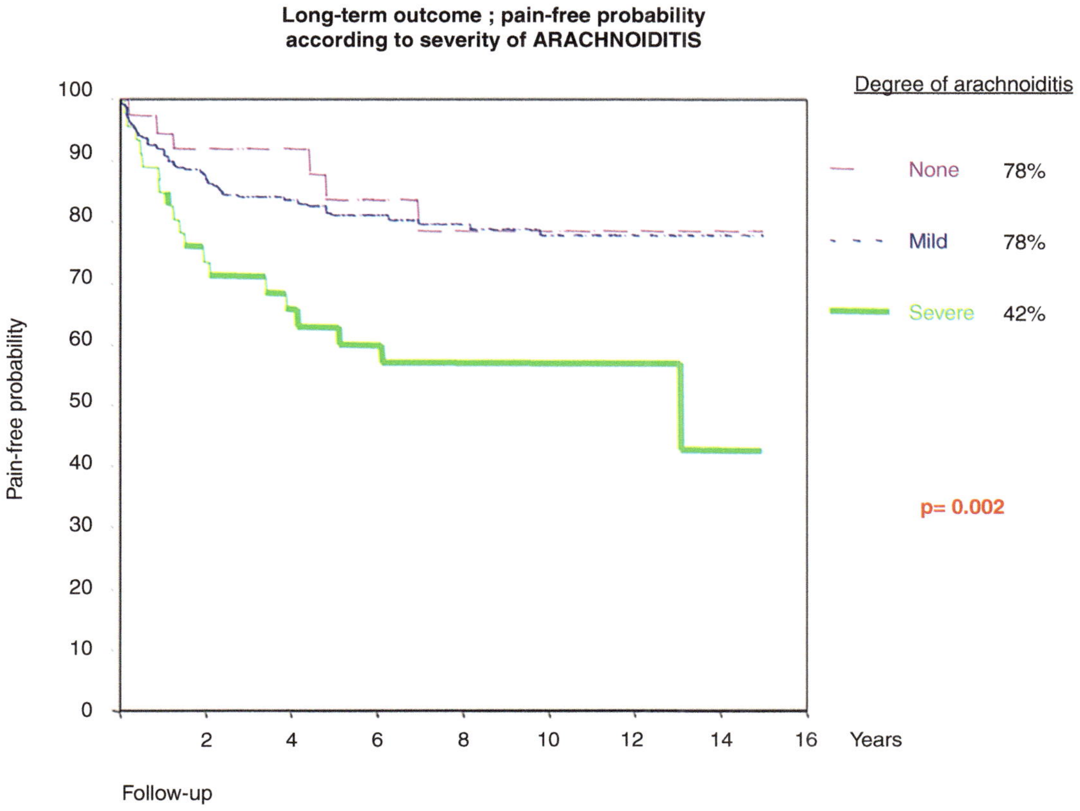


**Fig. 9.38** Long-term (15 years) probability of pain relief (BNI I or II) in classical trigeminal neuralgia after MVD *according to the presence or not of associated arachnoiditis* and its severity. A marked arachnoiditis manifested by a focally thickened membrane with adhesion to the root constitutes a significant pejorative prognostic factor ($p = 0.002$) (Sindou et al. 2007)

NVCs (Fig. 9.41), comparison of long-term outcomes after decompression of arterial and venous NVCs showing quasi-similarity between both of them (Fig. 9.42), outcome according to type of venous conflict: mixed or pure (Fig. 9.43), better outcome with high degree of compression by the vein (Fig. 9.44), and pejorative influence of the presence of a focal arachnoiditis (Fig. 9.45),

### 9.7.3 Complications

Mortality reported in literature ranged between 0 and 1.2% (0.3% as a reliable overall estimate), and at 0.3% in our series. Mortality was mainly related to cerebellar/brainstem infarction, either due to manipulations of cerebellopontine angle arteries or from venous sacrifices.

Persistent hearing loss was reported at 0.8–4.5% in the literature (1.2% on average), and amounted at 1.5% in our series.

Severe facial paresis was reported at 0.5–1.5% (0.9% on average), and occurred in 1.1% in our series. Permanent trochlear palsy was noted in 1.1% on average in the literature (0.5% in our series).

CSF leakage, manifested by a meningocele or a rhinorrhea, was observed in 2–17% according to published series. In our series this complica-

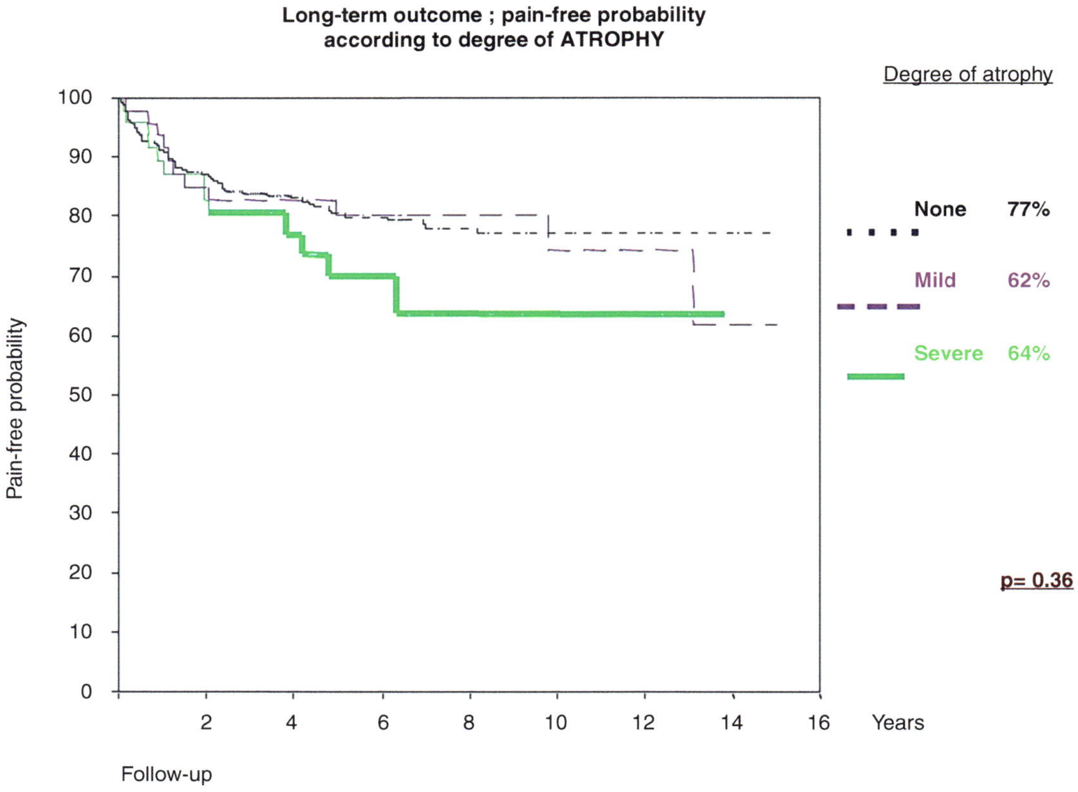


**Fig. 9.39** Long-term (15 years) outcome in classical trigeminal neuralgia after MVD *according to the presence or not of associated global atrophy of the root*. Although probability of pain relief was lesser in the group with a severely atrophic root, difference did not reveal statistically significant ($p = 0.36$) (Sindou et al. 2007)

tion amounted at 3% since systematic affixing of a piece of fat tissue in addition to a watertight dura closure.

Trigeminal sensory disturbances are uncommon with pure MVD; dysesthesias were reported in 2–5% in the literature (4%, mild, in our series).

Table 9.3 provides list of complication from some reported series.

### 9.7.4 Conclusions and Perspectives

1. Our 40-year experience led to the following estimations.

   Vascular decompression obtains a *high and stable rate of long-term relief* of the neuralgia, especially when the conflict exerts a *high degree of compression* to the trigeminal root.

In *Atypical trigeminal neuralgias*, relief can be obtained not only for the paroxysmal component but also for the continuous background of pain—albeit with a more or less delay linked to the neuropathic nature of the later component.

*Veins* can be the cause of NVCs, similarly to arteries, provided exerting a cross-compression effect—rather than coursing parallelly to the root—and of a high degree of compression.

Exploring and freeing the entire root from brainstem to porus of Meckel cave is wise, as the NVCs may be located not only at the TREZ but *also all along the root*, and are *multiple* in around one-third of cases.

Surgery should be as atraumatic as possible not to add a lesioning effect to the decom-

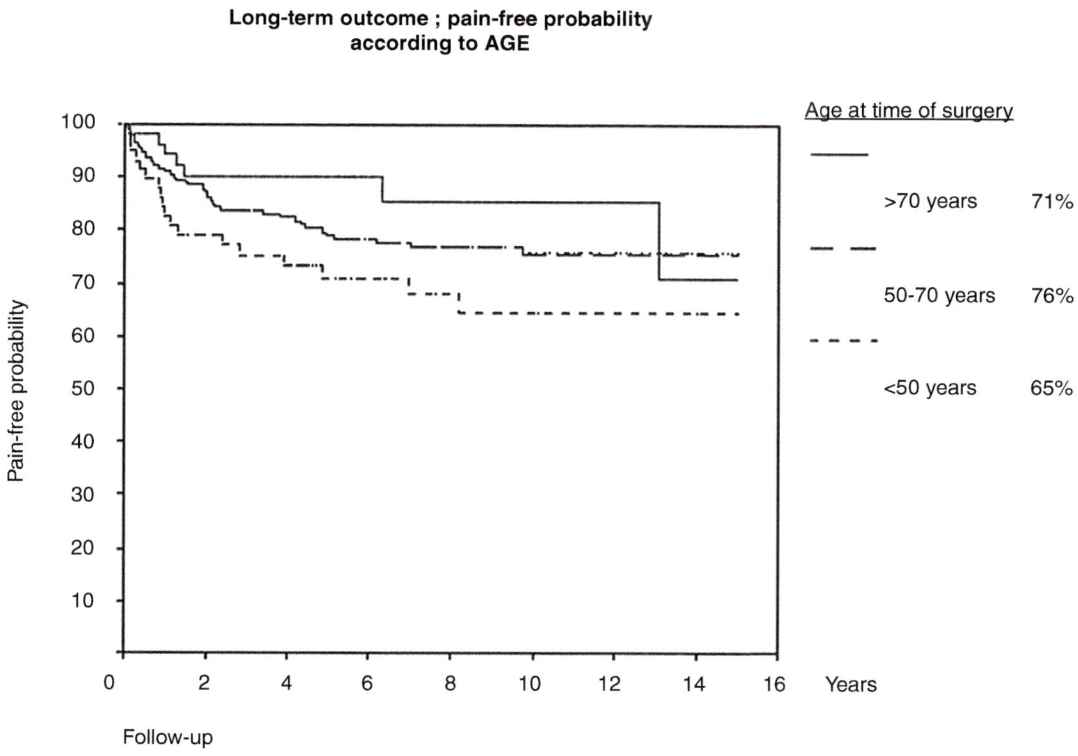


**Fig. 9.40** Study of the *influence of age* on probability of long-term outcome shows that pain relief was lesser in the group under 50 years of age. At the opposite the group of elder patients, that is, those above 70 years of age, had a high rate of pain relief. However, differences did not reach statistical significance (Sindou et al. 2007)

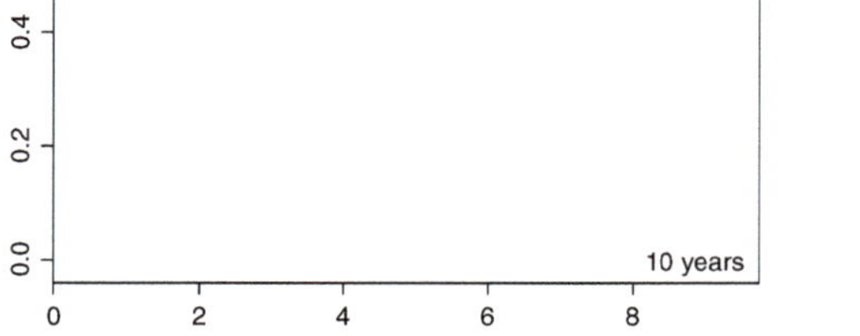


**Fig. 9.41** Long-term (10 years) outcome after MVD in the group of *patients with a venous conflict* (n: 55 pts). Study shows probability of pain relief (BNI I or II) at 8 years in 71.1% of the patients, of whom 52.8% with BNI I level (Dumot et al. 2017)

pression. Decompression should *not be neo-compressive*, and thus should favor the *Transposition* to the Interposition method.

Depiction of NVCs on *fine Imaging* and thus prediction of long-term prognosis are of prime importance for indication of surgery and the choice of the most appropriate technique. High-resolution MRI (preferentially with a 3-T machine) centered on the trigeminal nerves is reliable to ascertain the NVCs of high degrees of compression (II & III), but *not so for NVCs of grade I* (mere contact).

Perspective could be that in "difficult" cases to determine responsibility of the vessel in contact with the root, the *DTI methodology* could help to find out a local root alteration, testifying of a harmful effect of the vessel in contact with the root.

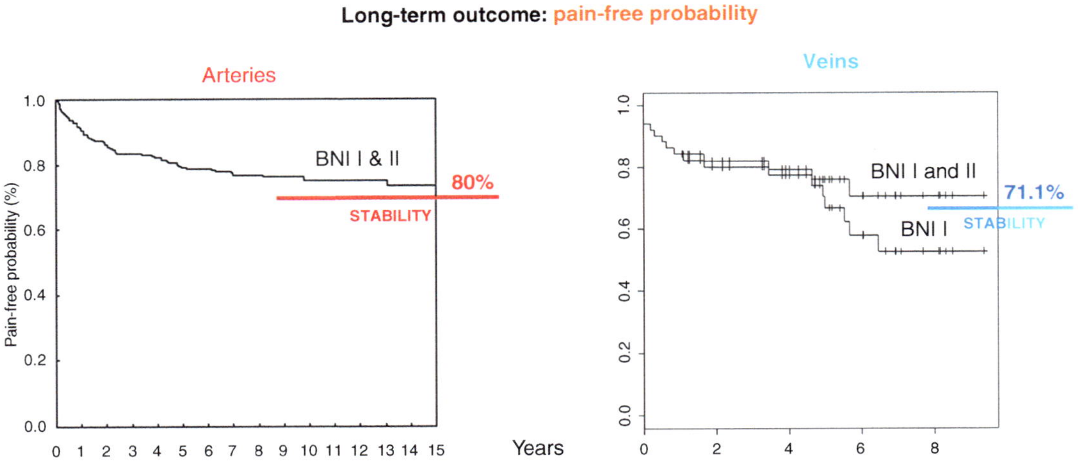


**Fig. 9.42** *Comparison* of probability of long-term outcomes after MVD between the groups of patients with classical *trigeminal neuralgia due to arterial (on the left) and to venous (on the right) Neuro-Vascular Conflicts* (NVCs). At 8 years probability of pain relief (BNI I or II) for the group with venous NVCs (71.1%) is almost as high as the one in the arterial NVCs group (80%) (Dumot et al. 2017)

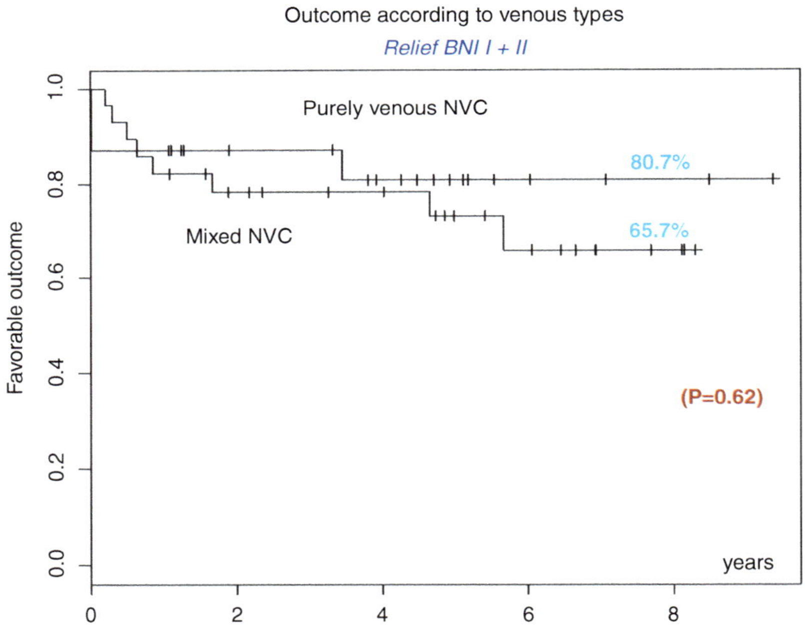


**Fig. 9.43** *Comparison* of probability of pain relief (BNI I or II) after MVD between the group of patients with *mixed venous* [vein associated to artery ($n = 29$ pts)] and the group of patients with *pure venous* [i.e., only a compressive vein ($n = 25$ pts)] *neurovascular conflicts*. Study shows no significant statistical difference between the two groups ($p = 0.62$) (Dumot et al. 2017)

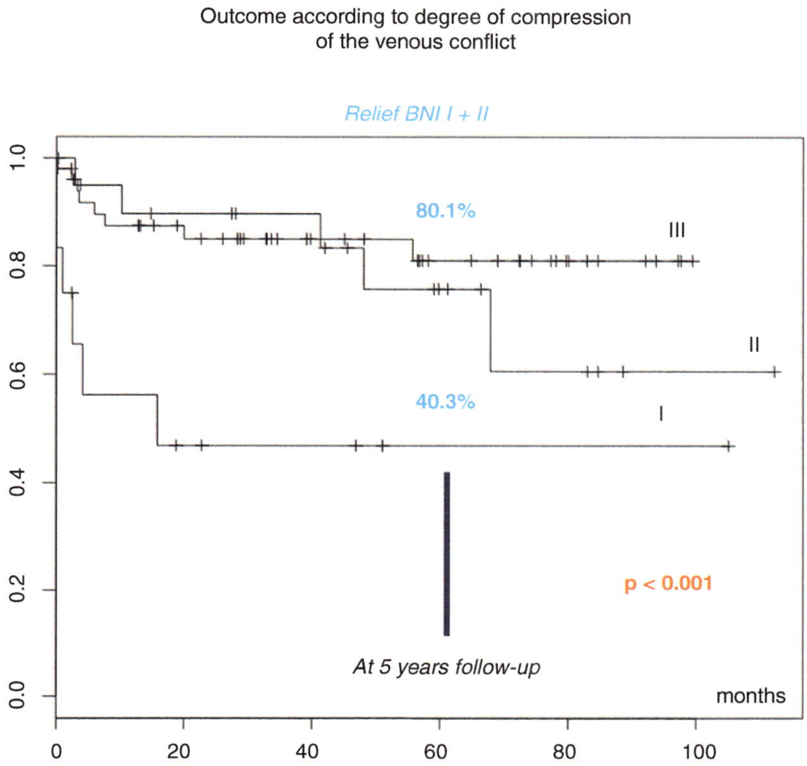


**Fig. 9.44** Statistical study of probability of MVD to obtain pain relief (BNI I or II) *according to the degree of compression by the venous conflict*. Probability is of 80.1% for grade III of compression (i.e., major compression) versus only 40.3% for grade I [i.e., only contact of the vessel to the root ($p = 0.001$)] (Dumot et al. 2017). NB: Values are quite similar to the ones observed with the arterial NVCs

2. Our findings are well in concordance with the data provided through the pioneering works of Jannetta and team (Jannetta 1967; Barker et al. 1997) (Fig. 9.46).
3. The Micro-Vascular Decompression (MVD) compared to the other techniques of the neurosurgical armamentarium has been recognized as the method with the optimal long-term effects to treat the refractory (classical) trigeminal neuralgias (TN), in other words, the real gold-standard. However, as not all situations can be solved satisfactorily by this method and because there are several effective alternatives, the implication of a suspected vascular compression in the mechanism of the TN in a particular patient should be critically considered, as pointed out by Burchiel in a sound editorial article (Burchiel 2016).

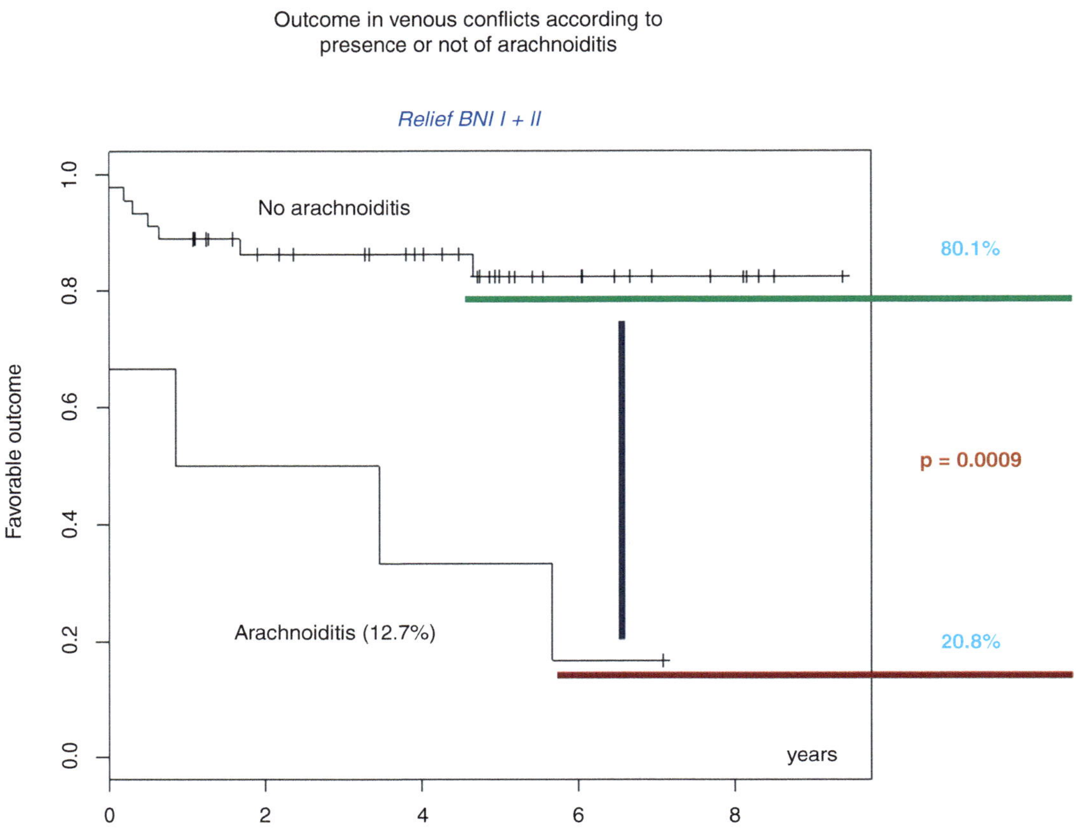


**Fig. 9.45** Statistical study of probability of MVD to obtain pain relief (BNI I or II), according to the absence or the presence of focal *arachnoiditis associated to the venous conflict*. Study shows a high probability of pain relief (80.1%) in the absence and a low probability (20.89%) in the presence of the arachnoiditis ($p = 0.0009$) (Dumot et al. 2017). NB: Presence of a marked arachnoiditis is a pejorative factor, similarly to what was observed in the group of arterial conflicts associated with arachnoiditis

**Table 9.3** Neurological complications in MVD Surgery[a]

| | |
|---|---|
| • *Mortality*: 2 pts/1800 (due to brainstem/cerebellar infarction) = 0.11% (1.1‰) | |
| • *Gait disturbances* (severe and permanent): 6 pts/1800 = 0.33% (3.3‰) | |
| • *CN Palsy* | Hearing loss (permanent): 39 pts/1800 = 2.1% (21‰) |
| | Facial Palsy (permanent) : 11 pts/1800 = 0.62% (6.2‰) |
| | Trochlear nerve palsy: 10 pts/1800 = 0.55% (5.5‰)<br>transient: 7 pts/1800 = 0.38% (3.8‰)<br>permanent: 3 pts/1800 = 0.17% (1.7‰) |
| • *Numbness (bothering) in trigeminal territory (permanent): 54 pts/1800 = 3.00% (30‰)* | |

[a]Data from retrospective study of overall personal series of 1800 patients affected with classical trigeminal neuralgia who underwent MVD

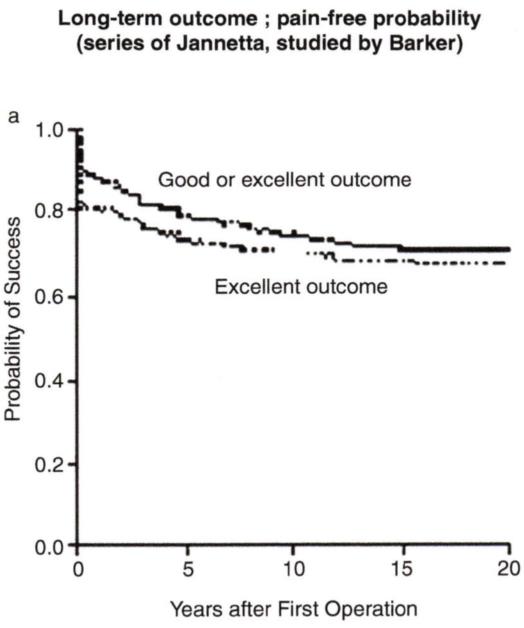


**Fig. 9.46** Long-term outcome after MVD: pain-free probability at 20 years calculated with Kaplan-Meier statistical study *in Jannetta's series* (Barker et al. 1997). Excellent outcome corresponds to BNI I, Good outcome to BNI or II

## 9.8 The Other Open Microsurgical Procedures

The conservative MVD method benefits the consensual agreement to be the favorite technique for treating the classical neuralgias, especially when the plausible NVC is estimated exerting a high degree (i.e., II or III) of compression on high-resolution MRI. When no clearcut vascular compression is found at surgery, an Internal neurolysis can be performed, or a Partial juxta-pontine rhizotomy of the rootlet(s) corresponding to the trigger-zone.

> **Key-Point**
> The Micro-Vascular Decompression procedure is the gold-standard to treat classical trigeminal neuralgia, but provided a sufficient probability of the suspected conflicting vessel to be compressive on preoperative MRI.

In other (very different) circumstances, like in secondary trigeminal neuralgias or some painful trigeminal neuropathies from tumor origin, for example, a Juxta-pontine partial rhizotomy can solve the pain problem. When the approach of the lesion allows direct access of the trigeminal nerve in the middle fossa, a Retrogasserian neurotomy can be preferred.

Both latter operations were widely performed for decades all over the world, and results extensively reported testifying of a remarkable effectiveness on the neuralgia. But both entail constant side effects, especially a more or less degree of facial numbness, and in a certain number of patients: anesthesia dolorosa.

### 9.8.1 The Sub-Temporal Trigeminal Retrogasserian Neurotomy

The first intracranial resection of the trigeminal ganglion and/or trigeminal root was attempted through a sub-temporal intradural approach by Horsley as soon as 1891 (Horsley 1891a, b). The approach was later refined and codified by Spiller and Frazier in 1925, achieving a retrogasserian selective resection of the sensory rootlets whilst sparing the first division fibers and the motor root (Frazier 1925). Thereafter, the procedure was

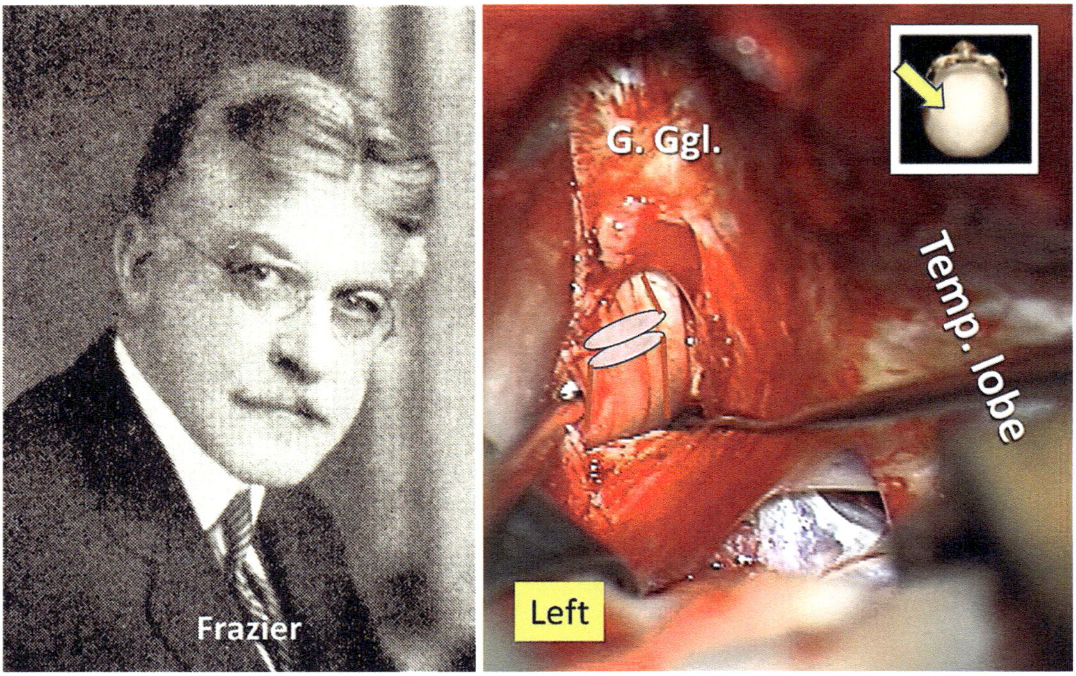


**Fig. 9.47** The Retrogasserian neurotomy procedure via sub-temporal approach was introduced by Charles Frazier. The neurotomy can be performed intradurally (as shown in the operative photography) or extradurally, a less invasive route. The operative view shows the sub-temporal intradural approach on left side, with the roof of the Meckel cave opened at level of the retrogasserian portion of the root on travelling over the upper petrous ridge. View also shows the four-fifths most lateral rootlets of the root cut. Such sectioning allows to spare the motor root and the $V_1$ rootlet(s) which corresponds to the corneal sensory territory of the root

widely adopted under the vocable of sub-temporal trigeminal (retrogasserian) neurotomy. The neurotomy can be performed intradurally, as shown in the operative photography (Fig. 9.47) or extradurally, a less invasive route.

### 9.8.2 The Juxta-Pontine Trigeminal Rhizotomy

This access of the trigeminal nerve in the posterior fossa was proposed by Dandy, also in1925 (Dandy 1925). The operation consisted via a retrosigmoid approach to partially section the sensory root at the pons. At this level the root has three components: the Pars Major, the Pars Intermediaris, and the Pars Minor which corresponds to the motor root. The sole cutting of the inferolateral two-thirds of the pars major allows analgesia/hypoesthesia of the V2 and V3 territories with conservation of the corneal sensation and the protector corneal reflex (Fig. 9.48).

**Key-Point**

Nowadays, these two operations keep a place in the neurosurgical armamentarium, especially in the frame of some refractory secondary TNs, particularly those observed in tumor cases. Juxta-pontine rhizotomy may also be the solution for TNs due to compression by huge megadolicho-VBAs when conservative decompression cannot be effectively performed.

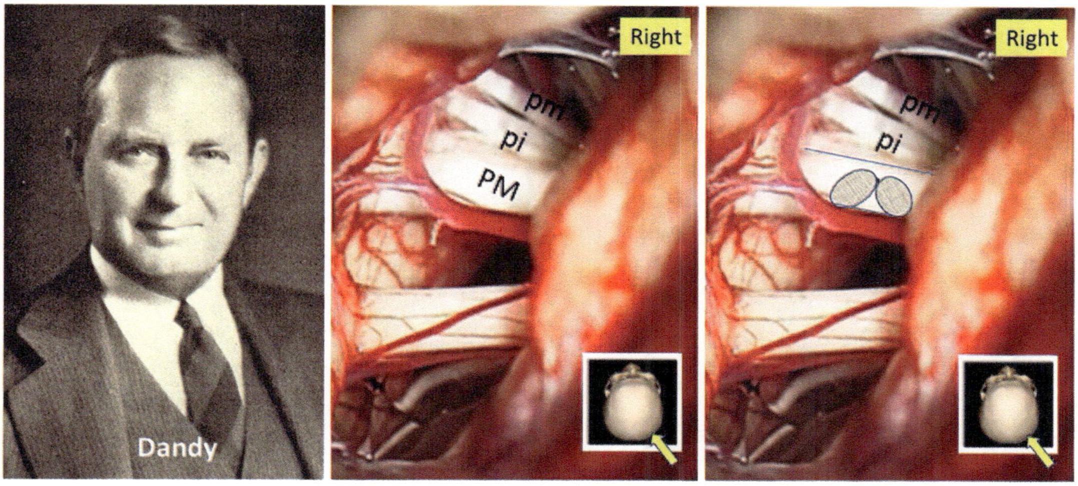


**Fig. 9.48** The Juxtapontine rhizotomy procedure via retrosigmoid approach was introduced by Walter Dandy. The operative view (center image) shows the Trigeminal Root Entry Zone (TREZ) on right side, with its three components: the Pars Major (PM) and the pars intermediaris (pi) of the sensory root, and the pars minor (pm) which corresponds to the motor root. The right image illustrates the partial (inferolateral) section of the PM in order to obtain analgesia of the $V_3$ and $V_2$ trigeminal sensory divisions, whilst sparing the sensory function in the $V_1$ division, especially in the corneal territory

### 9.8.3 Internal Neurolysis

Internal Neurolysis (IN) is a procedure in which all or portions of the trigeminal root are divided longitudinally along its fascicles between the pons and the porus of Meckel cave.

Literature compilation shows that facial numbness is the main side effect of the procedure (also named combing of nerve fibers): from 15 to 100%, 96% in the best documented series (Ko et al. 2015). This rate is comparable with the rate of numbness with other lesioning-techniques: 90.0–98.1% with the percutaneous balloon compression (PBC) (Stomal-Słowińska et al. 2011; Du et al. 2015) and 84.7–97.4% with the percutaneous radiofrequency thermocoagulation (PRT) (Son et al. 2011; Tang et al. 2015). However, on long-term FU facial numbness decreased or disappeared in most cases, so that it did not significantly impact quality of life (Ko et al. 2015) except in the 4% in whom anesthesia dolorosa developed.

Pain relief in the main reported series, at 3.6 years of average FU, was obtained in 72% of the patients (Manzoni and Torelli 2005).

IN is an option when no neurovascular conflict is found during surgery attempted for a plausible NVC.

# 10 Percutaneous Lesioning-Techniques for Trigeminal Neuralgias

Not all the primary trigeminal neuralgias are amenable to the (conservative) Micro-Vascular Decompression technique, especially those considered idiopathic. Therefore, lesioning-methods may be helpful to decrease the level of the pain, if not curing it totally. Purpose of those is to suppress the conduction of the trigeminal fibers that carry the neuralgic pain to the brainstem. Thanks to the modern interventional imaging techniques allowing to safely target the foramen ovale at skull base, the anesthesiologic means of modulating the patient's conscience level and the recently developed surgical refinements, a certain selectivity can be achieved.

## 10.1 Brief on the Evolution of the Surgical Treatments

*Improving techniques to become more effective and safer took a long period of time along decades, both for open surgery and the percutaneous lesioning-techniques.*

The first surgical intervention proposed for trigeminal neuralgia was the Gasserian ganglionectomy. Conceived by Wears in 1885 and pioneered in practice soon after by Rose (Rose 1890), the procedure was then performed by Hartley (Hartley 1893), Horsley (Horsley 1891a, b) and Cushing (Cushing 1900). But it was quickly abandoned due to the frequent occurrence of keratites and anesthesia dolora. In 1901 Frazier, at the instigation of Spiller, developed the extradural subtemporal Retrogasserian neurotomy (Spiller and Frazier 1901). Then in 1920 Dandy introduced the Juxtapontine radicotomy via suboccipital laterocerebellar route (Dandy 1925). Limited to the pars major, the section, especially if reduced to its inferolateral two-thirds, was able to obtain analgesia without complete anesthesia of the face, in particular of the cornea. In 1938 Sjoqvist performed the Trigeminal tractotomy by cutting the descending spinal trigeminal tract at level of the medulla, this tract being the vector of the fibers for the thermoalgesic sensation of the face (Sjoqvist 1938; Olivecrona 1942; Kunc 1959). This intervention was then refined and popularized by Kunc (Kunc 1964, 1977; Kunc et al. 1978).

In 1952 Taarnhoj, assuming that trigeminal neuralgia could be due to constriction of the Gasser ganglion by fibrosclerosis of the duramater of the trigeminal cave, proposed the Decompression of the ganglion by opening its dural roof (Taarnhøj 1952, 1982). This technique, which had the theoretical interest of being conservative, was later abandoned due to the frequent recurrences after surgery. Shortly after, Shelden in 1955, interpreting the immediate good


M. Sindou, A. Brinzeu, *Trigeminal Neuralgias: A Neurosurgical Illustrated Guide*,
https://doi.org/10.1007/978-3-031-25113-9_10

effect of the Taarnhoj's method due to an operative trauma to the ganglion and neighboring nerve fibers, proposed the Hammering of the ganglion through direct approach (Shelden et al. 1955). This gave rise to the more recent method of balloon compression by Mullan (Mullan and Lichtor 1983).

In parallel, to mitigate the risks of the interventions by direct approach, percutaneous techniques were developed on the principle of the "old" method of Alcoholization of the Gasserian ganglion, proposed as early as 1906 by Taptas (1911) and performed via lateral approach by Harris (1912a, b, 1940) then via the transforamen ovale approach by Hartel (1912). Instead of alcohol, Jaeger in 1957 proposed the Injection of hot water at the site of the ganglion (Jaeger 1959), and Jefferson in 1963 the Injection of phenol (at the concentration of 1/20th in glycerin) (Jefferson 1963). In 1941 Kirschner introduced the Electrocoagulation of the gasserian ganglion as the lesion-maker; surgery was performed under general anesthesia and using a stereotaxic percutaneous approach to the ganglion with penetration of the electrode through the foramen ovale (Kirschner 1933). The technique was then successively improved by Thiry who used a current of lower intensity in order to avoid the total loss of the tactile sensitivity (Thiry and Hotermans 1974), then by Schürmann who replaced general anesthesia by neuroleptanalgesia to control the effects of the coagulation in the patient awake (Schürmann et al. 1972).

In the early seventies, Sweet refined and popularized the technique under the name of Controlled differential thermocoagulation of the trigeminal ganglion and rootlets (Sweet and Wepsic 1974). A radio-frequency generator was used as the heat source, a thermistor to measure the temperature at the tip of the electrode, and short sequences of general anesthesia or neuroleptanalgesia—only during the painful steps of the intervention—to allow the patient's cooperation. The method is able to obtain analgesia without complete anesthesia and in the sole painful area, thanks to the somatotopy of the fibers at the targeted level.

Still within the framework of percutaneous techniques performed under fluoroscopic control, Hakanson introduced in 1981 the Neurolysis of the Gasser ganglion by injection of glycerol into the trigeminal cistern of the Meckel cave via the foramen ovale (Håkanson 1978), and Mullan in 1979 the Compression of the Gasser ganglion using the inflatable balloon of a Fogarty probe as the lesion-maker (Mullan and Lichtor 1983).

Besides, in the fifties, Leksell applied the technique of Stereotaxic gamma-knife radiosurgery to trigeminal neuralgia (Leksell 1971). But this method only lost its anecdotal character with the advent of high-resolution MRI, which made precise targeting of radiation possible.

Along with these lesioning methods, the conservative method of Microsurgical vascular decompression developed in successive stages. The method is based on the observation made by Dandy, of the frequent observation of vascular conflicts in patients operated on in the cerebellopontine angle for trigeminal neuralgia to perform a juxtapontine radicotomy (Dandy 1932). However, vascular decompression was not performed until 1956, when Gardner reported treatment by simple decompression of the trigeminal root (Gardner 1962). The method was then soon adopted and refined with the microsurgical techniques by Jannetta, who firstly used the subtemporal extradural transtentorial route (Jannetta and Rand 1966; Jannetta 1967), then the retromastoid approach (Jannetta 1977), the later after Hardy from Montreal University advised this route as the most appropriate for performing MVDs (Provost and Hardy 1970). Thanks to Jannetta, the method was popularized and became widely accepted as the first surgical option for treating conservatively the nowadays so-called classical trigeminal neuralgia (Cruccu et al. 2016).

## 10.2 The Percutaneous Hartel Route

The transjugal–transoval route was first described by Hartel in 1912 for alcohol injection at level of the gasserian ganglion to treat trigeminal neuralgia (Hartel 1912). Then this route was extensively used with the same indication for performing percutaneous destructive procedures of the trigeminal system by thermocoagulation, balloon compression, or glycerol injection. This route was also used for inserting EEG electrodes to explore patients with temporo-mesial epilepsy with the purpose of resective surgery (Wieser and Yaşargil 1982). Also more recently, it has been advised to use this approach to perform percutaneous biopsies of the Meckel cave and/or the petroclival regions, when imaging is insufficient to ascertain nature of the local occupying lesions before establishing therapeutic final decision (Sindou et al. 1997, 2012).

The anatomical region crossed by the trocar may be considered an inverted, three-sided, pyramidal volume, with its apex at a cheek cutaneous point, 3 cm lateral to the labial commissure. Its triangular base, located at skull base, is delineated by the three following landmarks. The supero-lateral one is a cutaneous point on the orbito-meatal line along the inferior border of the zygoma, 3 cm anterior to the tragus. The supero-mesial one corresponds to the pupilla. The deep-seated one is the Foramen Ovale (FO) itself (Fig. 10.1).

According to our team's description (Alvernia et al. 2010), this inverted pyramid can be subdivided into three segments (Fig. 10.2): an inferior

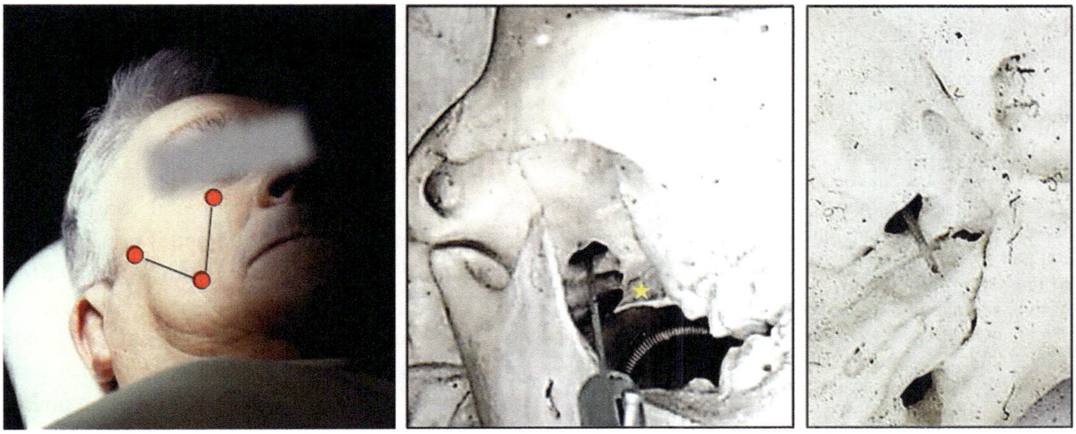

**Fig. 10.1** The transjugal-transoval Hartel route for percutaneous access to trigeminal cave and nerve. Left: Cutaneous landmarks: 30 ± 5 mm lateral to the labial commissure (60 mm from the middle of the inter-commisssural line). The foramen ovale is targeted by aiming: on lateral view, a point at 35 mm anterior to the anterior wall of the external auditory meatus (= tragus) on the orbito-meatal line along the inferior border of the zygoma; in frontal view, the medial border of the pupilla. Depth is guided by X-ray. Center: Exocranial view of the needle trajectory, successively transjugal and through the pterygomaxillary fossa, up to the foramen ovale. Note that trajectory passes close to the lateral pterygoid process (yellow star), which can be—if hypertrophied—an obstacle to access the foramen. Right: Endocranial view of a needle is place at level of the trigeminal cave

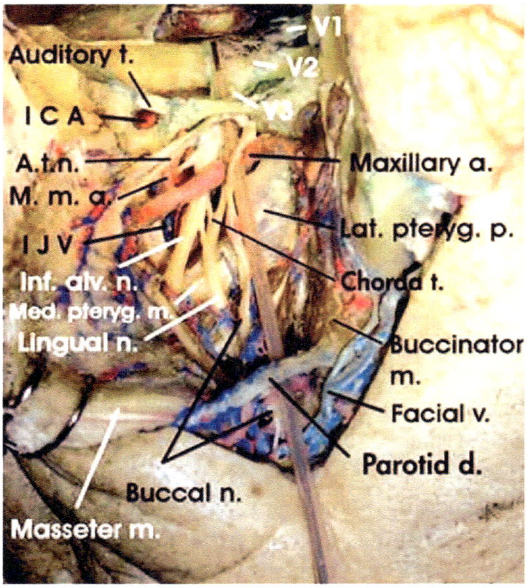


**Fig. 10.2** Anatomical dissection of transjugal-transoval Hartel trajectory. View of the right side of the face, with the zygomatic arch removed, the ascending branch of the mandible bone cut, and the lateral aspect of the middle fossa floor drilled off. In addition, a partial drilling of the petrous bone has been performed in order to show the intrapetrous portion of the internal carotid artery (ICA) and the Eustachian auditory tube. *Buccal n.* buccal nerve, *Buccinator m.* buccinator muscle, *Facial v.* facial vein, *IJV* internal jugular vein, *Inf. alv. n.* inferior alveolar nerve, *Chorda t* chorda tympani nerve, *Lat. Pteryg. p.* lateral pterygoid process, *Lingual n.* lingual nerve, *Masseter m.* masseter muscle, *Maxillary a.* maxillary artery, *Med. Pteryg. m.* medial pterygoid muscle, *M.m.a.* Middle meningeal artery, *A.t.n.* auriculotemporal nerve, *Parotid d.* parotid duct, *V3* mandibular branch of the trigeminal nerve, *V2* mandibular branch of the trigeminal nerve, *VI* ophthalmic branch of the trigeminal nerve (Alvernia et al. 2010). (*Dissection: courtesy of Dr. Jorge Alvernia*). Main structures in danger are successively: the parotid duct (hemosialorrhea), the maxillary artery (pterygo-maxillary fossa hematoma), the Eustachian auditory tube (transfixion with hearing disturbances), and above all the internal carotid artery

segment (of 13 mm long, on average). It comprises the portion from the apex of the pyramid where the trocar enters the cheek to the point where it contacts the parotid duct (PD); a middle segment (of 29 mm long on average). It consists of the portion from the parotid duct to the lateral pterygoid muscle (LPM), which is filled with fatty tissue and contains the lingual, the chorda tympani, the buccal, and the inferior alveolar nerves. In this portion, the trocar may encounter branches of the maxillary artery (MA) or its trunk if tortuous; and a superior segment. It starts from the LPM and ends at the FO. Within this portion, the MA runs posterior to the LPM, and may be in contact with the inserted needle. Also, pterygoid venous plexuses may be penetrated.

After passing through the Foramen Ovale under fluoroscopic guidance, the trocar enters the Trigeminal Cave and is in relation with the trigeminal system (Fig. 10.3).

At skull base the following structures can be endangered: the internal jugular vein located 27 mm postero-laterally to the trocar trajectory, the internal carotid artery at its entry into the petrous carotid canal (25 mm posterior to the needle axis), again the internal carotid artery at Foramen Lacerum if trajectory would be deviated of 10° medially from its correct pathway, and also the membranous portion of the Auditory tube if trajectory would be deviated of a 9° angle in the anteromedial direction. The inferior, then the superior, orbital fissure(s), and consequently the optic nerve, might be attained if needle would be placed 17° too anteriorly from its correct trajectory (Fig. 10.4).

Importantly, before any decision to use the percutaneous route, it is necessary to ensure by imaging of the base of the skull (CT scan and/or MRI) that there are no arterial structures at risk in the path of the trocar such as intracavernous aneurysm, megadolicho-carotid, and/or megadolicho-vertebrobasilar arteries, or persistent trigeminal artery (that may be found in 0.5% of the cases) (Fig. 10.5).

Knowledge of surgical anatomy and meticulous examination of imaging are of considerable help to understand the potential risks of the percutaneous Hartel approach. A wrong trajectory might lead to vital complications, especially if puncturing the internal carotid artery. Even with

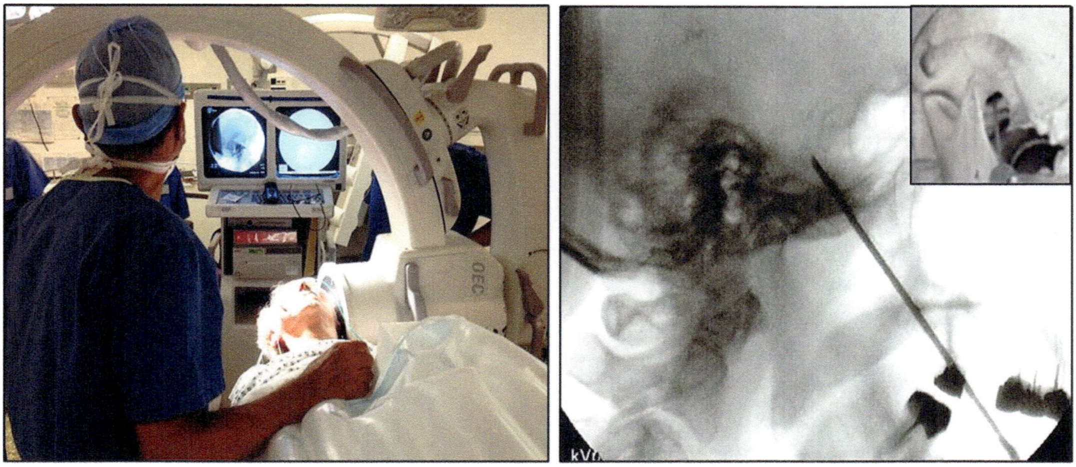

**Fig. 10.3** Percutaneous surgery via the *Hartel route performed under fluoroscopy*. The tip of the needle should target the intersection between the clivus and the upper petrous ridge

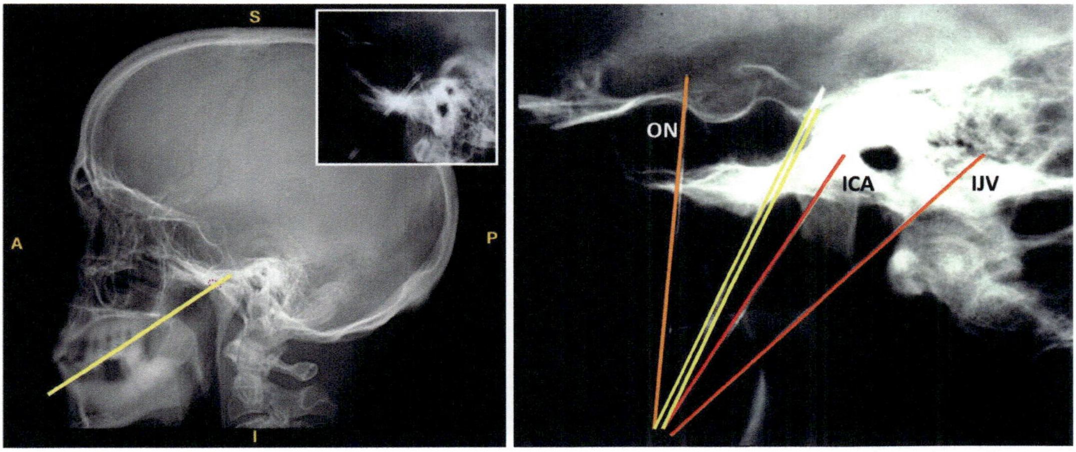


**Fig. 10.4** Wrong, dangerous, trajectories must be avoided when using the Hartel method. An excessive postero-lateral direction could puncture the internal jugular vein (IJV) at jugular foramen or the internal carotid artery at entrance into the petrous carotid canal. An excessive medial direction could enter the foramen lacerum and injure the internal carotid artery (ICA) at its C5 segment. An excessive anterior direction could penetrate the orbital apex through the inferior orbital fissure and injure the optic nerve (ON). The appropriate trajectory is yellow

a correct trajectory, the needle may encounter the parotid duct, the maxillary artery, the auditory tube, with the following respective consequences: hemosialorrhea, hematoma of the cheek and/or the pterygo-maxillary region, serous otitis, and so on.

Accessing and puncturing the foramen ovale may be difficult in some patients, especially those with a hypertrophic pterygoid process or those harboring platybasia. In such circumstances trajectory guided by neuro-navigation systems, or better by performing catheterization of the foramen under CT-control, can be helpful.

In well-trained hands, percutaneous-lesioning techniques may afford effective solutions for treating refractory trigeminal neuralgias (Fig. 10.6).

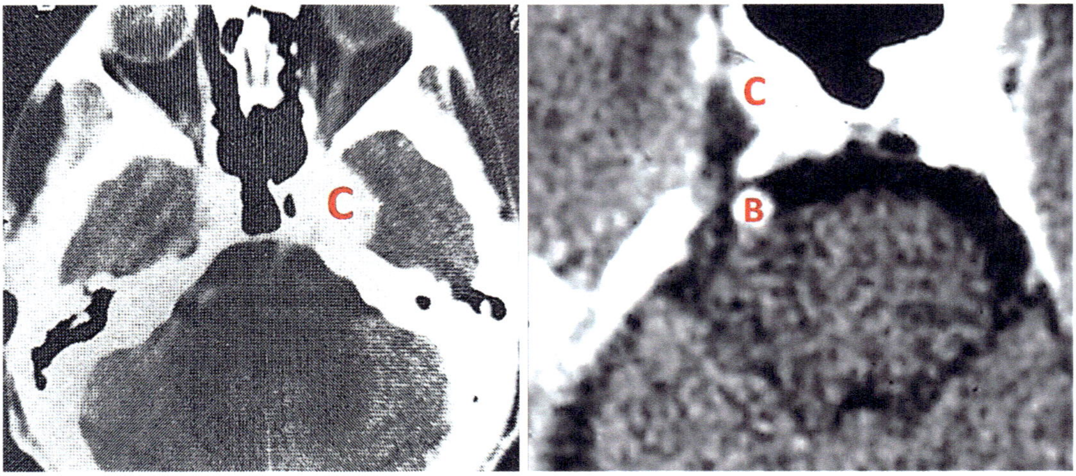


**Fig. 10.5** The percutaneous Hartel route: its intracranial risks. Because trocar could injure on its way important arterial structure(s), imaging (at least a CT-scan) should imperatively be performed prior using this method. Left: CT-image shows a giant aneurysm of the left internal carotid artery (C) bulging into the cavernous sinus and the Meckel trigeminal cave. Right: CT-image shows a megadolicho-vertebrobasilar artery (B) at level of the porus of the Meckel cave. Note that the carotid artery (C) has a normal location, medially to the Meckel's cave

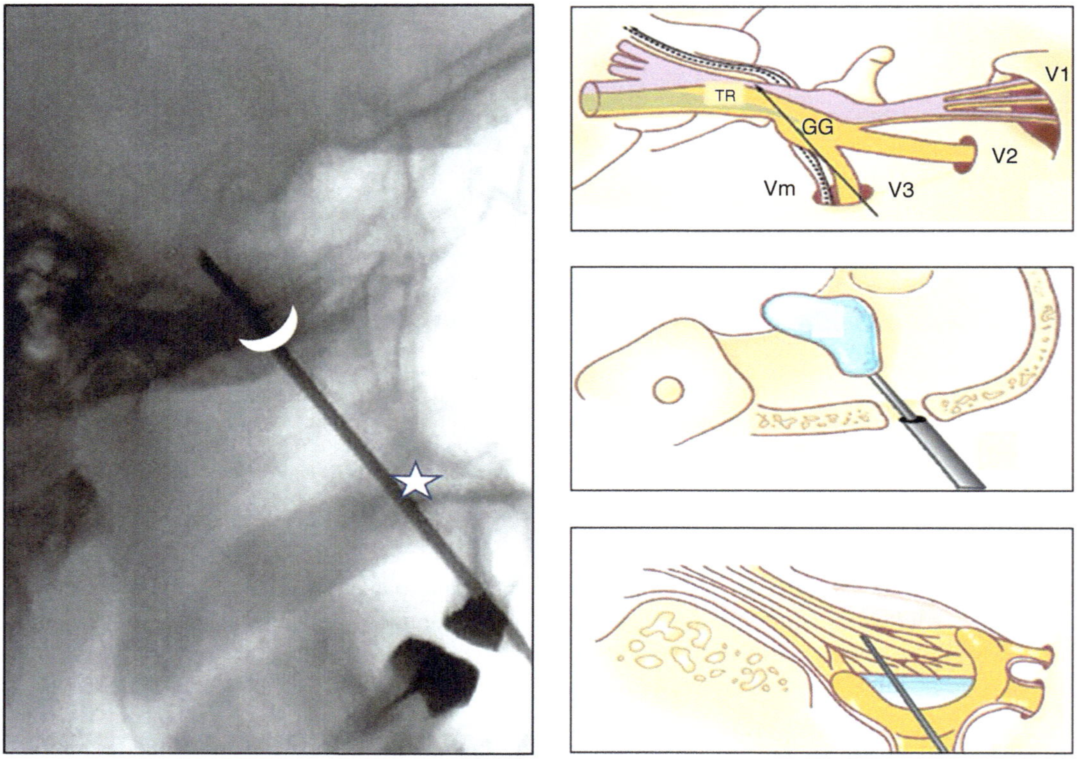


**Fig. 10.6** The various percutaneous lesioning-techniques performed using Hartel's transforaminal ovale route. Left: landmark of the maxillary sinus (star) and of the foramen ovale (semilunar shape). Right: The illustrated lesioning-techniques are from top to bottom: RF-Thermorhizotomy, Balloon Compression, Glycerol Injection

## 10.3 Radiofrequency-Thermorhizotomy

The Radiofrequency-Thermocoagulation technique was developed and popularized by William Sweet (Sweet and Wepsic 1974) since 1969, based on two anatomical-physiological principles (Fig. 10.7). A temperature of 60–70° C applied for several seconds to a few minutes is able to achieve analgesia without complete anesthesia of the covered area. The somatotopy of the sensory fibers at their retrogasserian location makes it possible to place the electrode so that the thermo-lesion preferentially targets those fibers corresponding to the painful territory and trigger-zone (Fig. 10.8).

### 10.3.1 Procedure

Patient is installed supine in a comfortable position, and equipped for safe anesthesiologic conditions and convenient X-ray control as well as easy surgical maneuvers (Fig. 10.9). The electrode is introduced through the cheek and foramen ovale following the Hartel percutaneous approach, then pushed to the upper ridge of the petrous bone, under X-ray fluoroscopic control and one or several brief intravenous anesthetic bolus/boli (initially Methohexital/Brevital, then Propanidide/Epontol, currently Propofol/Diprivan) (Fig. 10.10).

The uninsulated extremity of the active electrode is placed under lateral radio-fluoroscopy at the level the upper ridge of the petrous apex and just posterior to the clival plane. These landmarks were established to correspond to the triangular plexus, the optimal target for performing the thermo-lesion (Sindou and Keravel 1979). At this level, the fibers of the V3 (mandibular) division are located in an inferolateral position, those of the V2 (maxillary) division in an intermediate position, and those of the V1 (ophthalmic) division superomedially (Fig. 10.11). To be mentioned, the reference needle electrode (anode) is

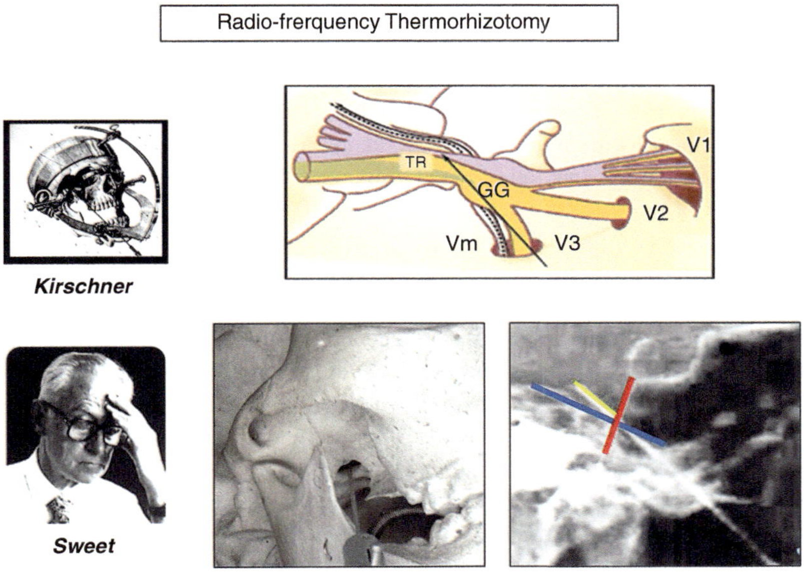


**Fig. 10.7** The Radiofrequency-Thermorhizotomy procedure was developed by William Sweet as a refinement of the procedure of electrocoagulation of the gasserian ganglion, performed under general anesthesia, introduced in 1933 by Kirschner (1933). The refinement by Sweet consisted in using a thermo-couple-electrode to measure the temperature delivered, and in controlling electrode location by performing the surgery under fluoroscopy, and the patient awake to assess the evoked paresthesias elicited by electrostimulation. This is especially important as the accuracy of the lesioning effect is based on the somatotopia of the sensory fibers in the retrogasserian rootlets (Sweet and Wepsic 1974)

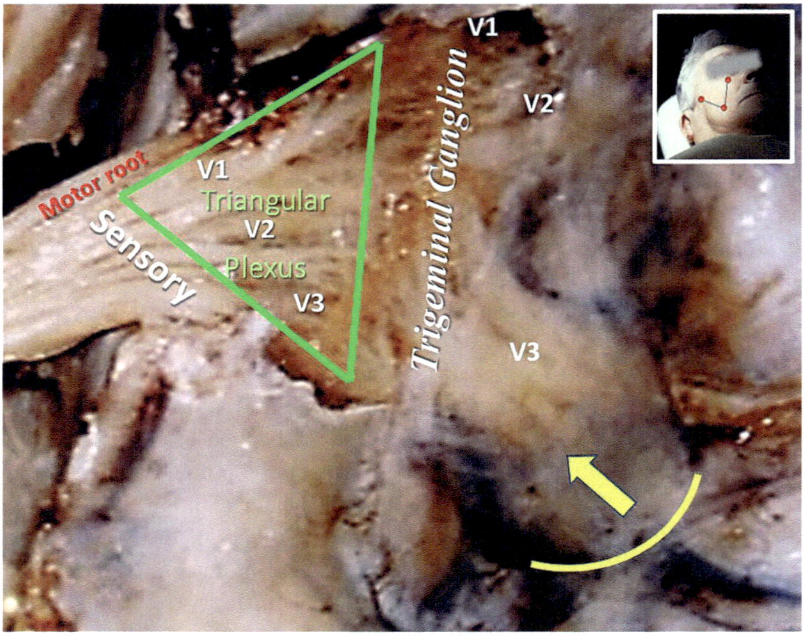


**Fig. 10.8** The anatomical basis for the RF-Thermorhizotomy procedure is the *somatotopia of the fibers at level of the Triangular plexus*. Photography shows trigeminal nerve dissection with roof of Meckel cave removed on right side. After penetrating the foramen ovale (yellow arciform shape), the uninsulated extremity of the electrode should be placed in retrogasserian location, that is, just posterior to the trigeminal ganglion, precisely at level of the triangular plexus where somatotopia of the fibers is well delineated according to their $V_3$, $V_2$, $V_1$ origin

inserted subcutaneously in the middle of the hairline at the forehead or at level of one shoulder.

After positioning the electrode in the estimated appropriate location on the radiological basis, stimulation for physiological localization is performed in an awake patient using an electrical current, at a frequency of 5 Hz in our technique (Tatli and Sindou 2008) (Fig. 10.12). The final placement of the electrode is adjusted until the evoked paresthesias correspond with the territory of pain, particularly its trigger-zone. Stimulation is delivered using a train lasting 3–5 s. When the intensity threshold to obtain paresthesias is greater than 0.4 V on first attempt(s), further trials with different trajectories of the electrode are made until the proper threshold (a lower one, ±0.3 V) is found. When stimulation provokes masticatory responses with a threshold below 0.3 V, relocation of the electrode away from the trigeminal motor fibers is attempted.

Noteworthy, at 5 Hz, electrical stimulation additionally produces muscle twitches in the facial nerve territory, clinically well-visible in approximately one-half of the patients (Fig. 10.13). These evoked muscular twitches, that we named facial Evoked Motor Responses (EMRs), and that we attributed to trigeminal-facial reflexes, could be evidenced by video-recordings and electromyographic recordings (Sindou et al. 1994) (Fig. 10.14).

Their localizing value was demonstrated by correlating the territory of the EMR with the location of the evoked paresthesias and the location of the postoperative hypoesthesia. It was established that EMRs in the orbicularis oculi indicate situation of the electrode in the V1 fibers, in levator labii in the V2 fibers, and in orbicularis oris in the V3 fibers. These clinically observable EMRs were hypothesized to be owing to trigeminofacial reflexes. The EMRs noted in the upper territory

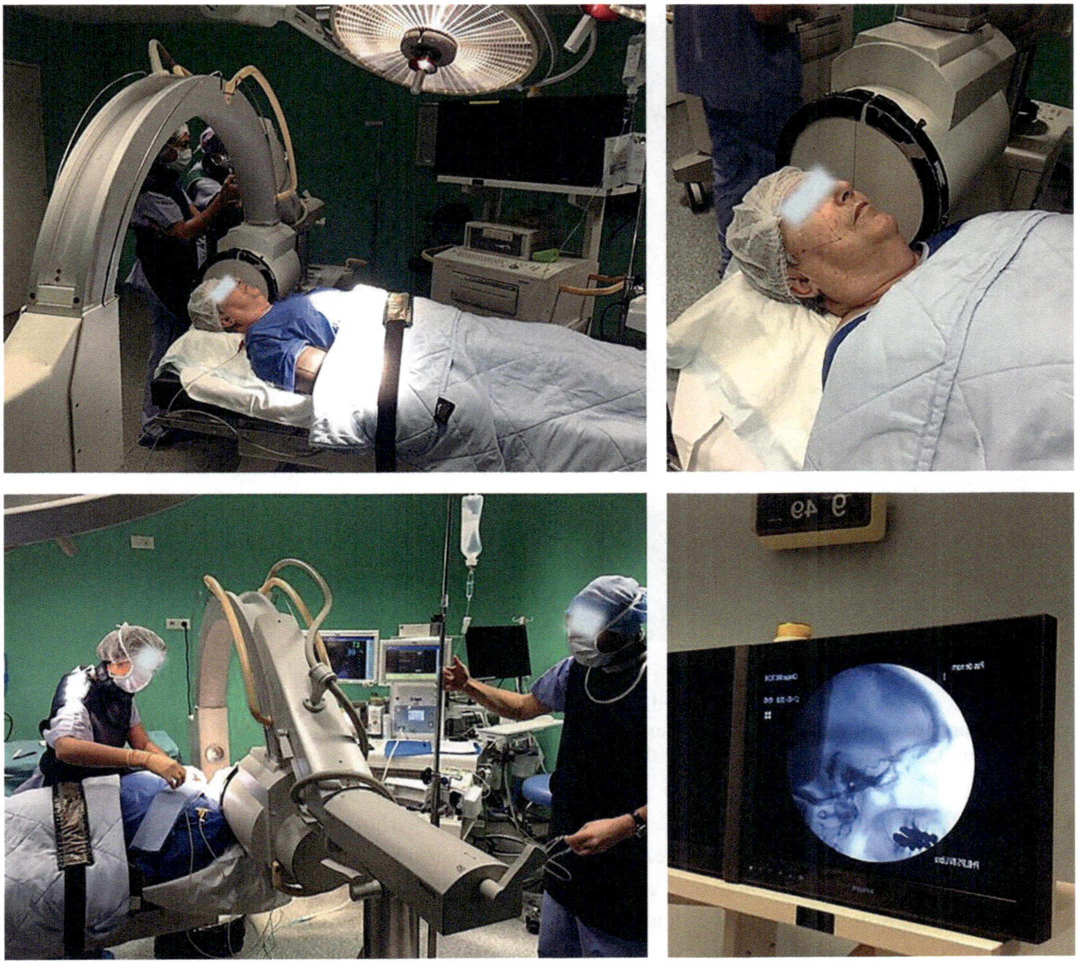

**Fig. 10.9** The patient is installed supine and *equipped for short-lasting IV sedation*. Patient is also equipped for blood pressure and EKG monitoring. Room is organized so that anesthesiologist and surgeon have easy access to the patient's head. A key-point is the accurate placement of the fluoroscopic equipment

resemble the classic blink reflex. Those observed in the lower territories reported (for the first time) were hypothesized—according to our electrophysiological studies—to be trigeminofacial reflexes generated in brainstem, similar to the aforementioned blink reflex. On these bases, we integrated the concept of "Neurophysiological navigation" guidance inside the protocol learned from Professor Sweet at MGH in Boston (Sindou 1999).

Then, to check the accurate location of the electrode before definitive lesioning, a minimal thermal lesion is added as a test. This thermal test is performed at the painful threshold of approximately 45–50 °C, and lasts—approximately 3–5 s—until the patient complains of a burning sensation., This thermal test, if not prolonged and surpassing 50 °C, produces only a very transient hypoesthesia. Good correlation of the site of the induced burning pain and the transient hypoesthesia with the territory of the neuralgia and the trigger zone are considered an additional indication of accurate electrode placement. Otherwise, attempts to reposition the electrode are made. After its final neurophysiological control, the location of the electrode is radiographically verified on lateral cranial X-ray.

Then, the therapeutic thermal lesioning is performed under (one or more frequently several)

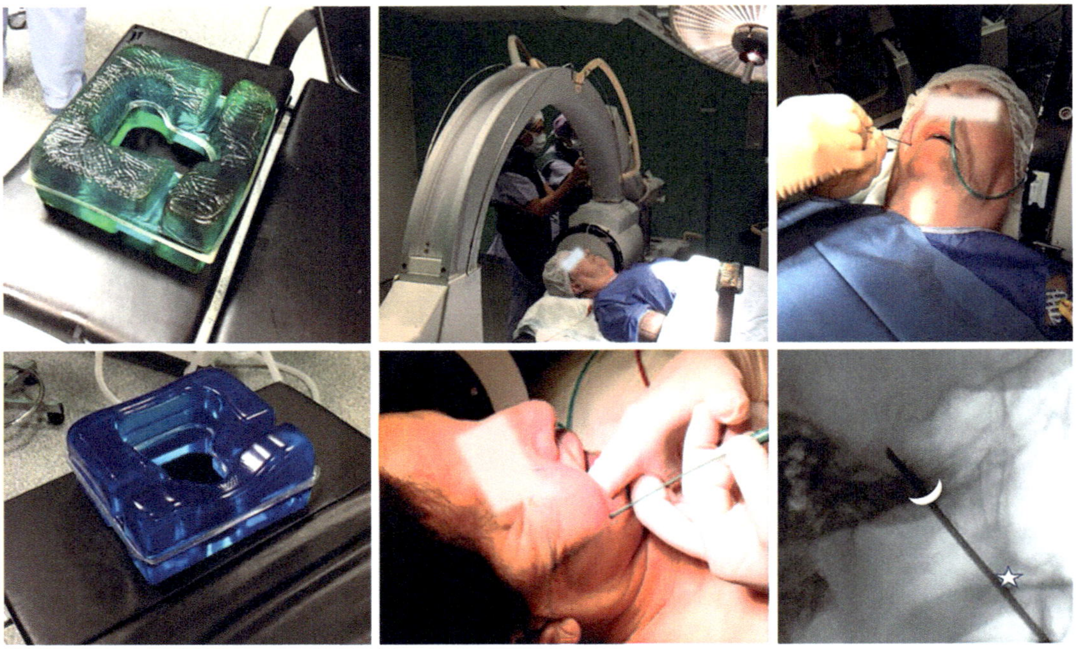

**Fig. 10.10** Puncturing and catheterisation of the (right) foramen ovale under fluoroscopic control need a comfortable and stable head cushion of the type shown. Upper row: puncturing under patient sedation. Note the catheter in the left nostril for oxygenation. Lower row: puncturing under patient sedation. Note the operator's index introduced in the mouth to prevent from piercing the buccal mucosa during cheek penetration

brief intravenous anesthesia(s), light enough to permit concomitant testing of the corneal reflex.

In our practice, we currently use a straight electrode, of 0.6 mm in diameter, with an uninsulated tip over 6 mm when all the three or two divisions of the trigeminal nerve are involved. Lesioning is usually made at a temperature of 55–75 °C. Temperature of heating is gradually increased by 5 °C increments, depending on the sensory loss produced after each lesion; a temperature of 75 °C is not exceeded during the procedure. Usually when the electrode tip is inside the trigeminal system, there is no need to exceed 70 °C. Paresthesias and EMRs elicited by an electrical stimulation of less than 0.5 V testify that the electrode tip is inside or in close contact with the trigeminal system.

The one or several thermo-lesion(s) are made until a marked hypoesthesia covers the entire area of pain. If the corneal reflex disappears, thermal lesioning is immediately stopped.

For us, the criterion for effectiveness of thermo-lesion is the obtention of analgesia to pinprick without complete loss of tactile sensation to for instance a pencil, and without alteration of the corneal reflex tested with a cotonoid. The analgesia/hypoesthesia should be centered on the trigger zone and cover the whole neuralgic territory.

A wise precaution is to prescribe, as soon as surgery is completed, eye drops of artificial tears, and if necessary to indicate a close ophthalmologic surveillance, which would be the more so important as the thermolesion has produced corneal hypoesthesia.

### 10.3.2 Outcome

1. A *retrospective analysis of an initial personal series of 583 patients* showed us that the best location of the electrode to perform the thermo-lesion was at the triangular plexus level, not only for achieving an optimal effect on pain (Fig. 10.15) but also for minimizing the side effects and complications (Fig. 10.16)

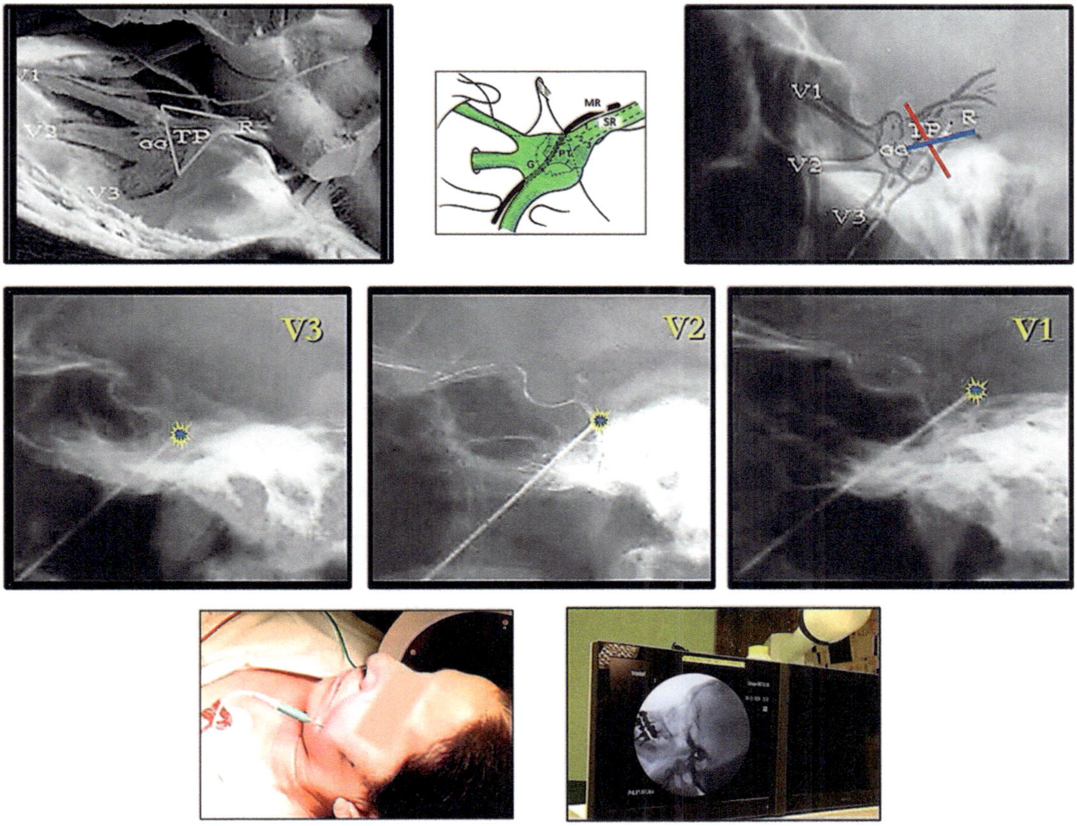


**Fig. 10.11** Fluoroscopic control of the electrode location. Upper row: landmarks of the gasserian ganglion (GG), of the triangular plexus (TP), and of the root (R). *MR* = motor root, *SR* = sensory root. Middle row: X-Ray projections of the $V_3$, $V_2$, $V_1$ components at triangular plexus level. Lower row: patient surgery in progress

(Sindou and Keravel 1979; Sindou and Tatli 2009). At this target, an effect qualified as "excellent"—that is, corresponding to the suppression of the neuralgia, with a strong analgesia at pin-prink testing and without complete loss of the tactile sensation, and covering the painful territory without trespassing the involved trigeminal divisions—was obtained in 70% of the patients. A result qualified of "good" (additionally 17% of the cases) was same, but not totally well-centered and/or not so well limited to the painful territory. At this triangular plexus target, the side effects and the complications were much less than at the neighboring locations of the electrode, as shown in the figure. Patients with dysesthesias amounted at 7% with 3% with a distressing anesthesia dolorosa; keratitis occurred in 5% of the patients of whom one case evolved to corneal ulcer with blindness (i.e., in 0.17% of the series).

In our *total series of 3250 cases* who had a thermo-rhizotomy procedure over a 40-year period of full-time activity, initial pain relief was achieved in 97% of the patients; overall, recurrent rate amounted at 7% with a survey of up to 28 years for the earliest patient operated on (17 years on average). This relatively low rate of recurrences can be put in relation to the fact that our aim was to create a noticeable hypoesthesia to nociception with only some degree of tactile hypoesthesia, in spite of a more or less (announced) bothering numbness, so as to minimize recurrence occurrence.

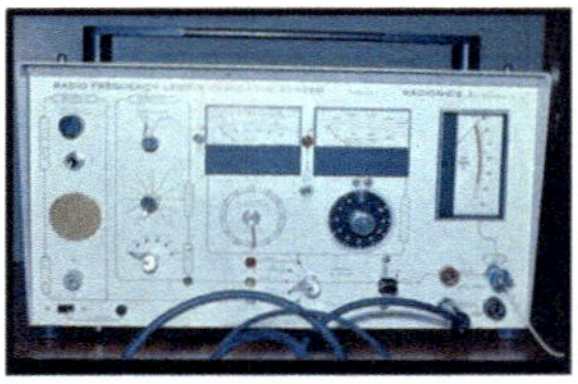

## Neurophysiological Testing

*Electrical stimulation ( 5c/sec)*

Threshold between 0.2-0.4 v to check

➡ **I** - Evoked Paresthesias in sensory territories (in awake patient)

➡ **II** - Muscle Twitches ( clinically-observable )

•1°) In masticatory muscles

***Stimulation of motor root ➡Direct muscle response***

•2°) In facial muscles

***Stimulation sensory root ➡Trigemino-facial reflex***

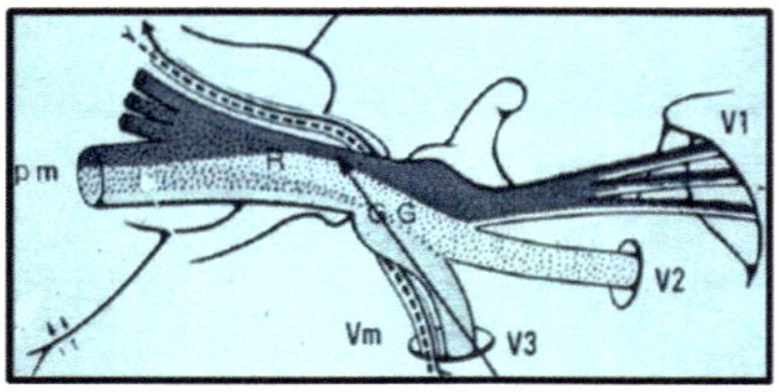


Meet Am Soc Stereotact Funct Neurosurg, Snowbird, Utah, 1999
Stereotact Funct Neurosurg 1999;73:117–121
Stereotactic and Functional Neurosurgery

**Neurophysiological Navigation in the Trigeminal Nerve: Use of Masticatory Responses and Facial Motor Responses Evoked by Electrical Stimulation of the Trigeminal Rootlets for RF-Thermorhizotomy Guidance**

M.P. Sindou
Department of Neurosurgery, Hôpital Neurologique, University of Lyon, France

**Fig. 10.12** Neurophysiological control of the electrode location by evoked paresthesias. Stimulation for physiological localization is performed in an awake patient using an electrical current at a frequency of 5 Hz. The placement of the electrode is adjusted until the evoked paresthesias correspond with the area of the pain. If intensity threshold to elicit paresthesias is greater than 0.4 V, a different trajectory of the electrode is searched until proper threshold (approximately 0.2 V) is found. When stimulation provokes masticatory responses with a threshold below 0.3 V, relocation of the electrode, away from the trigeminal motor fibers, is attempted

2. A review, that we carried out on *ten series totaling 7483 patients* and followed from 3 to 26 years depending on the series (9 years on average), showed an average rate with immediate pain relief of 94% of the cases (from 81 to 99% depending on the series) and an average rate with long-term efficacy of 60.4% (from 20 to 93% depending on the series) (Sindou and Tatli 2009). The side effects and neurological complications were reported at very different frequencies among the various publications reviewed: bothering facial hypoesthesia at 5–98% depending on the series and masticatory deficit at 4–24%, for the side effects, and keratitis (1–8%) and dysesthesias/anesthesia dolorosa (0.8–7% for the later), for the complications. The reported mortality was 0.1%, by carotid artery injury.
3. *A more recent review, in 2019*, which collected seven literature studies including 4533 patients

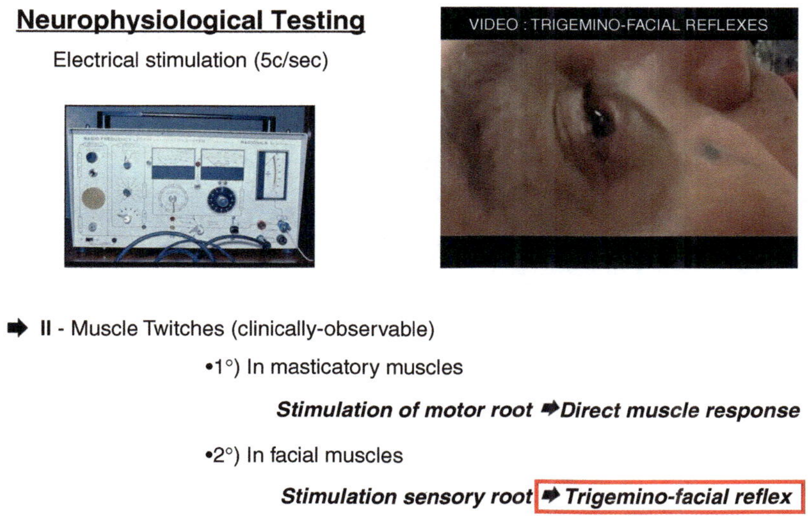


**Fig. 10.13** Neurophysiological control of the electrode location with evoked muscle responses (EMR). At 5 Hz, electrical stimulation of the root produces muscle twitches in the facial nerve territory; they are well-observable in approximately one-half of the patients. We named these evoked twitches: facial evoked motor responses (EMRs) (Sindou et al. 1994; Sindou 1999). These EMRs were demonstrated using electromyographic recordings, and video-recordings. By correlating these EMRs with the location of the evoked paresthesias and also with the territories of postoperative hypoesthesia, it could be established that the EMRs in the orbicularis oculi indicate electrode location in $V_1$, EMRs in the levator labii in $V_2$, and EMRs in the orbicularis location in $V_3$ (Sindou et al. 1994). Observation of these EMRs revealed useful in surgical practice due to their high localizing value, especially in drowsy and confused patients not cooperating (Sindou 1999)

with an average FU from 3 to 9.3 years according to series, reports pain-free and recurrence rates ranging from 26 to 82% and 16 to 74%, respectively (Bendtsen et al. 2019). In this review, mortality was none; patients with sequelae of hearing loss were 6, cranial nerve palsy 36, corneal hypoesthesia 300, keratitis 55, masticatory weakness 280, facial hypoesthesia 853, anesthesia dolorosa 29.

4. The *KM statistical curve* built by Kanpolat et al.—an expert in the procedure—is given in the joined figure as a valuable representative illustration of the current performance of the RF-thermo-rhizotomy method (Kanpolat et al. 2001) (Fig. 10.17).
5. *Disparity of the rates of the long-term relief* and recurrences among authors can be—logically—linked to the degree of the hypoesthesia left by the thermo-lesion. The important dilemma with this method is to decide between strong hypoesthesia with low probability of (early) recurrence, but bothersome numbness, and, mild hypoesthesia with less side effects, but high rate of pain return. Decision should be discussed with the patient, and clearly written down in the signed informed consent. Whatsoever, the method—which has almost no contraindication even in elderly patients—is very operator-dependent and requires specific training.
6. A list of important *documented reports from literature series* is presented in Table 10.1.

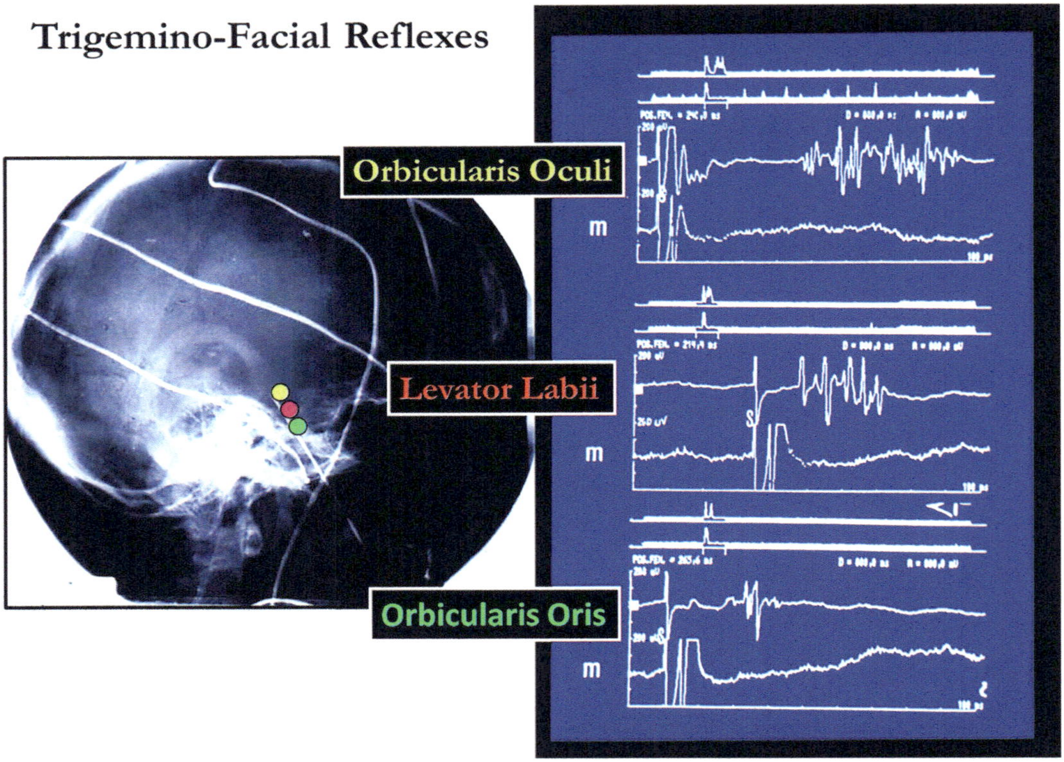


**Fig. 10.14** Trigemino-facial reflexes: localizing value. EMG-recordings showing facial evoked muscle responses (EMRs) under direct stimulation of the trigeminal root during RF-Thermohizotomy. EMRs are predominantly in orbicularis oris for stimulation of the fibers corresponding to the $V_3$ division of the root (green), in levator labii for stimulation of the $V_2$ fibers (red) and in orbicularis oculi for stimulation of the $V_1$ fibers (i.e., direct blink-reflex) (yellow) (Sindou et al. 1994). These responses were interpreted as trigemino-facial reflexes at brainstem level. Study of correlation with the territory of the hypoesthesia obtained by the thermolesion allowed to attribute to these EMR–clinically observable a practical localizing value for surgical guidance (Sindou 1999)

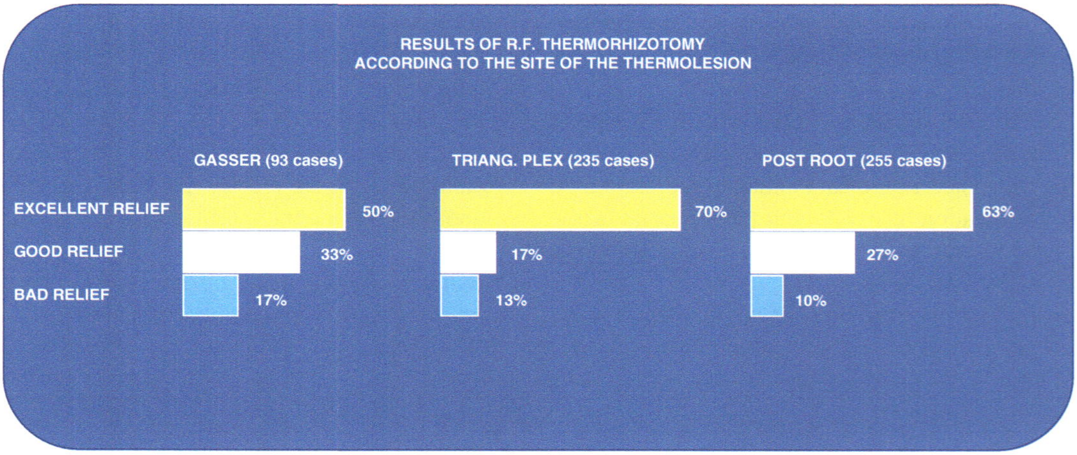


**Fig. 10.15** Results on pain after RF-Thermohizotomy, according to the site of the thermolesion. Pain relief was better achieved when the uninsulated tip of the electrode was located in the triangular plexus rather than in the gasserian ganglion or in the root in cerebello-pontine angle (Sindou and Keravel 1979)

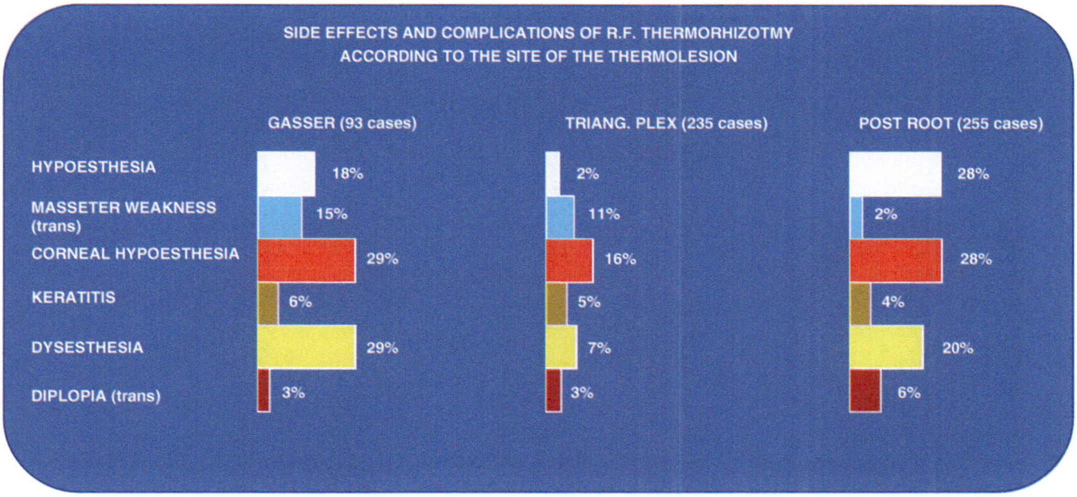


**Fig. 10.16** Side effects and complications of RF-Thermohizotomy according to the site of the thermolesion. Location of the thermolesion in the triangular plexus was safer than in root in the cerebello-pontine angle or in the ganglion (Sindou and Keravel 1979)

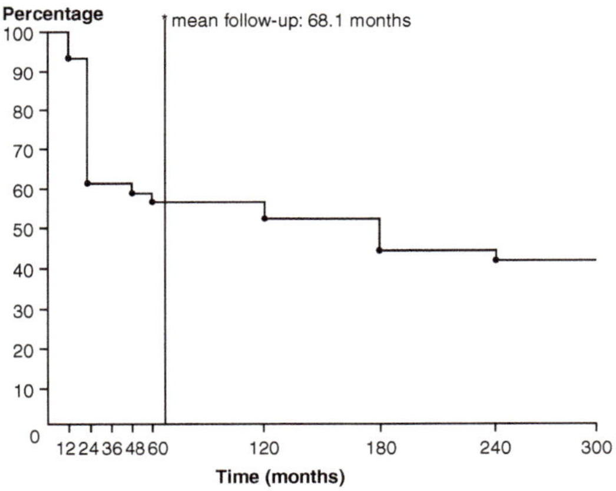


**Fig. 10.17** Kaplan-Meier statistical analysis of *long-term probability of pain relief with RF-Thermorhizotomy* in Kanpolat et al.'s series, as an example (Kanpolat et al. 2001)

**Table 10.1** Outcome after RF-Thermorhizotomy (literature review)

| | | | | RF - Thermorhizotomy | | | | | | |
|---|---|---|---|---|---|---|---|---|---|---|
| Nb. patients | Followup -Range- (mean) in year | Relief of the Neuralgia Initial (%) | Relief of the Neuralgia Late (%) | Side-effects Hypo-esthesia | Side-effects Hypo-esthesia (++) % | Side-effects Cornea Anesthesia | Side-effects Vth nerve motor weakness | Complications Dysesthesia (%) | Complications CN palsy (%) | Complications Permanent Severe Morbidy |
| 1000 | 5.5 | 98 | 75 | - | 24 | 3 | 25 | 3 | 4 | 0 |
| 235 | 1-2! | 99 | 93 | - | 15 | 20 | 25 | 5 | 6 | 0 |
| 533 | 6.5 | 97 | 75 | - | 15 | 3 | 16 | 15 | 0.2 | 0 |
| 702 | 5.6 | 99 | 63 | 6 | 2 | 9 | 25 | 9 | 0.4 | 0 |
| 1000 | 9 | 100 | 78 | - | 7.9 | 17 | 10 | 6.5 | 0.5 | 0 |
| 1070 | 4.7 | 87 | 73 | - | 6 | 3.5 | 25 | 6.5 | 0.2 | 0.2 |
| 265 | 3.8 | - | 71 | - | - | 9 | - | 8 | - | 0 |
| 1200 | 9 | 99 | 79 | - | 25 | 6 | 24 | 4 | 2.5 | 0 |
| 258 | 3 | - | 74 | - | - | 2.3 | 29 | 8 | 0 | 0 |
| 316 | 14 | - | 25 | - | 1 | 0 | - | 0.9 | 0.8 | 0.8 |
| 1600 | 5 | 97 | 58 | - | 9 | 5.7 | 401 | 1.8 | 0.14 | 0 |

Publications retained correspond to series with more than 100 operated cases, a follow-up of at least 1 year, and precise information on initial pain relief and outcome at last follow-up; in those, side-effects and/or complications were more or less detailed

Siegfried (1981), Sindou et al. (1987), Fraioli et al. (1989), Broggi et al. (1990), Sweet (1990), Nugent (1991), Zakrzewska and Thomas (1993), Tew and Taha (1995), Mathews and Scrivani (2000), Kanpolat et al. (2001), and Tronnier et al. (2001)

## 10.4 Balloon Compression

The technique of Percutaneous Balloon Compression (PBC), introduced in 1979 by John Mullan, consists in compressing the Gasser ganglion, under general anesthesia because of its painful nature, and using fluoroscopic control (Mullan and Lichtor 1983) (Fig. 10.18).

### 10.4.1 Procedure

The patient is placed in supine position, sedated and intubated. An additional local anesthetic is administered, and a 13-gauge trocar with a semi-sharp stylet is inserted through the percutaneous trans-ovale Hartel trajectory up to the level of the Meckel cave and trigeminal cistern (Fig. 10.19). Then the stylet is removed, and a Fogarty balloon catheter N°4 is introduced, protruding from the trocar of approximately 15 mm. When in place, the balloon is inflated with 0.5–1 ml of contrast-medium (iohexol at 300 mg/ml).

The effect is checked on lateral X-ray control. The ideal image is the classic "pear" deformation of the balloon which tail corresponds to the porus of the Meckel cave toward the cistern of the cerebellopontine angle (Fig. 10.20). The recommended duration of the compression is of 3 min (from 1 to 5 min depending on the team), so that the risk of disabling dysesthesias as a sequela be minimal. Finally, the contrast is aspirated, and the catheter and trocar are withdrawn.

### 10.4.2 Outcome

1. *A review of literature dated 2009 on ten series totalizing 1345 patients*, with a mean follow-up of 1–6 years according to the series and with an overall average of 4 years, reported an immediate sedation after PBC of 82–100% depending on the series (96% on average) and a long-term efficacy in 67% on average (from 54.5 to 91.3% depending on the series) (Keravel et al. 2009). Regarding the postoperative side effects and neurological complications, facial hypoesthesia was noted in 4–77% of the patients depending on the series, with an intensity and dysesthesia sequelae found quite correlated to the duration of the compression. A more or less lasting masticatory paralysis was reported in 50–66% of the patients depending on the series. A pterygomaxillary fossa hematoma complicated 2–5% of the cases. Mortality was of 0.2%, from carotid artery injury.
2. In 2016 the neurosurgical department at Umea University reported results its 82 patients, including a *detailed study of the sensory func-*

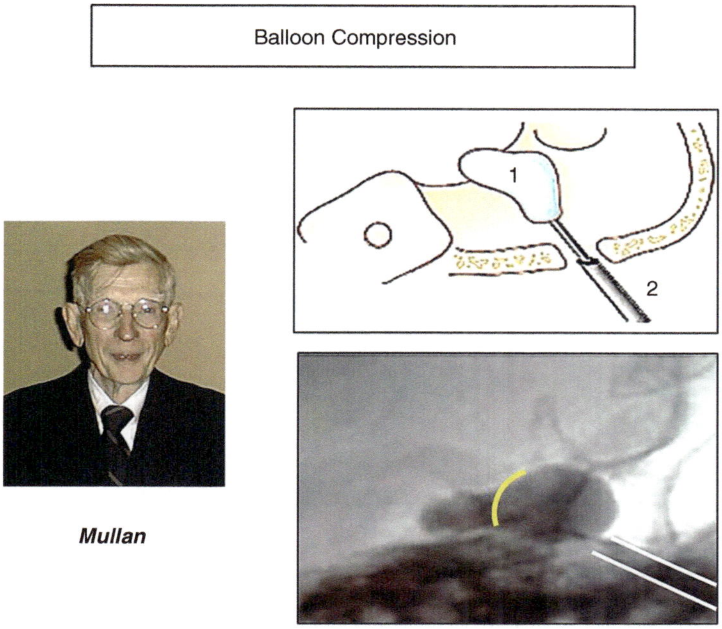


**Fig. 10.18** The percutaneous balloon compression method has been introduced in 1983 by John Mullan (Mullan and Lichtor 1983). The technique consists in the introduction, through the foramen ovale (2) via the Hartel trajectory, of a Fogarthy catheter into the trigeminal cave (1). The balloon is then inflated under fluoroscopic control, for usually 3 min, so as to compress the Gasserian ganglion and the triangular plexus. This results in a more or less important hypoesthesia depending on the cases, more often without corneal anesthesia. Note the piriform shape of the inflated balloon testifying its good location within the trigeminal cave and posteriorly the trigeminal porus

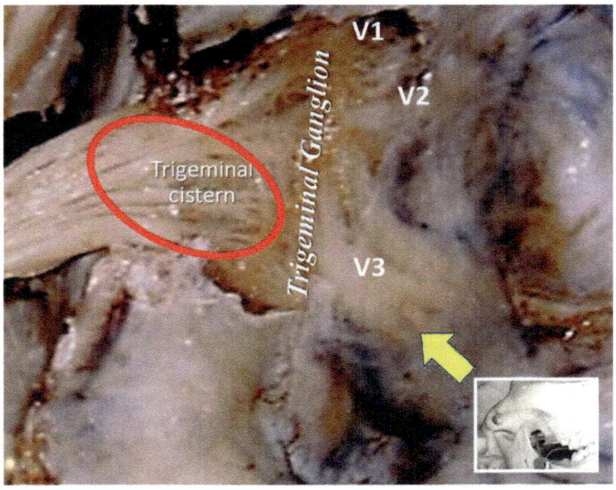


**Fig. 10.19** Anatomical dissection of the trigeminal system within the trigeminal cave of Meckel. Figure shows exposure of the trigeminal ganglion and the *trigeminal cistern*. Red ovale indicates the place where the inflated balloon should be located for efficacy and inocuity

*tion after PBC* (Asplund et al. 2016). Initial success rate was 82%; median pain-free time was 20 months; 30 patients (37%) were free of pain at the last follow-up. The perceptions for touch and pinprick were found significantly decreased immediately after PBC in most patients, but returned to close to normal at late follow-up. Complications were dysesthesias in 4%, masseter muscle weakness in 1%, diplopia in 3%, mild hearing loss in 3%, and herpes eruption in 4%. Corneal sensation was not significantly affected.

3. A report from the Mayo Clinic in 2008 about 222 patients followed up to 15 years with a median of 31 months paid a *particular attention to the timing of recurrences after PBC* (Grewal et al. 2018). Probability to remain pain-free at 15 years from the surgery was

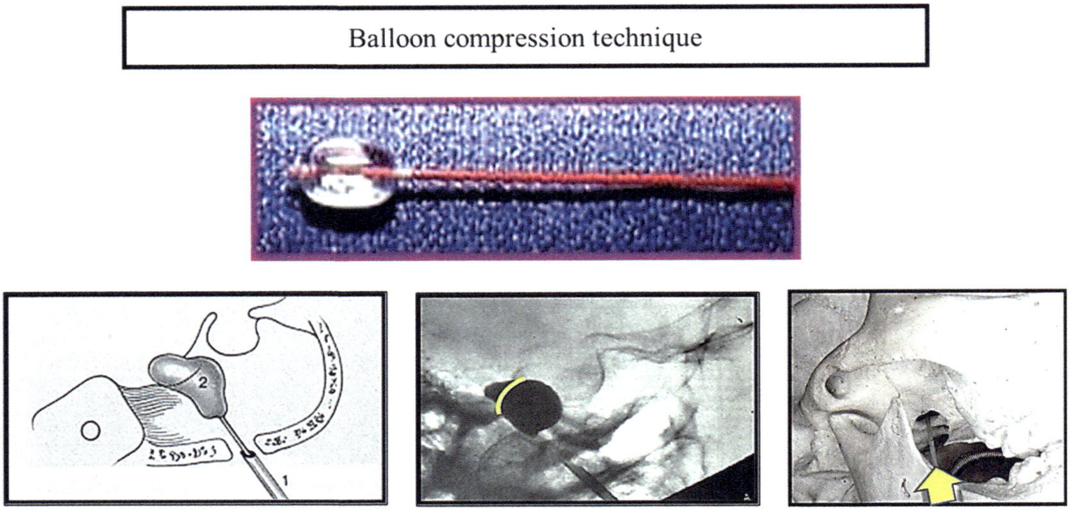


**Fig. 10.20** The percutaneous balloon compression technique is performed under general anesthesia due to the painful nature of the procedure. Using fluoroscopy and the landmarks of the Hartel trajectory, a trocar (most often of 14 gauge) is inserted into the foramen ovale up to the Meckel cave (lower row, right). A Fogarthy probe, currently a 4 Fr embolectomy catheter (upper image), is introduced through the cannula and beyond its extremity into the trigeminal cave (1, lower row, left). Then, under fluoroscopy, the balloon is inflated using an iodine contrast medium (2, lowest row, left) usually with 0.7–1 ml contrast. The balloon should have a pear-shape testifying of its adequate location inside the trigeminal cistern (lower row, center). In nowadays practice, the time of compression (i.e., the duration of inflation of the balloon) is between 1 and 5 min (3 min on average) for limiting the degree of hypoesthesia, potentially responsible for dysesthesias. The balloon is then deflated and trocar removed

only of 10% (Fig. 10.21). Recurrences occurred after a mean delay of 12 months. Further, a large proportion of patients complained of a certain degree of hypoesthesia (82%), but rather mild in most.

4. According to a *recent review in 2019* by the European Academy of Neurology which collected 5 studies regrouping 755 patients with a follow-up (F.U.) of 5–10.7 years, the initial rate of pain relief was of 95%, that then decreased to 54.5–80% (mean: 67%) at last FU. The recurrence or failure rate varied from 20 to 51.7%. The most important reported complications were facial hypoesthesia with paresthesias in 14.6% and trigeminal motor weakness in 4.5% (Bendtsen et al. 2019).
5. In conclusion and brief, less precise than the previously mentioned technique of RF-thermo-rhizotomy, and requiring general anesthesia, PBC has the *advantage of exposing to a lower risk of lasting corneal anesthesia* and therefore keratitis. However, it has the disadvantage of being followed by a high rate of failure or recurrences.
6. A list of important *documented reports from literature series* is presented in Table 10.2.

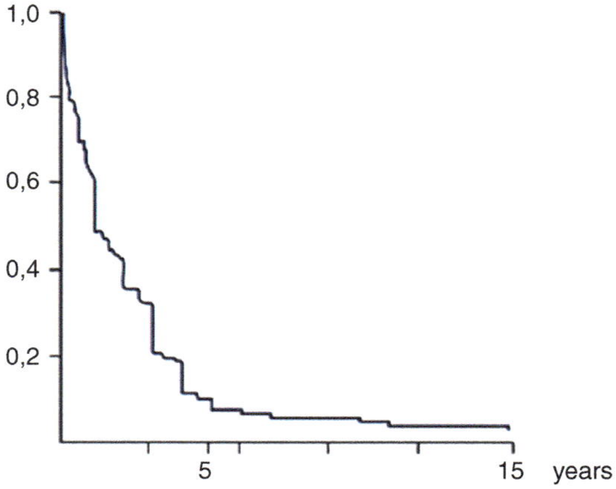


**Fig. 10.21** Probability (at 15 years) of long-term pain relief after Balloon compression; Kaplan-Meier statistical analysis of the MAYO CLINIC series (Grewal et al. 2018)

**Table 10.2** Outcome after balloon compression (literature review)

| | | | | Balloon Compression | | | | | | | |
|---|---|---|---|---|---|---|---|---|---|---|---|
| Nb. patients | Followup -Range- (mean) in year | Relief of the Neuralgia Initial (%) | Relief of the Neuralgia Late (%) | Side-effects Hypo-esthesia | Side-effects Hypo-esthesia (++) % | Side-effects Cornea Anesthesia | Side-effects Vth nerve motor weakness | Complications Dysesthesia (%) | Complications CN palsy (%) | Complications Others | Complications Permanent Severe Morbidy |
| 159 | 3.5 | 90 | 81 | 76 | 2.5 | - | 3 | 7.6 | 0 | - | 0 |
| 212 | 1-3 | - | 75 | - - | - | 0 | 9 | 0 | 0.9 | - | 0 |
| 100 | 1-10 | 100 | 72 | 17 | 12 | 0 | - | 4 | 1 | - | 0 |
| 144 | 1-4 | 90 | 83 | 4 | 40 | 0 | 12 | 3 | 2.8 | - | 0 |
| 141 | 1-2 | 92 | 68 | 83 | 11 | 0 | 24 | 6 | 0 | - | 0 |
| 200 | 1-4 | 96 | 68 | 93 | 10 | 3 | 7 | 10.6 | 1.5 | - | 0.5 |
| 158 | 1-5 | - | 70 | - | - | 0 | 33 | 15 | 1.9 | - | 0 |
| 496 | 1-12 | 99 | 68 | 89 | - | 0 | 3.4 | 3.8 | 1.6 | - | 0 |
| 127 | 7-10 | 93 | 52 | 31 | - | 2.3 | 6.2 | 3.3 | 1.6 | Herpes 33% | 0 |
| 105 | 1-6 | 99 | 84 | - | - | - | 50 | 5.2 | 7.6 | Herpes 44% | 0 |
| 206 | 1-4 | 93 | 85 | - | - | - | - | 0 | - | - | 0 |
| 100 | 1-5 | 90 | 40 | 31 | 7 | - | 4 | 4 | 3 | Herpes 4% | 0 |
| 400 | 4 | 88 | - | 24 | 6 | - | 11 | 6 | 5 | - | - |
| 138 | 1-5 | 98 | 72 | 98 | - | - | - | - | 0.7 | - | - |
| 222 | 2.5 | - | 54 | 82 | - | - | 5 | - | 3 | - | - |
| 131 | 3 | - | 41 | - | 20 | 20 | - | 20 | - | - | - |

Publications retained correspond to series with more than 100 operated cases, a follow-up of at least 1 year, and precise information on initial pain relief and outcome at last follow-up; in those, side effects and/or complications were more or less detailed

Fraioli et al. (1989), Frank and Fabrizi (1989), Lichtor and Mullan (1990), Lobato et al. (1990), Abdennebi et al. (1997), Brown and Gouda (1997), Corrêa and Teixeira (1998), Skirving and Dan (2001), Chen and Lee (2003), de Siqueira et al. (2006), Baabor and Perez-Limonte (2011), Bergenheim et al. (2013), Yadav et al. (2016), Ying et al. (2017), Grewal et al. (2018), and Kourilsky et al. (2022)

## 10.5 Glycerol Injection

The trigeminal ganglion neurolysis (GN) by glycerol injection was an incidental discovery. Leksell and his team in Stockholm for treating trigeminal neuralgia by stereotactic irradiation of the gasserian ganglion with gamma radiation, to facilitate the radiological location of the target, used an opaque medium diluted in glycerol injected inside the trigeminal cave. It was then observed that this single injection could make the pain cease, so that Sten Hakanson in 1981 proposed to treat neuralgia by the sole injection of glycerol into the trigeminal cistern (Håkanson 1981) (Fig. 10.22).

### 10.5.1 Procedure

For the procedure the patient, awake, is placed in a seated position with the head bent. A 22-gauge needle is introduced under local anesthesia into the foramen ovale following the Hartel trajectory, then pushed under fluoroscopic control into the trigeminal cave. As soon as the extremity of the trocar is in place, which results in the release of cerebrospinal fluid, a contrast medium (metrizamide) is injected to verify the correct needle position within the trigeminal cistern. After this cisternography, the contrast substance is drained, then glycerol is injected at small doses until satisfactory hypoesthesia is obtained in the painful area. The total dose of glycerol is as a rule of 0.2–0.4 ml. After withdrawal of the needle, the patient is kept seated for an hour or so.

This technique has the advantage of not being expensive, but the diffusion of glycerol to the subarachnoid spaces cannot be easily controlled, the method exposes to random neurotoxic effects.

### 10.5.2 Outcome

1. According a *review of the literature dated 2008 and totalizing 1310 cases* with follow-ups (FU) of 1–10 years according to the series (6.5 years on overall average), glycerol neurolysis resulted in immediate sedation in 42–84% of the cases with a maintenance of the long-term pain relief in 18–59% depending on the series (38.5% on average) (Tatli et al. 2008). The main reported complications were decrease in facial sensation with dyses-

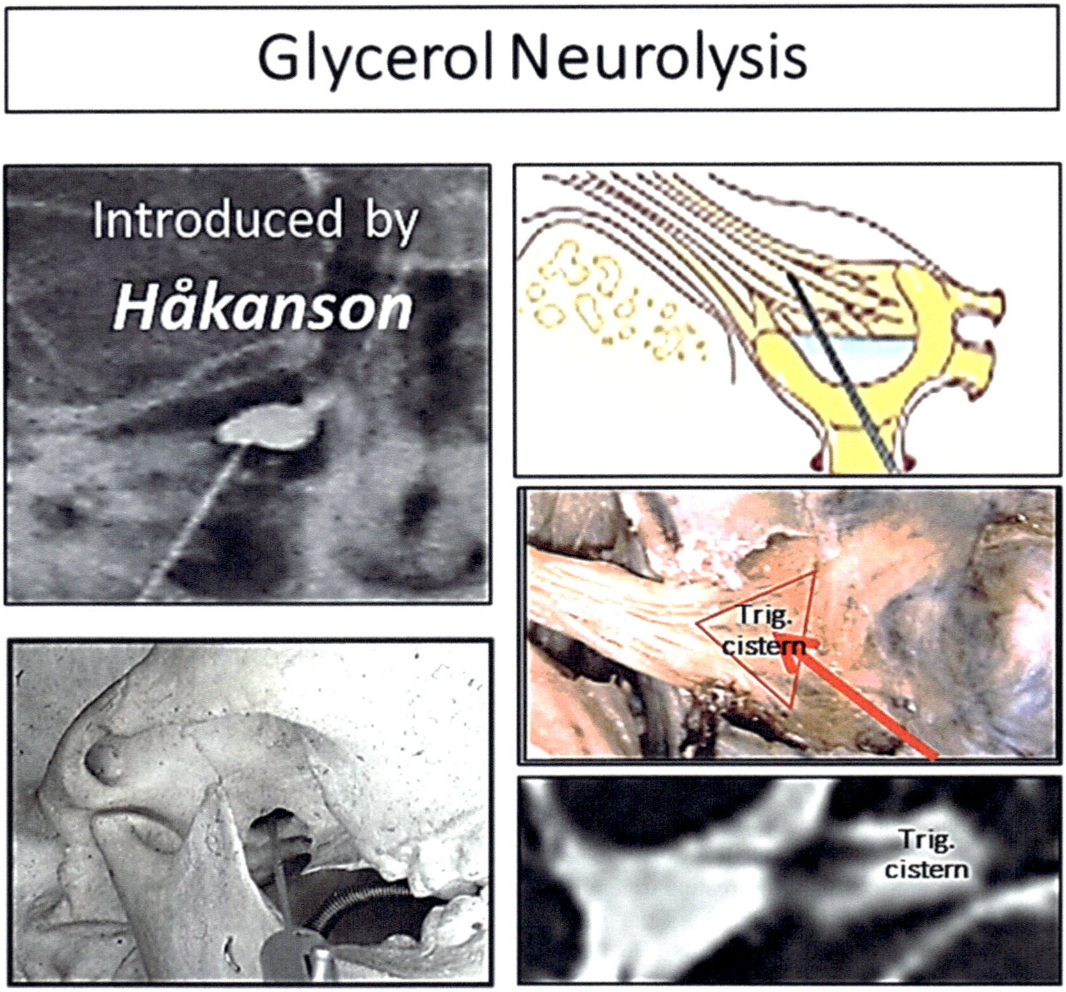


**Fig. 10.22** Neurolysis by glycerol injection was introduced by Sten Hakanson in 1981 (Håkanson 1978, 1981). After passing through the foramen ovale via the Hartel route, the tip of the needle is placed inside the Meckel cave. Cerebrospinal fluid is released. An injection of iodinated contrast medium should ensure that the needle is located in the trigeminal cistern itself, as detailed in the anatomical dissection and seen in $T_2$-MRI. Then a solution of the glycerol is injected, with the patient awake, until a (mild) hypoesthesia is obtained in the area of the trigeminal pain

thesias in 30%, keratitis in 5%, and herpetiform rashes in 50%.

2. A report from Umea University, with a *particular study of the postoperative sensory function in the face*, done in 124 patients who underwent Glycerol Neurolysis and were followed up to 5 years, mentioned an initial success rate at 85%, a median pain-free time of 21 months, with 47 patients (38%) free of pain at last FU (Asplund et al. 2016). Hypoesthesia with dysesthesias was present in 23% of the patients with a frequent association of a diminished corneal reflex. Herpes eruptions appeared in 3% and chemical meningitis also in 3%. In the authors' series according to a Kaplan-Meir statistical analysis, the probability to be pain-free at 5 years was less than 20% (Fig. 10.23).
3. According to the *2019 recent review* of the European Academy of Neurology based on

three studies regrouping 289 patients with a FU ranging from 4.5 to 8 years, an initial pain relief was achieved in 75% of the patients (Bendtsen et al. 2019). Pain relief at mean FU decreased to 18–59% according to the series (average: 40%), recurrence or failure rates varying from 41 to 84%. The most important complication in those series was facial hypoesthesia with more or less paresthesias/dysesthesias in 39%.

4. This technique has the advantage of *not needing special equipment*, but the neurotoxic effects of the glycerol due to difficulty to control diffusion to the subarachnoid spaces was exposed to harmful side effects and complications.
5. A list of important *documented reports from literature series* is presented in Table 10.3.

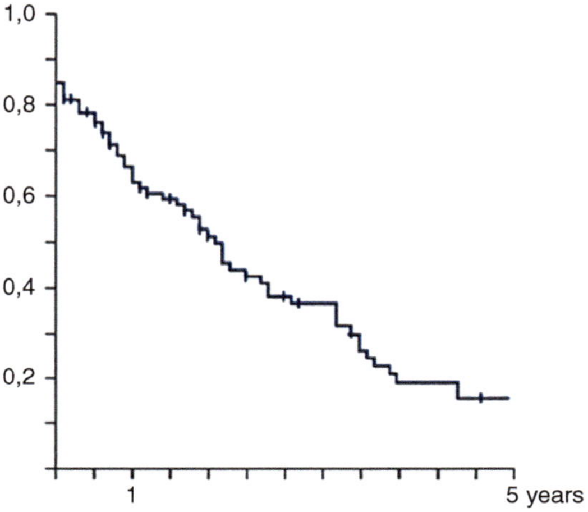


**Fig. 10.23** Probability at 5 years of long-term pain relief after Glycerol injection: Kaplan-Meier statistical study of the Umea series (Asplund et al. 2016)

**Key-Point**

*The Lesioning-techniques*, whatever their modality, are effective on pain transmission; but they generate side effects, of which numbness is the dominant component.

The lesser the postoperative hypoesthesia, the higher the risk of recurrence.

The stronger the hypoesthesia, the more risk of bothering paresthesias and secondary anesthesia dolorosa.

**Table 10.3** Outcome after glycerol neurolysis (literature review)

| | | | | | Glycerol Injection | | | | | | |
|---|---|---|---|---|---|---|---|---|---|---|---|
| Nb. patients | Follow-up -Range- in year | Relief of the Neuralgia Initial (%) | Relief of the Neuralgia Late (%) | Side-effects Hypo-esthesia | Side-effects Hypo-esthesia (++) % | Side-effects Cornea Anesthesia | Side-effects Vth nerve motor weakness | Complications Dysesthesia (%) | Complications CN palsy (%) | Complications Others | Complications Permanent Severe Morbidy |
| 100 | 5-10 | 96 | 57 | 60 | 0 | 0 | 0 | 0 | 0 | Herpes 50% | 0 |
| 100 | 2-3 | 95 | 90 | 13 | 0 | - | - | 0 | - | Herpes 10% | 0 |
| 252 | 2-5 | 91 | 63 | 20 | 1 | - | - | 2 | - | Herpes 77% | - |
| 550 | 1-6 | 76 | 17 | - | 5 | - | - | 11 | - | Herpes 3% | - |
| 162 | 1-6 | 90 | 63 | 72 | 12 | 2 | 0 | 3 | 0 | Herpes 38% | 0 |
| 200 | 2-6 | 73 | 53 | 37 | 7 | - | - | 2 | 0 | - | - |
| 122 | 3-5 | 80 | 22 | 67 | 29 | 0 | 0 | 13 | 0 | - | 0 |
| 112 | 1-5 | 92 | 73 | 32 | 0 | 8 | 0 | 3 | 0 | - | 0 |
| 122 | 1-8 | 84 | 41 | 59 | 0 | 16 | 4 | 13 | 0 | - | 0.8 |
| 191 | 1-7 | - | 70 | - | - | 10 | 6 | 0 | 0 | - | - |
| 523 | 1-11 | 90 | 46 | 32 | 6 | 0 | 0 | 2 | 0 | Herpes 37% | 0 |
| 139 | 1-11 | 95 | 50 | 47 | 45 | 5 | 0 | 7 | 0 | Herpes 3.8% | 0 |
| 117 | 1-11 | 90 | 60 | - | - | - | - | - | - | - | - |
| 152 | 1-2 | 71 | 15 | 64 | - | - | - | 9 | - | Herpes 19% | - |

Publications retained correspond to series with more than 100 operated cases, a follow-up of at least 1 year, and precise information on initial pain relief and outcome at last follow-up; in those, side effects and/or complications were more or less detailed

Lunsford (1982), Arias (1986), Dieckmann et al. (1987), Saini (1987), Young (1988), Waltz et al. (1989), Fujimaki et al. (1990), Ischia et al. (1990), Steiger (1991), Cappabianca et al. (1995), Jho and Lunsford (1997), Blomstedt and Bergenheim (2002), Kondziolka and Lunsford (2005), Asplund et al. (2016), Hakanson et al. (2016) and Noorani et al. (2016)

# Stereotactic Radiosurgery for Trigeminal Neuralgias

# 11

Radiosurgery was first attempted for trigeminal neuralgia in the early 1970s by Lars Leksell, who used the stereotactic technology and the gamma rays for irradiation of the trigeminal ganglion. The difficulties in locating the target, the lack of consensus on the doses to use and the success of other surgical treatments meant that this method remained anecdotal for a long time. New interest arose when resolution of MRI enabled the precise location of the trigeminal root. At present Stereotactic Radiosurgery had acquired a large place in the neurosurgical armamentarium for treating trigeminal neuralgia, due to its low degree of invasiveness. Its insertion in the long historical evolution of the neurosurgical methods is briefly mentioned in the following section.

## 11.1 Brief on the Evolution of the Surgical Treatments

*Improving techniques to become more effective and safer took a long period of time along decades, both for open surgery and the percutaneous lesioning-techniques.*

The first surgical intervention proposed for trigeminal neuralgia was the Gasserian ganglionectomy. Conceived by Wears in 1885 and pioneered in practice soon after by Rose (Rose 1890), the procedure was then performed by Hartley (Hartley 1893), Horsley (Horsley 1891a, b) and Cushing (Cushing 1900). But it was quickly abandoned due to the frequent occurrence of keratites and anesthesia dolora. In 1901 Frazier, at the instigation of Spiller, developed the extradural sub-temporal Retrogasserian neurotomy (Spiller and Frazier 1901). Then in 1920 Dandy introduced the juxtapontine radicotomy via suboccipital laterocerebellar route (Dandy 1925). Limited to the pars major, the section, especially if reduced to its inferolateral two-thirds, was able to obtain analgesia without complete anesthesia of the face, in particular of the cornea. In 1938 Sjoqvist performed the Trigeminal tractotomy by cutting the descending spinal trigeminal tract at level of the medulla, this tract being the vector of the fibers for the thermoalgesic sensation of the face (Sjoqvist 1938; Olivecrona 1942; Kunc 1959). This intervention was then refined and popularized by Kunc (Kunc 1964, 1977; Kunc et al. 1978).

In 1952 Taarnhoj, assuming that trigeminal neuralgia could be due to constriction of the Gasser ganglion by fibrosclerosis of the dura-mater of the trigeminal cave, proposed the Decompression of the ganglion by opening its dural roof (Taarnhøj 1952, 1982). This technique, which had the theoretical interest of being conservative, was later abandoned due to the frequent recurrences after surgery. Shortly after, Shelden in 1955, interpreting the immediate good effect of the Taarnhoj's method as due to an operative trauma to the ganglion and neighboring nerve fibers, proposed the Hammering of the ganglion through direct approach (Shelden et al. 1955).


M. Sindou, A. Brinzeu, *Trigeminal Neuralgias: A Neurosurgical Illustrated Guide*,
https://doi.org/10.1007/978-3-031-25113-9_11

This gave rise to the more recent method of balloon compression by Mullan (Mullan and Lichtor 1983).

In parallel, to mitigate the risks of the interventions by direct approach, percutaneous techniques were developed on the principle of the "old" method of Alcoholization of the Gasserian ganglion, proposed as early as 1906 by Taptas (1911) and performed via lateral approach by Harris (1912a, b, 1940) then via the transforamen ovale approach by Hartel (1912). Instead of alcohol, Jaeger in 1957 proposed the Injection of hot water at the site of the ganglion (Jaeger 1959), and Jefferson in 1963 the Injection of phenol (at the concentration of 1/20th in glycerin) (Jefferson 1963). In 1941 Kirschner introduced the Electrocoagulation of the gasserian ganglion as the lesion-maker; surgery was performed under general anesthesia and using a stereotaxic percutaneous approach to the ganglion with penetration of the electrode through the foramen ovale (Kirschner 1933). The technique was then successively improved by Thiry who used a current of lower intensity in order to avoid the total loss of the tactile sensitivity (Thiry and Hotermans 1974), then by Schürmann who replaced general anesthesia by neuroleptanalgesia to control the effects of the coagulation in the patient awake (Schürmann et al. 1972).

In the early seventies, Sweet refined and popularized the technique under the name of Controlled differential thermocoagulation of the trigeminal ganglion and rootlets (Sweet and Wepsic 1974). A radio-frequency generator was used as the heat source, a thermistor to measure the temperature at the tip of the electrode, and short sequences of general anesthesia or neuroleptanalgesia—only during the painful steps of the intervention—to allow the patient's cooperation. The method is able to obtain analgesia without complete anesthesia, and in the sole painful area, thanks to the somatotopy of the fibers at the targeted level.

Still within the framework of percutaneous techniques performed under fluoroscopic control, Hakanson introduced in 1981 the Neurolysis of the Gasser ganglion by injection of glycerol into the trigeminal cistern of the Meckel cave via the foramen ovale (Håkanson 1978), and Mullan in 1979 the Compression of the Gasser ganglion using the inflatable balloon of a Fogarty probe as the lesion-maker (Mullan and Lichtor 1983).

Besides, in the fifties, Leksell applied the technique of Stereotaxic gamma-knife radiosurgery to trigeminal neuralgia (Leksell 1971). But this method only lost its anecdotal character with the advent of high-resolution MRI, which made precise targeting of radiation possible.

Along with these lesioning methods, the conservative method of Microsurgical vascular decompression developed in successive stages. The method is based on the observation made by Dandy, of the frequent observation of vascular conflicts in patients operated on in the cerebellopontine angle for trigeminal neuralgia to perform a juxtapontine radicotomy (Dandy 1932). However, vascular decompression was not performed until 1956, when Gardner reported treatment by simple decompression of the trigeminal root (Gardner 1962). The method was then soon adopted and refined with the microsurgical techniques by Jannetta, who firstly used the sub-temporal extradural transtentorial route (Jannetta and Rand 1966; Jannetta 1967), then the retromastoid approach (Jannetta 1977), the later after Hardy from Montreal University advised this route as the most appropriate for performing MVDs (Provost and Hardy 1970). Thanks to Jannetta, the method was popularized and became widely accepted as the first surgical option for treating conservatively what is nowadays called classical trigeminal neuralgia (Cruccu et al. 2016).

Radiosurgery was first attempted for trigeminal neuralgia in the early 1970s by Lars Leksell, using its Gamma-knife system for irradiation of the Gasserian ganglion (Leksell 1971) (Fig. 11.1).

In 1993 Rand published a first series of 12 patients treated at the UCLA by the Gamma Knife (GK) system informing that 7 out of the 12 evolved well (Rand et al. 1993). This was

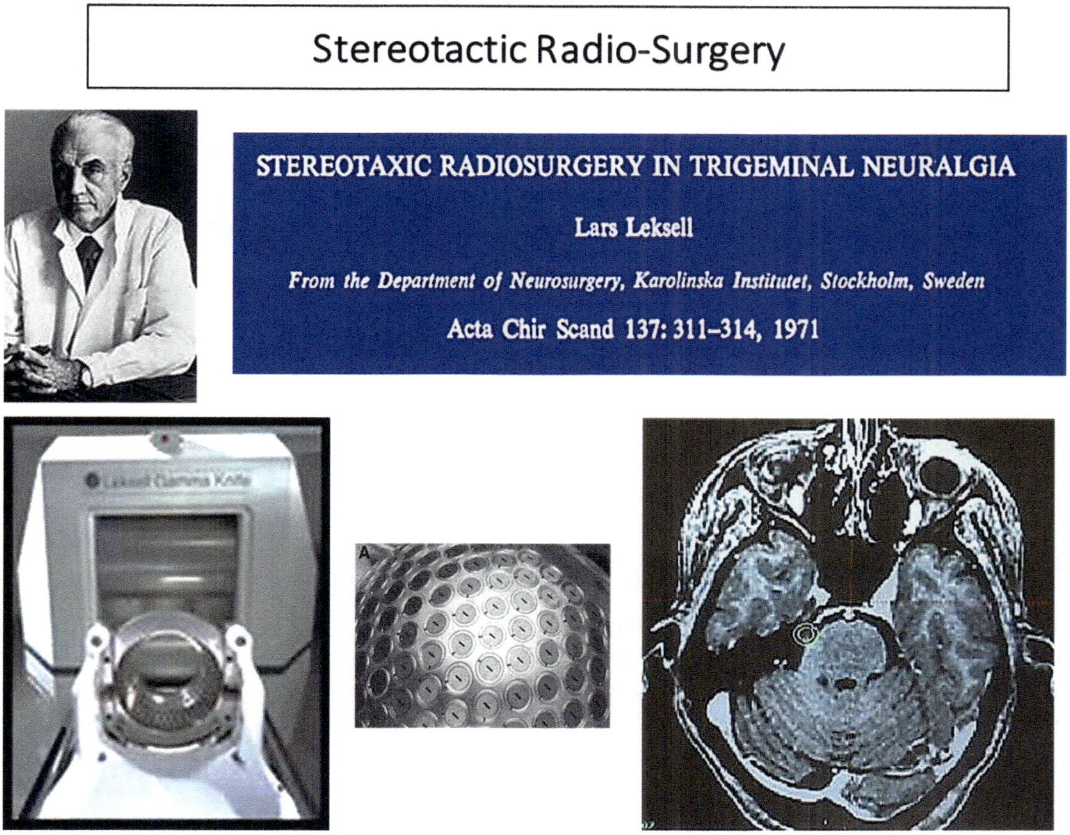


**Fig. 11.1** Introduction of radiosurgery occurred contemporaneously to the development of the stereotactic frames. This method was the major achievement of Lars Leksell from Karolinska Institute (Leksell 1951). The first patients with trigeminal neuralgia treated with the Gamma-Unit in Stockholm dated from 1953 and were reported in 1971 (Leksell 1971). However, the method only spread after modern imaging was developed, first the CT then high-resolution MRI

followed in 1995 by Regis from Marseilles who published a series of 20 patients (Régis et al. 1995) and next by Lunsford who published 51 patients treated in Pittsburg (Kondziolka et al. 1996a). The three pooled patients for a multi-institutional case series published in 1996 that definitively validated the use of the technique for the treatment of TN (Kondziolka et al. 1996b).

Radiosurgery can be done not only with Gamma-radiation, the Gamma-knife (GK) system, but also with photonic irradiation (LINAC/Cyber-knife) (Fig. 11.2). The procedures require putting on a stereotaxic frame, but being performed under simple local anesthesia they can be done on an outpatient basis. The procedures are quite standard and involve image acquisition and fusion, and obviously targeting and irradiation.

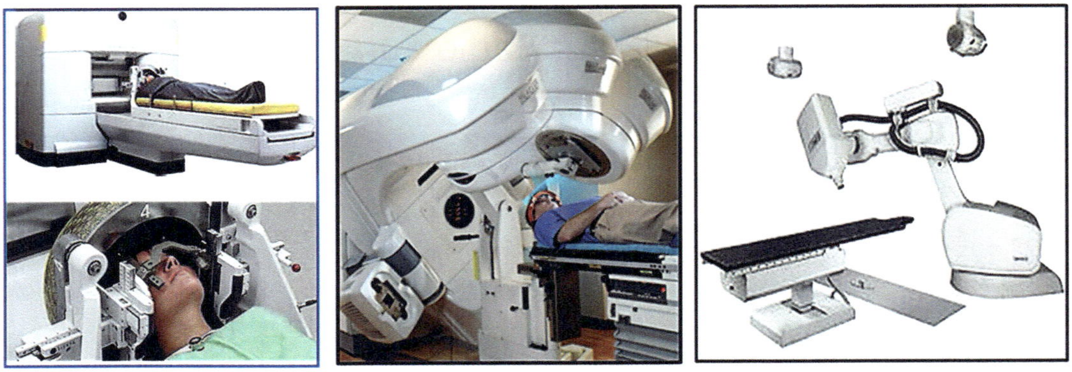

Gamma-knife Linac Cyber-knife

**Fig. 11.2** The main utilized stereotactic radiosurgical apparatus: Gamma-Kinfe, LINAC, and Cyberknife

## 11.2 Procedure

Radiosurgery is by definition irradiation through a single session. But much debate and research occurred concerning the precise details of the irradiation to be performed for best results.

An effect of radiation therapy on the trigeminal nerve is hypoesthesia. Pollock studied the relationship between radiation dose and hypoesthesia finding that there is a linear relationship between the two. He also found a direct and linear relationship between the dose and overall effect on pain sedation (Pollock 2006). The two lines appeared to be parallel and separated by 40 percentage points, adding weight to the choice of 90 Gy as a total dose since at this level about 20% of hypoesthesia occurs with 60% good long-term results. So, at present, there is a large consensus to recommend Stereotactic radiosurgery at a high dose of 80–90 Gy on radio-physical and radio-biological bases (Tuleasca et al. 2020) (Fig. 11.3).

The dose rate was also brought into question and higher dose rates appeared to be more effective (i.e., 2.5 Gy/min better than 1.5 Gy/min) (Lee et al. 2015). Further studies looked into the nerve volume being irradiated concluding that smaller irradiated volumes lead to better outcome with fewer side effects. Ultimately it appeared that the biological effect of radiation matters more than the strict physical characteristics of the beam and therefore a large dose in a concentrated volume at a high rate would lead to improved outcomes (Tuleasca et al. 2018).

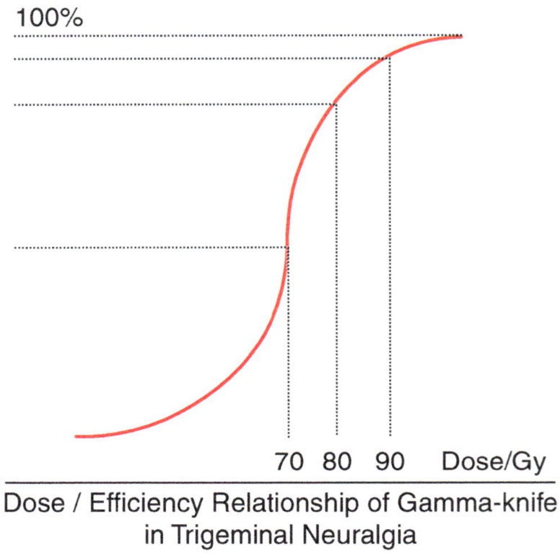


**Fig. 11.3** Schematic simplified representation of *Dose/Efficacy Relationship* of the Gamma-Knife radiosurgical modality for treating trigeminal neuralgia (Pollock 2006)

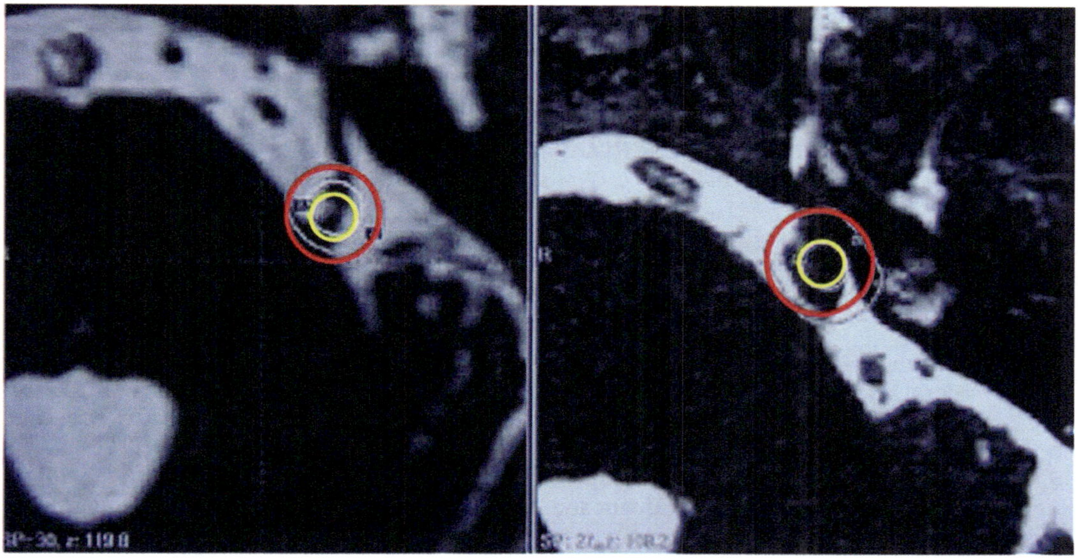


**Fig. 11.4** The two main targets for radiosurgical treatment of trigeminal neuralgia, represented in axial $T_2$-MRI of brainstem and trigeminal root, on left side. Left: target at Trigeminal Root Entry Zone Right: target at cisternal retrogasserian portion of the trigeminal root. Yellow cercle: isodose of 80 Gy; Red cercle: isodose of 30 Gy. According to literature, the TREZ target is more propicious for radiolesioning to endanger brainstem (Régis et al. 2006)

Concerning targets, at the beginning, the classical target was the Trigeminal Root Entry Zone (TREZ). More recently, the recommended target became the retrogasserian portion of the sensory root, with a single 4 mm isocenter on the cisternal path of the nerve, 7.5 mm from the emergence of the brainstem nerve. As a matter of fact, it is considered by most that the TREZ target exposes to more undesirable effects and complications, without obtaining a better effectiveness on the neuralgia. It is in fact not recommended to exceed a dose of 15 Gy at level of the brainstem (Régis et al. 1995, 2006; Régis 2002) (Fig. 11.4).

An inconvenience of radiosurgery is that it usually takes a few months to be effective. This is not, however, a major problem for most patients, with the exception of those referred in painful condition (Tuleasca et al. 2012) (Fig. 11.5a).

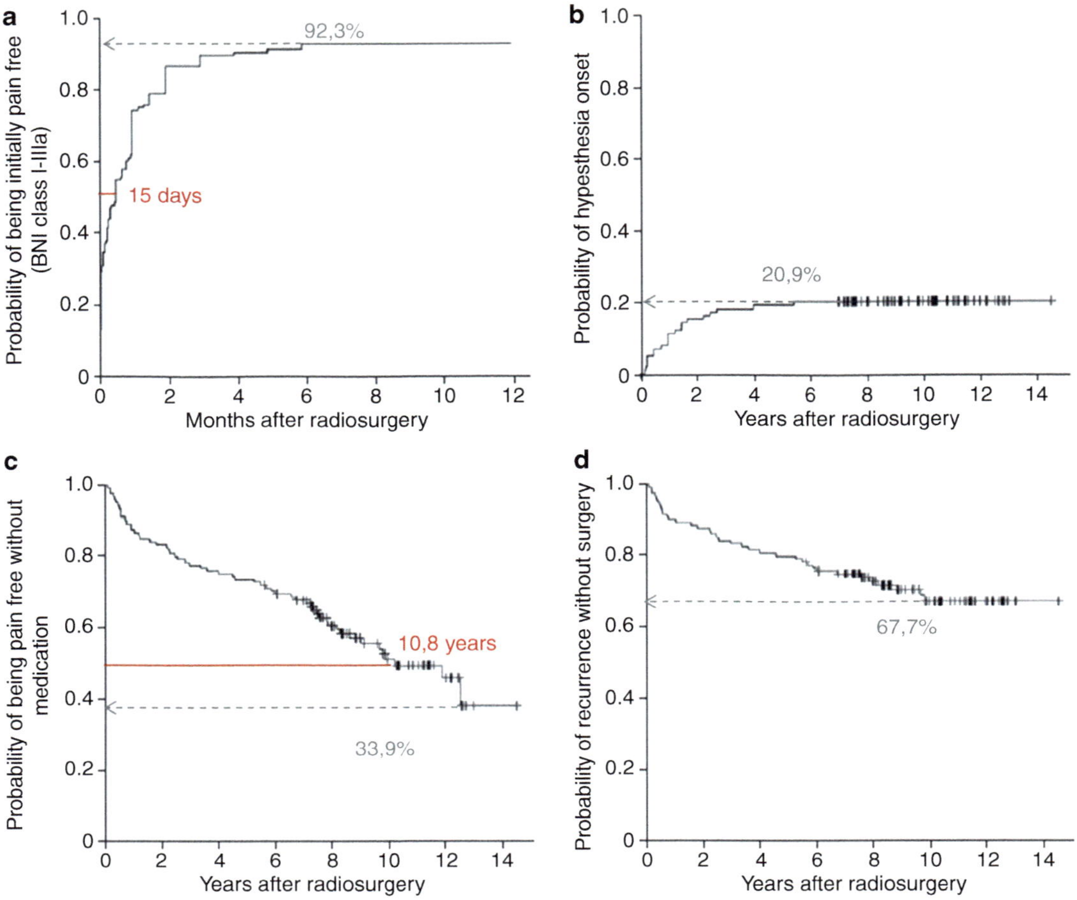


**Fig. 11.5** Long-term outcome after Gamma-Knife Radiosurgery (GK) for Trigeminal Neuralgia. In a 10-year median follow-up study Regis and Tuleasca studied the outcome of 130 patients treated for primary trigeminal neuralgia by GK. Success of therapy was considered if the patient could be classified as BNI I–IIIa (at worst no pain but continued medication) (Régis et al. 2016). A delay to the onset of pain sedation was constantly noted; it was estimated to be of a median of 15 days; however, this could occur up to 6 months after the treatment. 7.7 % of patients did not achieve significant pain control (**a**) A significant proportion of patients (up to 21%) showed clinically relevant hypoesthesia in the trigeminal territory, the onset of which could occur up to 6 years after the treatment. (**b**) Recurrence of pain after the treatment is frequent with only one-third of patients being pain-free and medication-free in the long run. Median time to pain recurrence was however almost 11 years. (**c**) On the other hand, only half of the recurring patients necessitated a second procedure with an overall probability of being BNI I–IIIa over 15 years of 67%. (**d**) Adapted from Régis et al. (2016)

## 11.3 Outcome

### 11.3.1 Main Published Series

Since the early 1990s, a large number of patient series have been published; most of them are simple retrospective case series, with outcome assessments quite variable. Latest series appear to illustrate somewhat more homogenous results at least for GK as the technique has stabilized. A couple of prospective series have been published as well as some comparative studies facing off radiosurgery with other techniques.

The current consensus by mainstream researchers is that outcome should be assessed according to the BNI scale considering good results as BNI I and II and acceptable ones BNI IIIa. Facial sensory disfunction must be regularly assessed as it frequently occurs, and this should also be performed using the BNI sensory disturbance scale.

The first large series using modern parameters for radiosurgery was that of Pollok et al. in 2002 describing 117 consecutive patients treated at the Mayo Clinic in Rochester Minnesota (Pollock et al. 2002). They considered a positive outcome only if pain relief was complete without medication (BNI I or II). Median follow-up duration was 26 months (range 1–48 months). The actuarial rate of achieving and maintaining this was 57 and 55% at 1 and 3 years. Sensory disturbance was noticed at doses of 90 Gy in the order of 25% of patients. Pollock also studied the relationship between sensory disturbance and effect (Fig. 11.6).

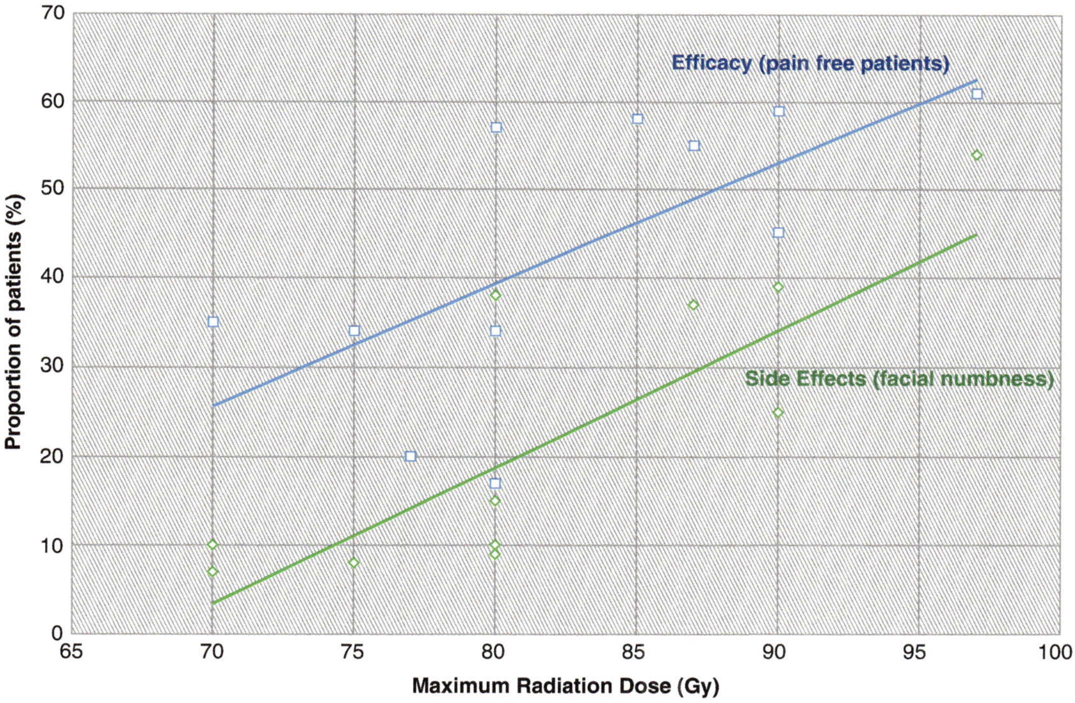


**Fig. 11.6** Relationship between radiation dose with Gamma-Knife Radiosurgery (GKR) and effect in terms of effectiveness on pain sedation and facial numbness. In a review of previously published studies Pollock analyzed the relationship between the administered focal radiation dose and efficacy on one hand and facial numbness on the other (Pollock 2006). This composite graph illustrates the regression line for efficacy according to radiation dosage in blue (individual study results shown as squares) in parallel to the regression line for facial numbness according to dosage in green (individual study results shown as diamonds). Both are directly correlated to dosage, the two lines being quasi parallel leading to the conclusion that for GK pain sedation in the neuralgia comes with the related encumbrance of hypoesthesia. Graph created from data published by B.E. Pollock (2006)

The largest published series to date is that of Tuleasca and Regis describing 497 patients treated at the Timone Hospital in Marseilles from 1992 to 2010 (Tuleasca et al. 2012). The series is formed of a total of 737 TN patients treated by GK out of which only 497 were considered to be classical. Exclusion criteria were obviously secondary TN but also megadolicho-basilar artery. The median follow-up period was 43.8 months (range 12–174.4 months). A 4-mm isocenter in the cisternal portion of the nerve was used with a median dose of 85 Gy (70–90 Gy). The series analyzed results according to the BNI scale over a median period of follow up of 43.8 months. BNI I–IIIa patients had an actuarial probability of 93.4%, 85.9%, 78.6%, 71.8%, 64.9%, 59.7%, and 45.3% at 0.5, 1, 2, 3, 5, 7, 10, 12, and 14 years, respectively.

This publication was followed by a subset analysis of 130 patients that were followed for a median of 7 years (Régis et al. 2016). This showed similar outcomes (for BNI I-IIIa) with the probability of remaining pain-free at 3, 5, 7, and 10 years of 77.9, 73.8, 68, and 51.5%, respectively.

Both publications analyzed time to pain sedation as well, concluding on a median time until pain relief from 10 to 15 days (1–180 days range). Hypoesthesia had a tendency to occur and was significant in 20% of patients with a median onset at 12 months. To be noted that no new facial hypoesthesia occurred after 7 years of FU.

The results described by Regis et al. from Marseilles constitute the largest series in the field (Fig. 11.5b–d). Globally the Marseille team reports a 5-year cure rate of 60% and the presence of hypoesthesia at 5 years in 17%. There are however other significant series with results that deserve to be considered in particular for the details of their conclusions.

However, the difficulty to have a definitive appraisal from the literature of the capacity of SRS to reliably control the disease comes from the diversity of the results and of their assessment from one publication to another: from 22 to 89% after average setbacks ranging from 10 to 60 months, a reported recurrence rate of 0–46%, a hypoesthesia from 0 to 54%, depending on the series. This lack of homogeneity is explained by the disparity of the radio-surgical equipment, that of targets, that of doses, variable setbacks, and also the way of evaluating the results according to the authors.

A list of important *documented reports from literature series* is presented in Table 11.1.

**Table 11.1** Outcome after stereotactic radio-surgery (literature review)

| | | | Stereotactic Radiosurgery | | | | | |
|---|---|---|---|---|---|---|---|---|
| **Author(s) NB. pts** | **Followup (mean in year)** | **Mean Age** | **Device** | **Mean Dose, Gy** | **Time to Pain Response, weeks** | **Relief of the Neuralgia Initial (%)** | **Relief of the Neuralgia Late (%)** | **Side-effects Facial Numbness(%)** |
| 136 | 1 | 68 | GKRS | 80 | 3 | 90 | 70 | 51 |
| 107 | 5 | 75 | GKRS | 75 | 12 | 81 | 58 | 20 |
| 106 | 1 | 72 | GKRS | 80 | 4 | 90 | 60 | 4 |
| 160 | 1 | 63 | GKRS | 85 | 7 | 90 | 61 | 0 |
| 112 | 5.6 | 64 | GKRS | 75 | 2 | 69 | 34 | 6 |
| 503 | 2 | 72 | GKRS | 80 | 5 | 80 | 71 | 11 |
| 365 | 2.5 | 65 | GKRS | 80 | 4 | 75 | 60 | 6.5 |
| 130 | 3.2 | 68 | GKRS | 90 | 3 | 80 | 66 | 24 |
| 179 | 2 | 74 | LINAC | 90 | 9 | 79 | 60 | 50 |
| 448 | 2 | 67 | GKRS | 90 | - | 86 | 46 | 25 |
| 250 | 5.5 | 71 | GKRS | 90 | 8 | 90 | 79 | 33 |
| 497 | 5 | 68 | GKRS | 85 | 4 | 91 | 64 | 21 |

Publications retained correspond to series with more than 100 operated cases, a follow-up of at least 1 year, and precise information on initial pain relief and outcome at last follow-up; in those, side effects and/or complications were more or less detailed

Sheehan et al. (2005), Urgosik et al. (2005), Fountas et al. (2007), Longhi et al. (2007), Dhople et al. (2009), Kondziolka et al. (2010), Verheul et al. (2010), Hayashi et al. (2011), Smith et al. (2011), Marshall Hayashi et al. (2012), Young et al. (2013), Regis et al. (2016)

### 11.3.2 Comparisons Between GK & LINAC & CK

Studies for radiosurgery using LINAC and Cyber-Knife have been published though in lesser numbers than those using GK (Kubicek et al. 2004; De La Peña et al. 2022). Figure 11.7 gives a perspective on such outcomes (Fig. 11.7).

Recently (2018) Tuleasca, Regis, and Levivier performed a systematic review of all published series until 2015 (Tuleasca et al. 2018). They found 65 studies including 6461 patients. Out of these series 45 used GammaKnife (GK), 11 LINAC, and 9 CyberKnife (CK). The review gives a broad range for outcomes according to the technique used. Recurrence rates ranged from 0 to 52.2% (mean 24.6%, median 23%) for GK, from 19 to 63% (mean 32.2%, median 29%) for LINAC, and from 15.8 to 33% (mean 25.8%, median 27.2%) for CK.

More importantly, they assessed complication rates in specific detail. Hypoesthesia, ranged from 0 to 68.8% (mean 21.7%, median 19%) for GKS, from 11.4 to 49.7% (mean 27.6%, median 28.5%) for LINAC, and from 11.8 to 51.2% (mean 29.1%, median 18.7%) for CKR. Other complications included dysesthesias, paresthesias, dry eye, deafferentation pain, and keratitis.

Hypoesthesia and paresthesia occurred as complications only when the anterior retrogasserian portion of the trigeminal nerve was targeted, whereas the other listed complications occurred when the root entry zone was targeted.

More recently (2019) the European Academy of Neurology reviewed all published series up to 2018 in order to give recommendations (Bendtsen et al. 2019). Criteria for inclusion were more stringent since studies had to have independent outcome assessment and with more than 25 patients and that were followed for more than 3 years. In this comparative review, a group of eight studies were found relating experience with stereotactic radiosurgery, namely GK. These studies comprised 1168 patients. In the selected series, the radiation dose varied from 75 to 95 Gy. Six of the eight studies reported more than 20% of patients that had prior surgical procedures before GK. The average FU varied from 3.2 to 5.6 years. Immediate pain relief was achieved in less than 80%. The pain relief rate at mean FU decreased to 36–91.7%

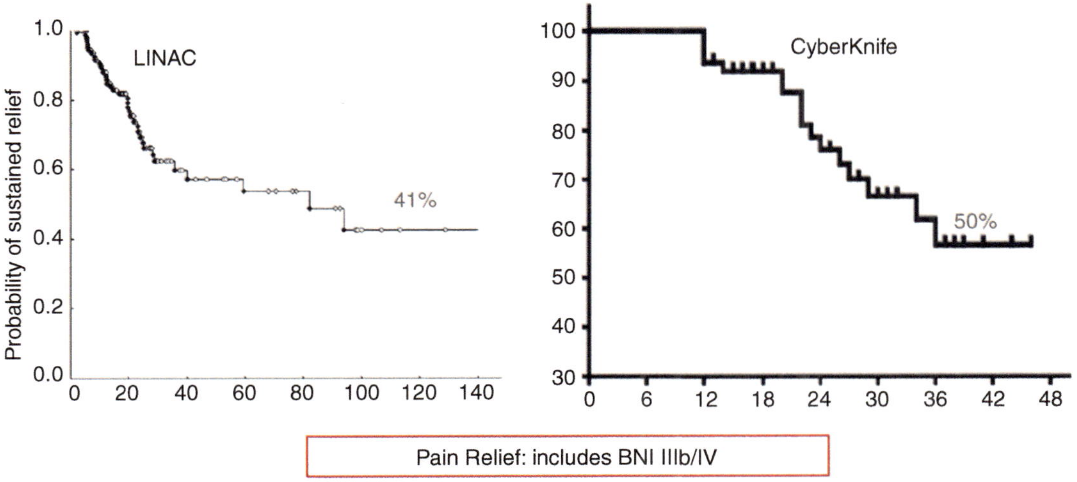


**Fig. 11.7** Probability of Long-term outcome after LINAC radiosurgery and Cyber-Knife radiosurgery. The shown Kaplan-Meir curves are from independent studies: LINAC (on the left) at 11 years (Smith et al. 2011) and Cyber-Knife (on the right) at 4 years (Villavicencio et al. 2008). In both these and other studies using LINAC and Cyber-Knife, results qualified: pain relief included all patients that showed "improvement" after radiosurgery, even those with benefit graded BNI III b or IV. To be noted, inclusion of patients that qualify BNI III b or IV are generally not considered successes with other techniques; therefore, results are difficult to compare, even to those from GKR series. Adapted from Smith et al. (2011) and Villavicencio et al. (2008)

(mean: 60%) and recurrence or failure rates varied from 18 to 52.2%. The time to pain relief varied from 1 day to 24 months. In those series the major complication was facial hypoesthesia with more or less paresthesias (184/1168 patients: 15.8%, from 6 to 72% according to series) with other complications being only sporadic.

### 11.3.3 Results After Second and Third Surgeries

Given that there is no technical reason not to perform repeated surgeries after a first procedure and that many if not most patients do recur after a first procedure of radiosurgery, investigators were encouraged to try a second and even third procedures.

In 2005 Pollock published a series of 19 patients who underwent repeat radiosurgery for trigeminal neuralgia after a median of 16 months after the first surgery with a median additive dose of 163 Gy (Pollock et al. 2005). At 2 years, 61% of them were pain-free and medication-free, but 58% described facial hypoesthesia which was correlated with good outcome.

Another series of 119 patients with repeat SRS was published by the Pittsburg team led by Lunsford and Kondziolka. The median received dose for repeat GK SRS was 70 Gy (range 50–90 Gy), and the median cumulative dose was 145 Gy (range 120–170 gY). THe median follow-up was 48 months (range 6-187) after repeat GK SRS. Pain relief was 44.2% at 5 years (BNI I-IIIa). Facial sensory disfunction occurred in 21% of patients within 18 months after GK SRS (Park et al. 2012).

Tuleasca and Regis analyzed the repeat surgeries in their large series of 497 patients (Tuleasca et al. 2012, 2014). Even if 157 experienced a recurrence only 13 were considered for repeat surgery which was performed at a median of 72 months with a median dose of 90 Gy. The team describes a probability for a good result (at least BNI IIIa) of 75% but with the price of hypoesthesia in more than 50% of patients that were followed for 3 years and over.

One study analyzed the results of a third attempt at radiosurgery for trigeminal neuralgia (Tempel et al. 2015). All patients treated three times by the North American Gamma Knife Consortium from 1995 to 2012 were included. There was a total of 17 patients followed for 24 months with a reported probability of BNI I of 35%. Unfortunately, the series reported the rest of the patients in the category BNI II–IIIb.

### 11.3.4 Comparisons with Other Techniques

Few comparative series exist that estimate the results of radiosurgery in comparison with other techniques. Several of them compared microvascular decompression with radiosurgery. These were reviewed by the European Academy of Neurology in 2019 including (separately) prospective and retrospective series (Bendtsen et al. 2019). They were all considered low or very low quality of evidence. The first and well-known study is that by Pollock comparing posterior fossa exploration with a TREZ target for GKRS (Pollock and Schoeberl 2010). All prospective studies favored MVD and the meta-analysis yielded a group of 287 patients for MVD and 274 patients for GK with a probability of a good outcome of 61–80% for MVD and 33–56% respectively for GK (Fig. 11.8).

Other comparative studies exist for glycerol for example published by Henson et al. in 2005 (Henson et al. 2005). Advantages of glycerol are related to the rapidity of the effect but efficacy seems to be better for GK. This is probably true for many other percutaneous techniques.

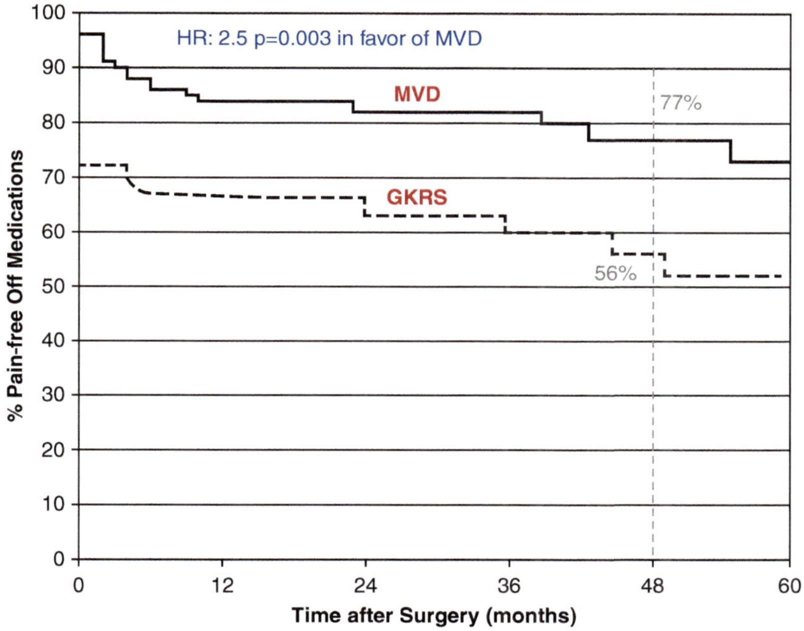


**Fig. 11.8** Comparison of long-term outcomes after Micro-Vascular Decompression (MVD) and Gamma-Knife Radiosurgery (GKRS) for Trigeminal Neuralgia. Prospective comparative study, from a single center, between a series of 91 patients treated with MVD (solid line) and a series of 49 patients who benefited from GKRS (dotted line), all followed up over 4 years (Pollock and Schoeberl 2010). Hazards ratio in favor of MVD were 2.5 with an overall pain-free probability for patients treated by MVD of 77%. Adapted from Pollock and Schoeberl (2010)

## 11.4 Conclusions

Radiosurgery is possible for trigeminal neuralgia and now a large body of literature exist detailing results, especially with the GK system. A correlation between hypoesthesia rates and effect is rather well established although more research is warranted on dosing and targeting given that the absorbed dose seems to be more important than its physical characteristics of the radiation. Repeat surgery is possible, even a third time but this increases the rates of hypoesthesia. Overall results seem as good as those of percutaneous techniques but less so than those of microvascular decompression. Although studies are heterogenous in assessment, good outcome probability after GK in the very long run seems to be just below 50% with 20% probability of facial numbness. LINAC and Cyber-Knife have been also used but are less extensively studied.

**Key-Point**

The low incidence of severe morbidity is the greatest advantage of SRS compared with the other surgical methods. For certain teams, among them the Marseilles team, the presence of hypoesthesia is not necessary to obtain a good analgesic result. For others on the contrary, in particular the one at the Mayo Clinic, the duration of the pain sedation is correlated with the presence of postoperative hypoesthesia and consequently with a certain degree of dysesthesia ($p = 0.02$).

A wait for pain relief, often for "months," is clinically impractical in patients with intense pain. However, in patients benefiting from a quiescent period this is not a major obstacle.

# 12 Decision-Making and Conclusions

Confronted to facial pain, first step is to ascertain the diagnosis of Trigeminal Neuralgia (TN) and define to which category pain belongs: secondary, classical, or idiopathic, according to the recent classification established by Cruccu et al. (2016) and the Classification Committee of the International Headache Society (IHS) (2018) (Fig. 12.1).

Secondary TNs are most often easily identifiable by imaging and laboratory investigations. Their management should be directed to respective etiologies; however, when specific treatments fail or are not available, a neurosurgical operation belonging to the frame of functional neurosurgery is considered.

Classical TNs and Idiopathic TNs come of course under the pharmacological treatments as the first step, firstly, the antalgic anticonvulsants. If the neuralgia reveals refractory to all medications or if medications are not well tolerated, a neurosurgical treatment should be considered (Fig. 12.2).

There are several neurosurgical interventions that can be offered. The choice of the most appropriate may be difficult, each one having its own advantages, disadvantages, and risks.

Referring to literature publications to access objective information on the various neurosurgical methods in use is not full warranty of having strictly comparable data. There had been, as quite understandable, no randomized prospective controlled studies. The (few) comparative studies between techniques were for most retrospective studies. The abundant publications on single methods report respective clinical results of corresponding cohorts, but with more or less long-term follow-ups. Further, they are tainted of frequent disparities between criteria for indication, between ways of doing the surgery, and in between the criteria of assessing the results. However, some reviews published in the recent literature, as the one by the European Academy of Neurology, may be of help to compare methods (Bendtsen et al. 2019) as well as a personal meta-analysis of the main publications which appeared in the three past decades (Tatli et al. 2008), a summary of which is presented in the following figure (Fig. 12.3). It emerges that MVD affords the optimal pain relief with the minimum of side effects, but as an open surgical procedure with some potentially severe complications. Regarding the lesioning-techniques including stereotactic radiosurgery, it also emerges that duration of the pain relief tends to be related to the importance of the created hypoesthesia, with consequently a certain degree of numbness induced.

Figures 12.4 and 12.5 illustrate the decision-making process that we adopted along our neurosurgical practice for the choice of the procedure. For (suspected) classical TN, when imaging was in favor of a clearcut NVC, that is, grade II or III of compression in our classification, patient was preferentially offered the MVD procedure


M. Sindou, A. Brinzeu, *Trigeminal Neuralgias: A Neurosurgical Illustrated Guide*,
https://doi.org/10.1007/978-3-031-25113-9_12

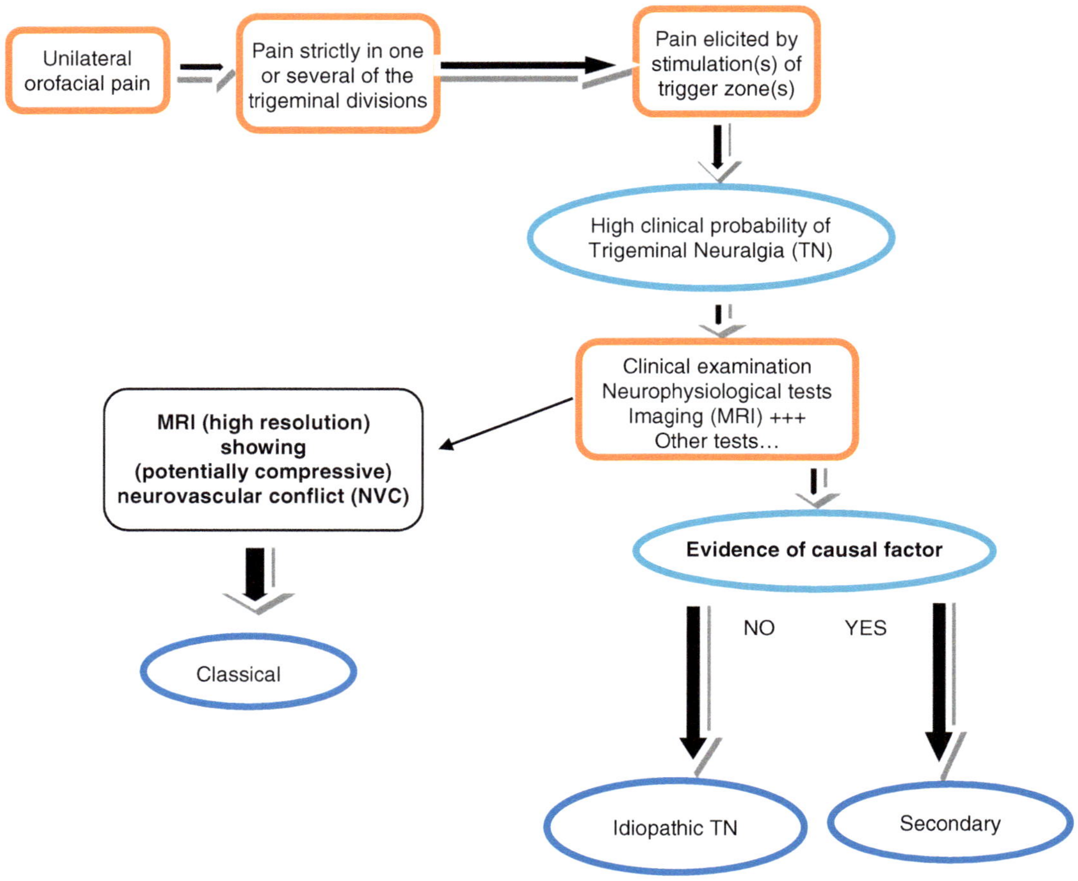


**Fig. 12.1** Algorithm for diagnosis of trigeminal neuralgias, summarized from Cruccu et al. (2016)

(Fig. 12.4); if not, a lesioning-technique was considered. For idiopathic TNs, a lesioning-method was systematically proposed. Same applied for patients with multiple sclerosis.

Regarding the percutaneous lesioning-techniques, albeit we most often used the RF-thermo-rhizotomy, in most recent period when pain predominated in the V1 (often associated with V2) territory we favored the balloon compression modality—known to expose to a lesser rate of corneal hypoesthesia (Fig. 12.5).

Based on an overall experience of more than 5000 of surgically treated patients with TNs, our proposal for (suspected) Classical TNs is MVD as the first option. A lesioning-procedure would be proposed for patients in precarious conditions or if the high-definition MRI does not evidence a clearcut NVC (Fig. 12.6).

A major problem is the predictability on the preoperative MRI of the responsibility of the (suspected) vessel in the genesis of the neuralgia. As previously demonstrated, the degree of compression of vessels is significantly correlated with the probability of long-term pain relief, so that its prediction is of paramount importance to take the decision to propose MVD as the first option for surgical treatment (Sindou et al. 2007) (Fig. 12.7).

Consequently, an important practical question arises: "Is MRI reliable to predict the degree or compression of a suspected NVC?" As previously pointed out in an above chapter, high-resolution MRI has an overall good reliability to predict the presence of a (potential) Neuro-Vascular Conflict. But, if prediction value is excellent for the high grades of compression, some apparent low-grade of compression revealed as false positives at surgical exploration. Therefore, indication of MVD for patients with estimated low grade of compression (Grade I:

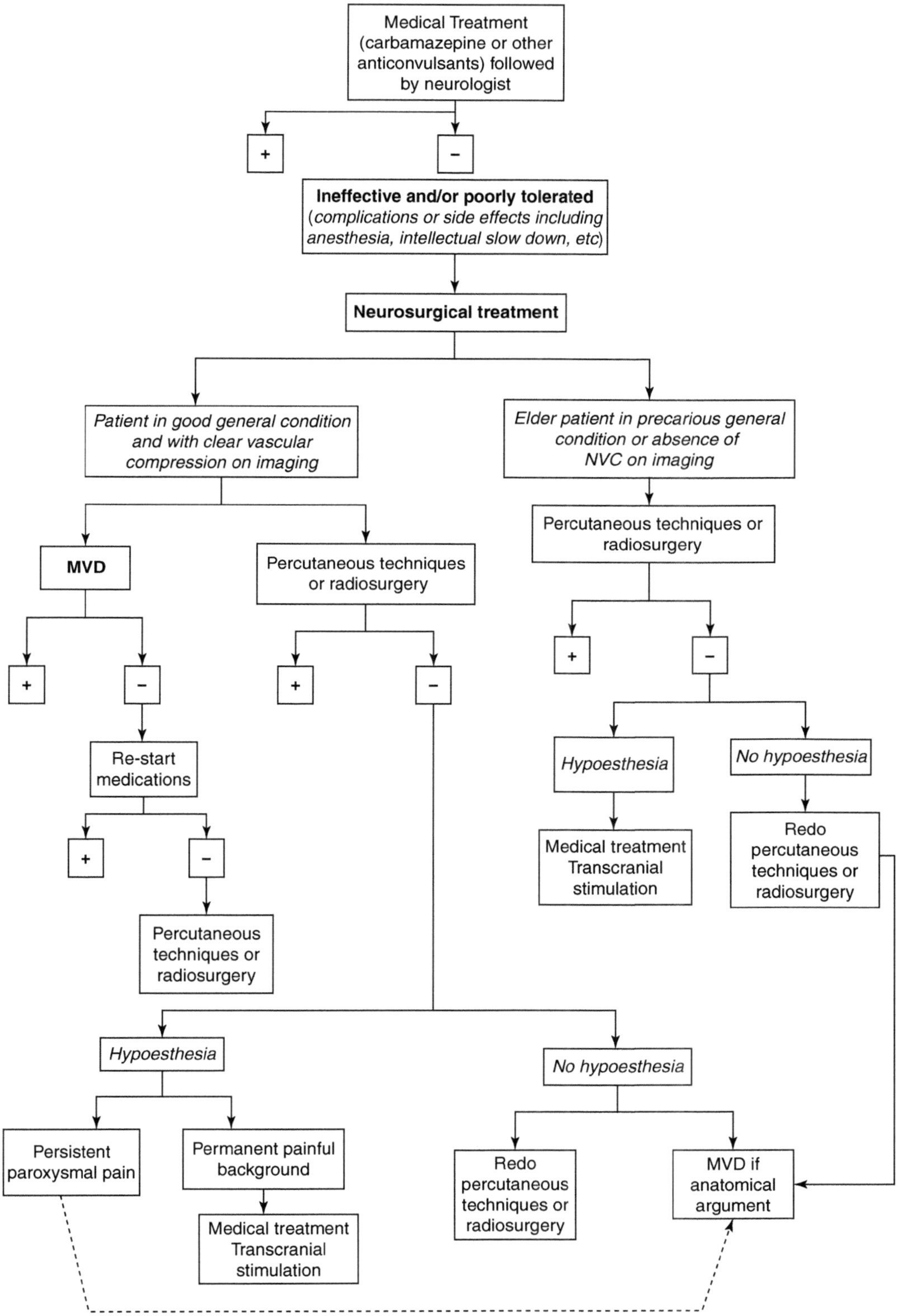


**Fig. 12.2** Our current management of trigeminal neuralgias: from pharmacological to surgical treatments (Sindou et al. 2020). In the eventuality of a (first) surgical failure, the decisions depends on the existence or not of a secondary hypoesthesia and of the type of the persistent pain (paroxysmal or permanent)

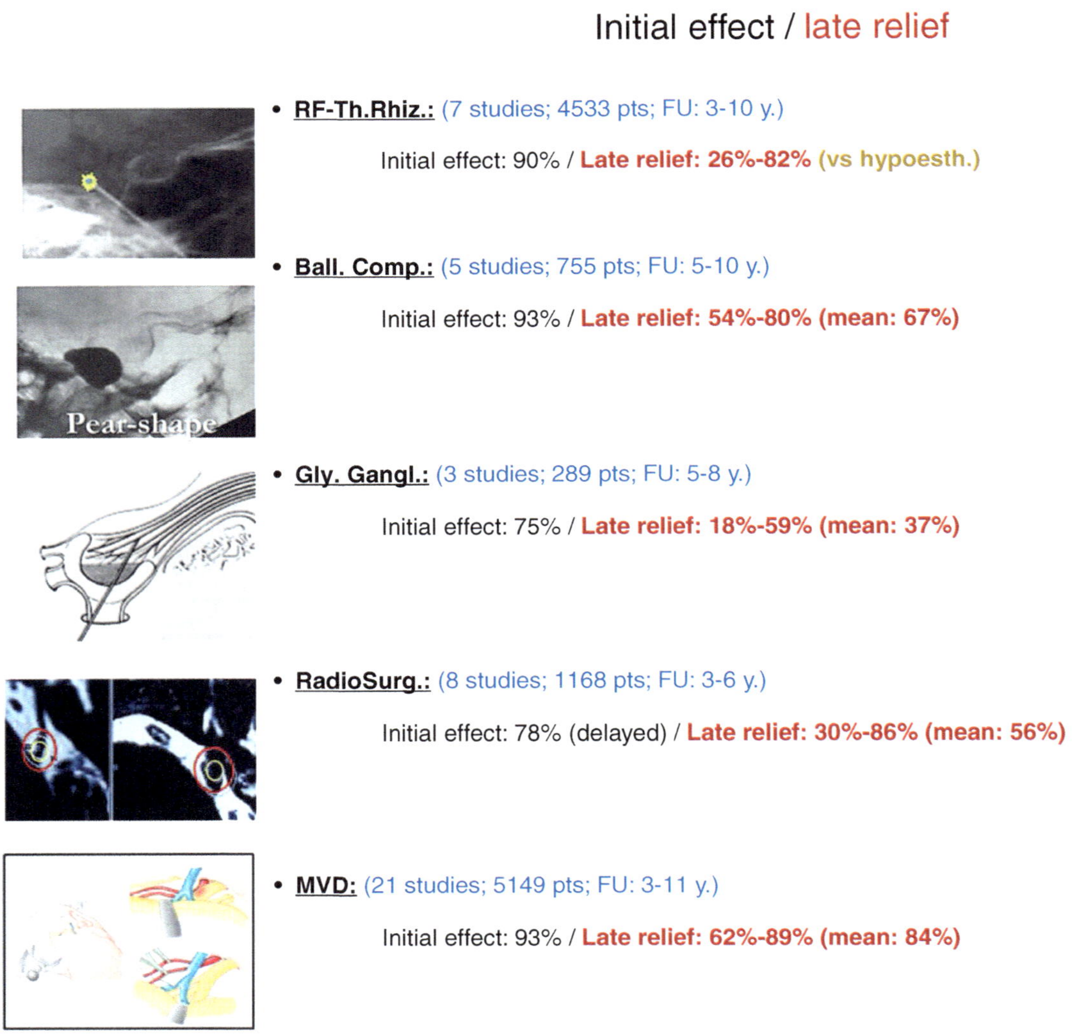


**Fig. 12.3** Summary of main literature data on initial and long-term pain relief after the various neurosurgical procedures (Tatli et al. 2008; Sindou et al. 2021). Regarding the Lesioning-methods, most authors stress on the fact that duration of the pain relief along years is proportional to the intensity of the sensory loss, with the consequence of some more or less degree of "bothering" numbness

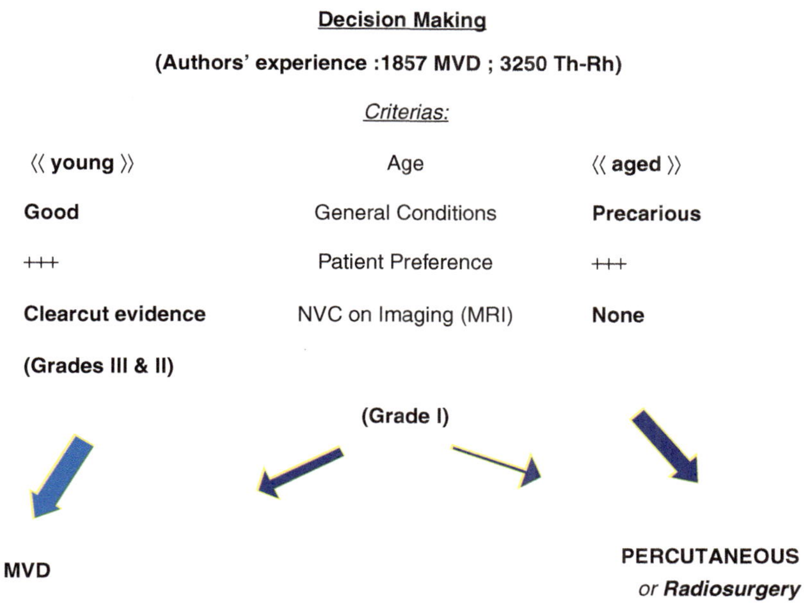


**Fig. 12.4** Decision-making process for the choice of the neurosurgical procedure, personal experience (Sindou and Brinzeu 2018)

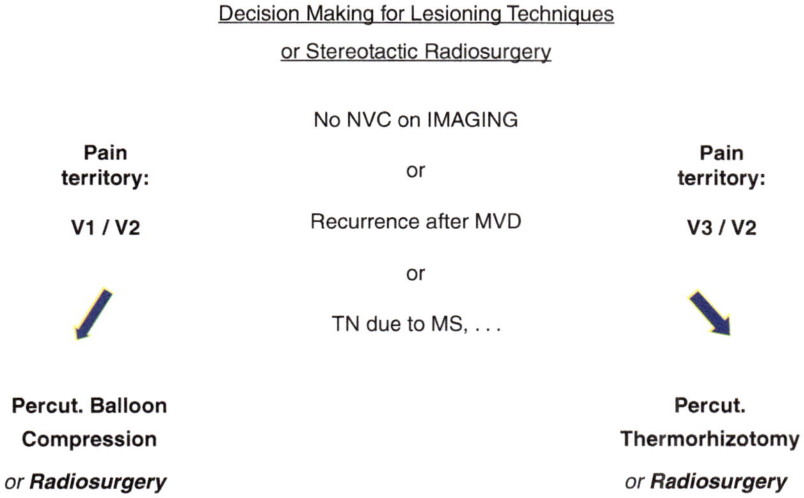


**Fig. 12.5** Decision-making process for the choice of the lesioning neurosurgical procedure, personal experience (Sindou and Brinzeu 2018). Although secondary neuralgias are off topic, their severe neuralgic forms, especially those due to multilocular sclerosis, are amenable to thermo-rhizotomy; this procedure is most often effective on the paroxystic component but at the cost of a marked hypoesthesia sequela

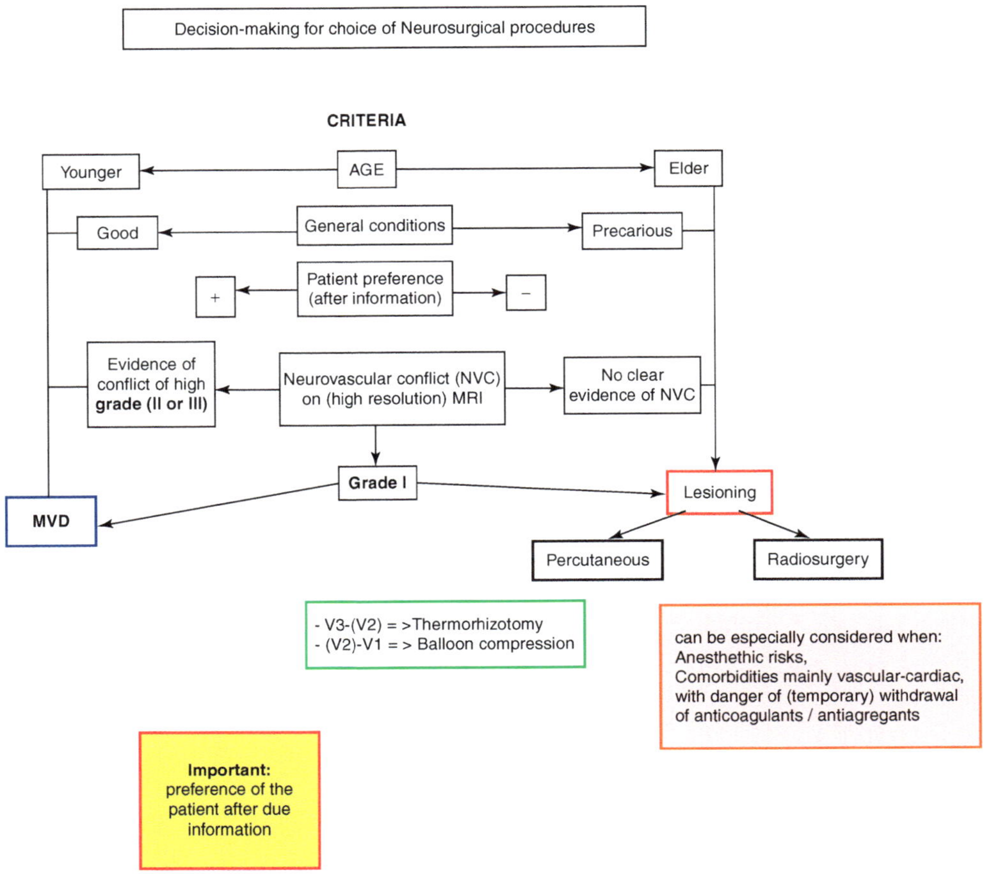


**Fig. 12.6** Proposal for treating the Classical trigeminal neuralgias. Importance of the patient information (Sindou and Brinzeu 2018)

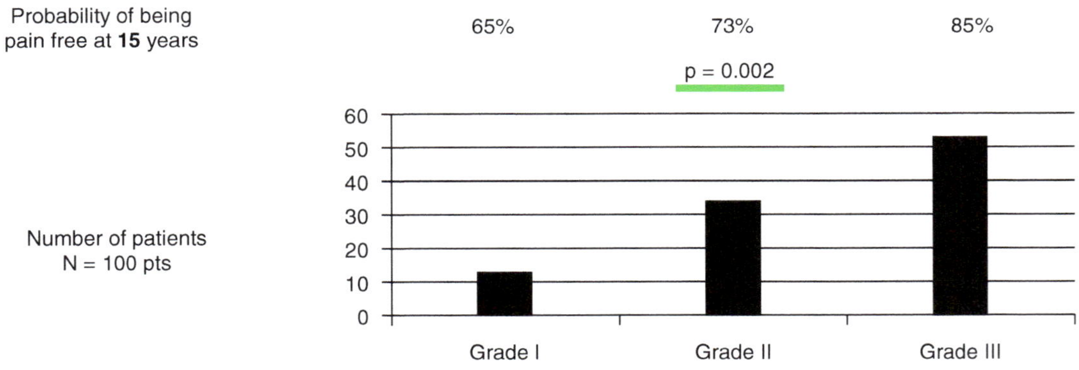


**Fig. 12.7** Probability of being pain-free after MVD according to grade of compression (Sindou et al. 2007). The degree of compression is of paramount importance to predict the probability of long-term pain relief, and thus to take the decision to propose MVD as the first choice of surgical treatment

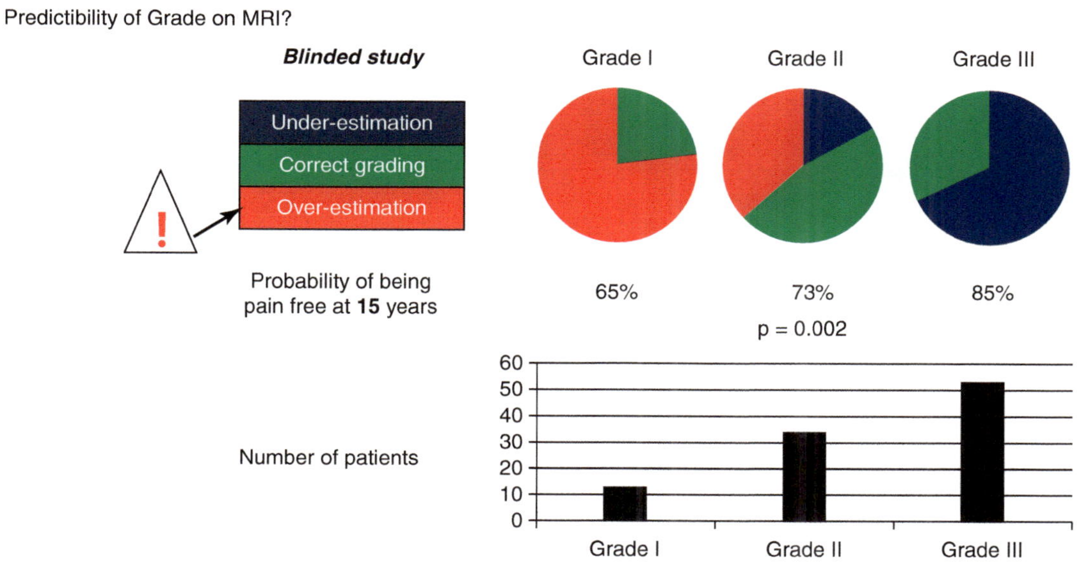


**Fig. 12.8** Predictability of the grade of the neurovascular conflict from MRI: reliability? (Brinzeu et al. 2018a). Study shows an overall good reliability of MRI to predict the existence of a Neuro-Vascular Conflict. The prediction value is excellent for the high grades of compression. But some apparent low-grade compressions on MRI may be revealed as false positives at surgical exploration. Indication of MVD for patients with estimated Grade I of compression on MRI should be "prudently" if not critically discussed

simple contact with the root) on MRI should be "prudently" if not critically discussed (Leal et al. 2010; Brinzeu et al. 2018a) (Fig. 12.8). Further research is needed in Imaging techniques for improving accuracy and reliability for prediction of the pathological anatomy responsible of the disease, and thus reduces the rate of failures of the corresponding surgery. Use of fine measurements of the cross-section area of the trigeminal root at the site of a suspected NVC and also DTI methodologies have already demonstrated their usefulness for evidencing neural tissue alteration and so ascertaining the harmfulness of suspected conflicting vessels.

*In conclusion*, the neurosurgical armamentarium offers a large spectrum of surgical opportunities with for each intrinsic advantages and disadvantages. The choice of the most appropriate procedure for a particular patient should depend on the specific features of his/her neuralgia, and his/her general and psychological conditions, as well as the patient's personal wishes after precise information. Among the several factors conditioning outcome, no doubt that the most important one is the pathological anatomy of the trigeminal pathways. No doubt that from a practical point of view, Imaging is the key for taking decision. Although the nowadays technology attained a relatively good accuracy, there is still the need for further refinements (and consequently research) to reach a high degree of reliability for safe predictability.

# Epilogue

The purpose of this book was to provide practitioners with readily available information that the authors harvested from the literature and tested constantly in clinical practice with an experience of over 5000 patients operated on for trigeminal neuralgia. The aim is to provide practical advice so as to limit failures and complications in particular through an optimized selection process.
Critical analysis of long-term results and complications should be considered before deciding which treatment might be best for each of the patients. One always must take into account patients own expectations and wishes, as well as the neuralgia peculiarities.

Not every technical modality has the possibility to obtain an optimal effect, but all have a role in the spectrum of possible treatments for trigeminal neuralgia. Thus microvascular decompression is considered the first option for what is now considered classical trigeminal neuralgia; however affirming the responsibility of the incriminated vessel might not always be possible. We strongly advocate that the indication and choice of the treatment method should be firstly based on the anatomy-pathological apparent cause, thus targeting the supposed etiology of the disease. Of course, this implies that most indications are based mainly on imaging. Because of that there is still a considerable amount of work to be performed in order to increase the reliability of imaging in selecting patients for the appropriate method of treatment.

There is also a need to create a consensus as to what way is best to achieve root decompression and obtain reestablishment of trigeminal function as there is a need for refinements in the lesioning methods in order to improve their effectiveness and limit their side effects.

The book is an analysis of what the surgical state of the art is at this point in its evolution. Surgery is not the first option for trigeminal neuralgia patients but has been one from before the time medical treatments were available and has marked neurosurgery for almost 150 years, and we are certain it will continue to do so for a while to come. We leave it in this point after decades of work on the subject both practical and scientific that we hope have improved the patients and physicians options as we try to show in the book and emphasize in the presented selection algorithm.


M. Sindou, A. Brinzeu, *Trigeminal Neuralgias: A Neurosurgical Illustrated Guide*,
https://doi.org/10.1007/978-3-031-25113-9

# References

Abdennebi B, Mahfouf L, Nedjahi T. Long-term results of percutaneous compression of the gasserian ganglion in trigeminal neuralgia (series of 200 patients). Stereotact Funct Neurosurg. 1997;68(1–4 Pt 1):190–5.

Adams CB. Microvascular compression: an alternative view and hypothesis. J Neurosurg. 1989;70(1):1–12.

Alvernia JE, Sindou MP, Dang ND, Maley JH, Mertens P. Percutaneous approach to the foramen ovale: an anatomical study of the extracranial trajectory with the incorrect trajectories to be avoided. Acta Neurochir. 2010;152(6):1043–53.

Antherieu P, Vassal F, Sindou M. Vagoglossopharyngeal neuralgia revealed through predominant digestive vagal manifestations. Case report and literature review. Neurochirurgie. 2016;62(3):174–7.

Arias MJ. Percutaneous retrogasserian glycerol rhizotomy for trigeminal neuralgia. A prospective study of 100 cases. J Neurosurg. 1986;65(1):32–6.

Asplund P, Blomstedt P, Bergenheim AT. Percutaneous balloon compression vs percutaneous retrogasserian glycerol rhizotomy for the primary treatment of trigeminal neuralgia. Neurosurgery. 2016;78(3):421–8. discussion 428

Baabor MG, Perez-Limonte L. Percutaneous balloon compression of the gasserian ganglion for the treatment of trigeminal neuralgia: personal experience of 206 patients. Acta Neurochir Suppl. 2011;108:251–4.

Barker FG 2nd, Jannetta PJ, Bissonette DJ, Larkins MV, Jho HD. The long-term outcome of microvascular decompression for trigeminal neuralgia. N Engl J Med. 1996;334(17):1077–83.

Barker FG 2nd, Jannetta PJ, Bissonette DJ, Jho HD. Trigeminal numbness and tic relief after microvascular decompression for typical trigeminal neuralgia. Neurosurgery. 1997;40(1):39–45.

Basser PJ, Pierpaoli C. Microstructural and physiological features of tissues elucidated by quantitative-diffusion-tensor MRI. 1996. J Magn Reson. 2011;213(2):560–70.

Bederson JB, Wilson CB. Evaluation of microvascular decompression and partial sensory rhizotomy in 252 cases of trigeminal neuralgia. J Neurosurg. 1989;71(3):359–67.

Bendtsen L, Zakrzewska JM, Abbott J, Braschinsky M, Di Stefano G, Donnet A, Eide PK, Leal PRL, Maarbjerg S, May A, Nurmikko T, Obermann M, Jensen TS, Cruccu G. European Academy of Neurology guideline on trigeminal neuralgia. Eur J Neurol. 2019;26(6):831–49.

Bendtsen L, Zakrzewska JM, Heinskou TB, Hodaie M, Leal PRL, Nurmikko T, Obermann M, Cruccu G, Maarbjerg S. Advances in diagnosis, classification, pathophysiology, and management of trigeminal neuralgia. Lancet Neurol. 2020;19(9):784–96.

Bergenheim AT, Asplund P, Linderoth B. Percutaneous retrogasserian balloon compression for trigeminal neuralgia: review of critical technical details and outcomes. World Neurosurg. 2013;79(2):359–68.

Bergouignan M. [Fifteen years of trial therapy of essential trigeminal neuralgia: the place of diphenylhydantoin and its derivatives]. Rev Neurol (Paris). 1958;98(5):414–6.

Bergouignan M. [Anti-epileptic drugs in the treatment of essential trigeminal neuralgia]. Presse Med (1893). 1970;78(42):1832–4.

Bergouignan M, D'Aulnay N. [Effect of diphenylhydantoinate salt on essential trigeminal neuralgia]. Rev Otoneuroophtalmol. 1951;23(7):427–31.

Bernard F, Mercier P, Sindou M. Morphological and functional anatomy of the trigeminal triangular plexus as an anatomical entity: a systematic review. Surg Radiol Anat. 2019;41(6):625–37.

Blom S. Trigeminal neuralgia: its treatment with a new anticonvulsant drug (G-32883). Lancet. 1962;1(7234):839–40.

Blomstedt PC, Bergenheim AT. Technical difficulties and perioperative complications of retrogasserian glycerol rhizotomy for trigeminal neuralgia. Stereotact Funct Neurosurg. 2002;79(3–4):168–81.

Bobek MP, Sagher O. Aseptic meningitis caused by Teflon implantation for microvascular decompression. Case report. J Neurosurg. 1999;90(1):145–7.

Bond AE, Zada G, Gonzalez AA, Hansen C, Giannotta SL. Operative strategies for minimizing hearing loss and other major complications associated with microvascular decompression for trigeminal neuralgia. World Neurosurg. 2010;74(1):172–7.


M. Sindou, A. Brinzeu, *Trigeminal Neuralgias: A Neurosurgical Illustrated Guide*,
https://doi.org/10.1007/978-3-031-25113-9

Brinzeu A, Drogba L, Sindou M. Reliability of MRI for predicting characteristics of neurovascular conflicts in trigeminal neuralgia: implications for surgical decision making. J Neurosurg. 2018a:1–11. https://doi.org/10.3171/2017.8.JNS171222.

Brinzeu A, Dumot C, Sindou M. Role of the petrous ridge and angulation of the trigeminal nerve in the pathogenesis of trigeminal neuralgia, with implications for microvascular decompression. Acta Neurochir. 2018b;160(5):971–6.

Broggi G, Franzini A, Lasio G, Giorgi C, Servello D. Long-term results of percutaneous retrogasserian thermorhizotomy for "essential" trigeminal neuralgia: considerations in 1000 consecutive patients. Neurosurgery. 1990;26(5):783–6. discussion 786–787

Broggi G, Ferroli P, Franzini A, Servello D, Dones I. Microvascular decompression for trigeminal neuralgia: comments on a series of 250 cases, including 10 patients with multiple sclerosis. J Neurol Neurosurg Psychiatry. 2000;68(1):59–64.

Brown JA, Gouda JJ. Percutaneous balloon compression of the trigeminal nerve. Neurosurg Clin N Am. 1997;8(1):53–62.

Burchiel KJ. Abnormal impulse generation in focally demyelinated trigeminal roots. J Neurosurg. 1980a;53(5):674–83.

Burchiel KJ. Ectopic impulse generation in focally demyelinated trigeminal nerve. Exp Neurol. 1980b;69(2):423–9.

Burchiel KJ. Ectopic impulse generation in demyelinated axons: effects of PaCO2, pH, and disodium edetate. Ann Neurol. 1981;9(4):378–83.

Burchiel KJ. Facial pain syndromes: practical considerations. Clin Neurosurg. 2000;46:435–45.

Burchiel KJ. A new classification for facial pain. Neurosurgery. 2003;53(5):1164–6. discussion 1166–1167

Burchiel KJ. Trigeminal neuralgia: new evidence for origins and surgical treatment. Neurosurgery. 2016;63(Suppl 1):52–5.

Calvin WH, Devor M, Howe JF. Can neuralgias arise from minor demyelination? Spontaneous firing, mechanosensitivity, and afterdischarge from conducting axons. Exp Neurol. 1982;75(3):755–63.

Cappabianca P, Spaziante R, Graziussi G, Taglialatela G, Peca C, De Divitiis E. Percutaneous retrogasserian glycerol rhizolysis for treatment of trigeminal neuralgia. Technique and results in 191 patients. J Neurosurg Sci. 1995;39(1):37–45.

Chen JF, Lee ST. Comparison of percutaneous trigeminal ganglion compression and microvascular decompression for the management of trigeminal neuralgia. Clin Neurol Neurosurg. 2003;105(3):203–8.

Chen J, Sindou M. Vago-glossopharyngeal neuralgia: a literature review of neurosurgical experience. Acta Neurochir. 2015;157(2):311–21. discussion 321

Chen J, Lee S, Lui T, Yeh Y, Chen T, Tzaan W. Teflon granuloma after microvascular decompression for trigeminal neuralgia. Surg Neurol. 2000;53(3):281–7.

Cho DY, Chang CG, Wang YC, Wang FH, Shen CC, Yang DY. Repeat operations in failed microvascular decompression for trigeminal neuralgia. Neurosurgery. 1994;35(4):665–9. discussion 669-670

Corrêa CF, Teixeira MJ. Balloon compression of the Gasserian ganglion for the treatment of trigeminal neuralgia. Stereotact Funct Neurosurg. 1998;71(2):83–9.

Cruccu G, Finnerup NB, Jensen TS, Scholz J, Sindou M, Svensson P, Treede RD, Zakrzewska JM, Nurmikko T. Trigeminal neuralgia: new classification and diagnostic grading for practice and research. Neurology. 2016;87(2):220–8.

Cushing H. Landmark article April 28, 1900: A method of total extirpation of the Gasserian ganglion for trigeminal neuralgia. By a route through the temporal fossa and beneath the middle meningeal artery. By Harvey Cushing. JAMA. 1983;250(4):519–28. https://doi.org/10.1001/jama.250.4.519. PMID: 6345823.

Cutbush K, Atkinson RL. Treatment of trigeminal neuralgia by posterior fossa microvascular decompression. Aust N Z J Surg. 1994;64(3):173–6.

Drake CG, Mckenzie KG. Mesencephalic tractotomy for pain: experience with six cases. J Neurosurg. 1953;10(5):457–62. https://doi.org/10.3171/jns.1953.10.5.0457. PMID: 13097205.

Dandy W. Section of the sensory root of the trigeminal nerve at the pons.; Preliminary report of the operative procedure. Baltimore: Bulletin of the Jhons Hokins Hospital; 1925.

Dandy WE. The treatment of trigeminal neuralgia by the cerebellar route. Ann Surg. 1932;96(4):787–95.

De La Peña NM, Singh R, Anderson ML, Koester SW, Sio TT, Ashman JB, Vora SA, Patel NP. High-dose frameless stereotactic radiosurgery for trigeminal neuralgia: a single-institution experience and systematic review. World Neurosurg. 2022; https://doi.org/10.1016/j.wneu.2022.08.038.

De Ridder D, Møller A, Verlooy J, Cornelissen M, De Ridder L. Is the root entry/exit zone important in microvascular compression syndromes? Neurosurgery. 2002;51(2):427–33. discussion 433–424

de Siqueira SR, da Nóbrega JC, de Siqueira JT, Teixeira MJ. Frequency of postoperative complications after balloon compression for idiopathic trigeminal neuralgia: prospective study. Oral Surg Oral Med Oral Pathol Oral Radiol Endod. 2006;102(5):e39–45.

DeSouza DD, Davis KD, Hodaie M. Reversal of insular and microstructural nerve abnormalities following effective surgical treatment for trigeminal neuralgia. Pain. 2015;156(6):1112–23.

DeSouza DD, Hodaie M, Davis KD. Structural magnetic resonance imaging can identify trigeminal system abnormalities in classical trigeminal neuralgia. Front Neuroanat. 2016;10:95.

Devor M, Amir R, Rappaport ZH. Pathophysiology of trigeminal neuralgia: the ignition hypothesis. Clin J Pain. 2002a;18(1):4–13.

Devor M, Govrin-Lippmann R, Rappaport ZH. Mechanism of trigeminal neuralgia: an ultrastructural analysis of trigeminal root specimens obtained during microvascular decompression surgery. J Neurosurg. 2002b;96(3):532–43.

Di Stefano G, La Cesa S, Truini A, Cruccu G. Natural history and outcome of 200 outpatients with classical trigeminal neuralgia treated with carbamazepine or oxcarbazepine in a tertiary centre for neuropathic pain. J Headache Pain. 2014;15(1):34.

Di Stefano G, Truini A, Cruccu G. Current and innovative pharmacological options to treat typical and atypical trigeminal neuralgia. Drugs. 2018;78(14): 1433–42.

Di Stefano G, De Stefano G, Leone C, Cruccu G, Tardioli S, Cartocci G, Fiorelli M, Truini A, Caramia F. Concomitant continuous pain in patients with trigeminal neuralgia is associated with trigeminal nerve root atrophy. Cephalalgia. 2020;40(13):1502–10.

Di Stefano G, De Stefano G, Leone C, Di Lionardo A, Di Pietro G, Sgro E, Mollica C, Cruccu G, Truini A. Real-world effectiveness and tolerability of carbamazepine and oxcarbazepine in 354 patients with trigeminal neuralgia. Eur J Pain. 2021;25(5):1064–71.

Dieckmann G, Bockermann V, Heyer C, Henning J, Roesen M. Five-and-a-half years' experience with percutaneous retrogasserian glycerol rhizotomy in treatment of trigeminal neuralgia. Appl Neurophysiol. 1987;50(1–6):401–13.

Dhople AA, Adams JR, Maggio WW, Naqvi SA, Regine WF, Kwok Y. Long-term outcomes of Gamma Knife radiosurgery for classic trigeminal neuralgia: implications of treatment and critical review of the literature. Clinical article. J Neurosurg. 2009;111(2):351–8.

Du Y, Yang D, Dong X, Du Q, Wang H, Yu W. Percutaneous balloon compression (PBC) of trigeminal ganglion for recurrent trigeminal neuralgia after microvascular decompression (MVD). Ir J Med Sci. 2015;184(4):745–51.

Dumot C, Sindou M. Trigeminal neuralgia due to neurovascular conflicts from venous origin: an anatomical-surgical study (consecutive series of 124 operated cases). Acta Neurochir. 2015;157(3):455–66.

Dumot C, Sindou M. Veins of the cerebellopontine angle and specific complications of sacrifice, with special emphasis on microvascular decompression surgery. A review. World Neurosurg. 2018;117:422–32.

Dumot C, Brinzeu A, Berthiller J, Sindou M. Trigeminal neuralgia due to venous neurovascular conflicts: outcome after microvascular decompression in a series of 55 consecutive patients. Acta Neurochir. 2017;159(2):237–49.

Emmons WF, Rhoton AL Jr. Functional subdivision of the trigeminal sensory root. Surg Forum. 1968;19:440–1.

Fertleman CR, Baker MD, Parker KA, Moffatt S, Elmslie FV, Abrahamsen B, Ostman J, Klugbauer N, Wood JN, Gardiner RM, Rees M. SCN9A mutations in paroxysmal extreme pain disorder: allelic variants underlie distinct channel defects and phenotypes. Neuron. 2006;52(5):767–74.

Fish CJ, Blakemore WF. A model of chronic spinal cord compression in the cat. Neuropathol Appl Neurobiol. 1983;9(2):109–19.

Fountas KN, Smith JR, Lee GP, Jenkins PD, Cantrell RR, Sheils WC. Gamma-Knife stereotactic radiosurgical treatment of idiopathic trigeminal neuralgia: long-term outcome and complications. Neurosurg Focus. 2007;23(6):E8. PMID: 18081485.

Fraioli B, Esposito V, Guidetti B, Cruccu G, Manfredi M. Treatment of trigeminal neuralgia by thermocoagulation, glycerolization, and percutaneous compression of the gasserian ganglion and/or retrogasserian rootlets: long-term results and therapeutic protocol. Neurosurgery. 1989;24(2):239–45.

Frank F, Fabrizi AP. Percutaneous surgical treatment of trigeminal neuralgia. Acta Neurochir. 1989;97(3–4):128–30.

Frazier CH. Subtotal resection of sensory root for relief of major trigeminal neuralgia. Arch Neurol Psychiatry. 1925;13(3):378–84.

Fromm GH, Graff-Radford SB, Terrence CF, Sweet WH. Pre-trigeminal neuralgia. Neurology. 1990;40(10):1493–5.

Fujimaki T, Fukushima T, Miyazaki S. Percutaneous retrogasserian glycerol injection in the management of trigeminal neuralgia: long-term follow-up results. J Neurosurg. 1990;73(2):212–6.

Fujimaki T, Hoya K, Sasaki T, Kirino T. Recurrent trigeminal neuralgia caused by an inserted prosthesis: report of two cases. Acta Neurochir. 1996;138(11):1307–9. discussion 1310

Gardner WJ. Concerning the mechanism of trigeminal neuralgia and hemifacial spasm. J Neurosurg. 1962;19:947–58.

Gledhill RF, Harrison BM, McDonald WI. Demyelination and remyelination after acute spinal cord compression. Exp Neurol. 1973;38(3):472–87.

Grewal SS, Kerezoudis P, Garcia O, Quinones-Hinojosa A, Reimer R, Wharen RE. Results of percutaneous balloon compression in trigeminal pain syndromes. World Neurosurg. 2018;114:e892–9.

Guclu B, Sindou M, Meyronet D, Streichenberger N, Simon E, Mertens P. Cranial nerve vascular compression syndromes of the trigeminal, facial and vago-glossopharyngeal nerves: comparative anatomical study of the central myelin portion and transitional zone; correlations with incidences of corresponding hyperactive dysfunctional syndromes. Acta Neurochir. 2011;153(12):2365–75.

Gudmundsson K, Rhoton AL Jr, Rushton JG. Detailed anatomy of the intracranial portion of the trigeminal nerve. J Neurosurg. 1971;35(5):592–600.

Gybels JM, Sweet WH. Neurosurgical treatment of persistent pain. Physiological and pathological mechanisms of human pain. Pain Headache. 1989;11:1–402.

Ha SM, Kim SH, Yoo EH, Han IB, Shin DA, Cho KG, Chung SS, Park YS. Patients with idiopathic trigeminal neuralgia have a sharper-than-normal trigeminal-pontine angle and trigeminal nerve atrophy. Acta Neurochir. 2012;154(9):1627–33.

Håkanson S. Transoval trigeminal cisternography. Surg Neurol. 1978;10(2):137–44.

Håkanson S. Trigeminal neuralgia treated by the injection of glycerol into the trigeminal cistern. Neurosurgery. 1981;9(6):638–46.

Han PP, Shetter AG, Smith KA, Fiedler JA, Rogers CL, Speiser B, Feiz-Erfan I. Gamma knife radiosurgery for trigeminal neuralgia: experience at the Barrow Neurological Institute. Stereotact Funct Neurosurg. 1999;73(1–4):131–3.

Harris W. Alcohol injection of the gasserian ganglion for trigeminal neuralgia. Lancet. 1912a;179(4613): 218–21.

Harris W. Three cases of alcohol injection of the gasserian ganglion for trigeminal neuralgia. Proc R Soc Med. 1912b;5(Clin Sect):115–9.

Harris W. An analysis of 1,433 cases of paroxysmal trigeminal neuralgia (trigeminal-tic) and the end-results of gasserian alcohol injection. Brain. 1940;63(3):209–24.

Hartel F. Die Leitungsanasthese und Injecktionbehandlung des Ganglion gasseri und der Trigeminusstamme. Arch Klin Chir. 1912;100:627–38.

Haskel RBL, Berry MM, Standing SM. Nervous system. In: Williams PL, editor. Gray's anatomy. 38th ed. London: Churchill Livingstone; 1995. p. 1158–60.

Hayashi M, Chernov M, Tamura N, Takakura K. Stereotactic radiosurgery of essential trigeminal neuralgia using Leksell Gamma-knife model C with automatic system. Neurosurg Rev. 2011;34(4):497–508.

Henson CF, Goldman HW, Rosenwasser RH, Downes MB, Bednarz G, Pequignot EC, Werner-Wasik M, Curran WJ, Andrews DW. Glycerol rhizotomy versus gamma knife radiosurgery for the treatment of trigeminal neuralgia: an analysis of patients treated at one institution. Int J Radiat Oncol Biol Phys. 2005;63(1):82–90.

Hartley FI. Intracranial neurectomy of the fifth nerve. Ann Surg. 1893;17(5):511–26.1. https://doi.org/10.1097/00000658-189301000-00120. PMID: 17859915; PMCID: PMC1492970.

Hilton DA, Love S, Gradidge T, Coakham HB. Pathological findings associated with trigeminal neuralgia caused by vascular compression. Neurosurgery. 1994;35(2):299–303. discussion 303

Honey CR, Gooderham P, Morrison M, Ivanishvili Z. Episodic hemilaryngopharyngeal spasm (HELPS) syndrome: case report of a surgically treatable novel neuropathy. J Neurosurg. 2017;126(5):1653–6.

Horsley V. Remarks on the various surgical procedures devised for the relief or cure of trigeminal neuralgia (tic douloureux). Br Med J. 1891c;2(1615):1249–52. https://doi.org/10.1136/bmj.2.1615.1249. PMID: 20753459; PMCID: PMC227394.

Horsley V. Remarks on the Various Surgical Procedures Devised for the Relief or Cure of Trigeminal Neuralgia (Tic Douloureux). Br Med J. 1891a;2(1615):1249–52. https://doi.org/10.1136/bmj.2.1615.1249. PMID: 20753459; PMCID: PMC2273941.

Horsley V. Remarks on the Various Surgical Procedures Devised for the Relief or Cure of Trigeminal Neuralgia (Tic Douloureux). Br Med J. 1891b;2(1613):1139–43. https://doi.org/10.1136/bmj.2.1613.1139. PMID: 20753444; PMCID: PMC2273522.

Huang J, Han C, Estacion M, Vasylyev D, Hoeijmakers JG, Gerrits MM, Tyrrell L, Lauria G, Faber CG, Dib-Hajj SD, Merkies IS, Waxman SG. Gain-of-function mutations in sodium channel Na(v)1.9 in painful neuropathy. Brain. 2014;137(Pt 6):1627–42.

IHS. Headache Classification Committee of the International Headache Society (IHS) The International Classification of Headache Disorders, 3rd edition. Cephalalgia. 2018;38(1):1–211.

Illingworth NM. Trigeminal neuralgia treated by microvascular decompression: a long-term follow-up study. Br J Neurosurg. 1995;9(1):13–20.

Ischia S, Luzzani A, Polati E. Retrogasserian glycerol injection: a retrospective study of 112 patients. Clin J Pain. 1990;6(4):291–6.

Jaeger R. The results of injecting hot water into the gasserian ganglion for the relief of tic douloureux. J Neurosurg. 1959;16:656–63.

Jannetta PJ. Arterial compression of the trigeminal nerve at the pons in patients with trigeminal neuralgia. J Neurosurg. 1967;26(Suppl 1):159–62.

Jannetta PJ. Treatment of trigeminal neuralgia by suboccipital and transtentorial cranial operations. Clin Neurosurg. 1977;24:538–49.

Jannetta PJ, Rand RW. Transtentorial retrogasserian rhizotomy in trigeminal neuralgia by microneurosurgical technique. Bull Los Angel Neurol Soc. 1966;31(3):93–9.

Jefferson A. Trigeminal root and ganglion injections using phenol in glycerine for the relief of trigeminal neuralgia. J Neurol Neurosurg Psychiatry. 1963;26(4):345–52.

Jho HD, Lunsford LD. Percutaneous retrogasserian glycerol rhizotomy. Current technique and results. Neurosurg Clin N Am. 1997;8(1):63–74.

Joo W, Yoshioka F, Funaki T, Mizokami K, Rhoton AL Jr. Microsurgical anatomy of the trigeminal nerve. Clin Anat. 2014;27(1):61–88.

Kanpolat Y, Savas A, Bekar A, Berk C. Percutaneous controlled radiofrequency trigeminal rhizotomy for the treatment of idiopathic trigeminal neuralgia: 25-year experience with 1,600 patients. Neurosurgery. 2001;48(3):524–32. discussion 532–524

Karol EA, Sanz OP, Rey RD. Sensory and motor trigeminal evoked potentials to localize the position of trigeminal electrodes. Acta Neurochir. 1991;108(3–4):110–5.

Katusic S, Williams DB, Beard CM, Bergstralh EJ, Kurland LT. Epidemiology and clinical features of idiopathic trigeminal neuralgia and glossopharyngeal neuralgia: similarities and differences, Rochester, Minnesota, 1945–1984. Neuroepidemiology. 1991;10(5–6):276–81.

Keravel Y, Gaston A, Ciampi de Andrade D, Mencattini G, Le Guérinel C. [Balloon compression for the

treatment of trigeminal neuralgia]. Neurochirurgie. 2009;55(2):197–202.
Kerr FW. Evidence for a peripheral etiology of trigeminal neuralgia. J Neurosurg. 1967a;26(Suppl 1):168–74.
Kerr FW. Pathology of trigeminal neuralgia: light and electron microscopic observations. J Neurosurg. 1967b;26(Suppl 1):151–6.
Kerr FW, Miller RH. The pathology of trigeminal neuralgia. Electron microscopic studies. Arch Neurol. 1966;15(3):308–19.
Kirschner M. The puncturing technique and the electrocoagulation of the Ganglion Gasseri: transferred. operations (DiePunktiostechnik und die Elektrocoagulation des Ganglion Gasseri: übergez Operationen) German. Arch Klin Chir. 1933;176:620.
Klun B. Microvascular decompression and partial sensory rhizotomy in the treatment of trigeminal neuralgia: personal experience with 220 patients. Neurosurgery. 1992;30(1):49–52.
Klun B, Prestor B. Microvascular relations of the trigeminal nerve: an anatomical study. Neurosurgery. 1986;19(4):535–9.
Ko AL, Ozpinar A, Lee A, Raslan AM, McCartney S, Burchiel KJ. Long-term efficacy and safety of internal neurolysis for trigeminal neuralgia without neurovascular compression. J Neurosurg. 2015;122(5):1048–57.
Kondo A. Follow-up results of microvascular decompression in trigeminal neuralgia and hemifacial spasm. Neurosurgery. 1997;40(1):46–51. discussion 51–42
Kondziolka D, Lunsford LD. Percutaneous retrogasserian glycerol rhizotomy for trigeminal neuralgia: technique and expectations. Neurosurg Focus. 2005;18(5):E7.
Kondziolka D, Flickinger JC, Lunsford LD, Habeck M. Trigeminal neuralgia radiosurgery: the University of Pittsburgh experience. Stereotact Funct Neurosurg. 1996a;66(Suppl 1):343–8.
Kondziolka D, Lunsford LD, Flickinger JC, Young RF, Vermeulen S, Duma CM, Jacques DB, Rand RW, Regis J, Peragut JC, Manera L, Epstein MH, Lindquist C. Stereotactic radiosurgery for trigeminal neuralgia: a multiinstitutional study using the gamma unit. J Neurosurg. 1996b;84(6):940–5.
Kondziolka D, Zorro O, Lobato-Polo J, et al. Gamma Knife stereotactic radiosurgery for idiopathic trigeminal neuralgia. J Neurosurg. 2010;112(4):758–65.
Kotecha M, Cheshire WP, Finnigan H, Giblin K, Naik H, Palmer J, Tate S, Zakrzewska JM. Design of phase 3 studies evaluating vixotrigine for treatment of trigeminal neuralgia. J Pain Res. 2020;13:1601–9.
Kourilsky A, Palpacuer C, Rogers A, Chauvet D, Wiart C, Bourdillon P, Le Guérinel C. Multivariate models to predict pain recurrence and sensitive complications after percutaneous balloon compression in trigeminal neuralgia. J Neurosurg. 2022:1–10. https://doi.org/10.3171/2022.2.JNS212644.
Kubicek GJ, Hall WA, Orner JB, Gerbi BJ, Dusenbery KE. Long-term follow-up of trigeminal neuralgia treatment using a linear accelerator. Stereotact Funct Neurosurg. 2004;82(5–6):244–9.
Kunc Z. [Sjoqvist's tractotomy]. Rozhl Chir. 1959;38:733–44.
Kunc Z. [Some anatomical problems in the spinal trigeminal tract and its nucleus]. Cesk Neurol. 1964;27:353–60.
Kunc Z. [Modification of trigeminal tractotomy by partial vertical nucleotomy]. Cesk Neurol Neurochir. 1977;40(4):201–5.
Kunc Z, Fuchsová M, Novák M. Excision of the spinal trigeminal tract. Electron microscopy. Acta Neurochir. 1978;41(1–3):233–41.
Kureshi SA, Wilkins RH. Posterior fossa reexploration for persistent or recurrent trigeminal neuralgia or hemifacial spasm: surgical findings and therapeutic implications. Neurosurgery. 1998;43(5):1111–7.
Le Bihan D. Molecular diffusion, tissue microdynamics and microstructure. NMR Biomed. 1995;8(7–8):375–86.
Leal PR, Hermier M, Froment JC, Souza MA, Cristino-Filho G, Sindou M. Preoperative demonstration of the neurovascular compression characteristics with special emphasis on the degree of compression, using high-resolution magnetic resonance imaging: a prospective study, with comparison to surgical findings, in 100 consecutive patients who underwent microvascular decompression for trigeminal neuralgia. Acta Neurochir. 2010;152(5):817–25.
Leal PR, Hermier M, Souza MA, Cristino-Filho G, Froment JC, Sindou M. Visualization of vascular compression of the trigeminal nerve with high-resolution 3T MRI: a prospective study comparing preoperative imaging analysis to surgical findings in 40 consecutive patients who underwent microvascular decompression for trigeminal neuralgia. Neurosurgery. 2011a;69(1):15–25. discussion 26
Leal PR, Roch JA, Hermier M, Souza MA, Cristino-Filho G, Sindou M. Structural abnormalities of the trigeminal root revealed by diffusion tensor imaging in patients with trigeminal neuralgia caused by neurovascular compression: a prospective, double-blind, controlled study. Pain. 2011b;152(10):2357–64.
Leal PRL, Roch J, Hermier M, Berthezene Y, Sindou M. Diffusion tensor imaging abnormalities of the trigeminal nerve root in patients with classical trigeminal neuralgia: a pre- and postoperative comparative study 4 years after microvascular decompression. Acta Neurochir. 2019;161(7):1415–25.
Lee KH, Chang JW, Park YG, Chung SS. Microvascular decompression and percutaneous rhizotomy in trigeminal neuralgia. Stereotact Funct Neurosurg. 1997;68(1–4 Pt 1):196–9.
Lee JY, Sandhu S, Miller D, Solberg T, Dorsey JF, Alonso-Basanta M. Higher dose rate Gamma Knife radiosurgery may provide earlier and longer-lasting pain relief

for patients with trigeminal neuralgia. J Neurosurg. 2015;123(4):961–8.

Leksell L. The stereotaxic method and radiosurgery of the brain. Acta Chir Scand. 1951;102(4):316–9. PMID: 14914373.

Leksell L. Sterotaxic radiosurgery in trigeminal neuralgia. Acta Chir Scand. 1971;137(4):311–4.

Leal PR, Barbier C, Hermier M, Souza MA, Cristino-Filho G, Sindou M. Atrophic changes in the trigeminal nerves of patients with trigeminal neuralgia due to neurovascular compression and their association with the severity of compression and clinical outcomes. J Neurosurg. 2014;120(6):1484–95. https://doi.org/10.3171/2014.2.JNS131288. Epub 2014 Apr 18. PMID: 24745706.

Li S-T, Sun H. Surgical techniques of microvascular decompression for hemifacial spasm. In: Li S-T, Zhong J, Sekula JRF, editors. Microvascular decompression surgery. Dordrecht: Springer Netherlands; 2016. p. 79–93.

Liao JJ, Cheng WC, Chang CN, Yang JT, Wei KC, Hsu YH, Lin TK. Reoperation for recurrent trigeminal neuralgia after microvascular decompression. Surg Neurol. 1997;47(6):562–8. discussion 568–570

Lichtor T, Mullan JF. A 10-year follow-up review of percutaneous microcompression of the trigeminal ganglion. J Neurosurg. 1990;72(1):49–54.

Lobato RD, Rivas JJ, Sarabia R, Lamas E. Percutaneous microcompression of the gasserian ganglion for trigeminal neuralgia. J Neurosurg. 1990;72(4):546–53.

Loeser JD. Tic douloureux and atycial facial pain. In: Wall PD, editor. Textbook of pain. New York: Churchill Livingstone; 1994. p. 1.

Love S, Coakham HB. Trigeminal neuralgia: pathology and pathogenesis. Brain. 2001;124(Pt 12):2347–60.

Love S, Hilton DA, Coakham HB. Central demyelination of the Vth nerve root in trigeminal neuralgia associated with vascular compression. Brain Pathol. 1998;8(1):1–11. discussion 11-12

Longhi M, Rizzo P, Nicolato A, Foroni R, Reggio M, Gerosa M. Gamma knife radiosurgery for trigeminal neuralgia: results and potentially predictive parameters—part I: idiopathic trigeminal neuralgia. Neurosurgery. 2007;61(6):1254–60 PMID: 18162905.

Lunsford LD. Treatment of tic douloureux by percutaneous retrogasserian glycerol injection. JAMA. 1982;248(4):449–53.

Maarbjerg S, Gozalov A, Olesen J, Bendtsen L. Concomitant persistent pain in classical trigeminal neuralgia—evidence for different subtypes. Headache. 2014a;54(7):1173–83.

Maarbjerg S, Gozalov A, Olesen J, Bendtsen L. Trigeminal neuralgia—a prospective systematic study of clinical characteristics in 158 patients. Headache. 2014b;54(10):1574–82.

Maarbjerg S, Sørensen MT, Gozalov A, Bendtsen L, Olesen J. Field-testing of the ICHD-3 beta diagnostic criteria for classical trigeminal neuralgia. Cephalalgia. 2015a;35(4):291–300.

Maarbjerg S, Wolfram F, Gozalov A, Olesen J, Bendtsen L. Significance of neurovascular contact in classical trigeminal neuralgia. Brain. 2015b;138(Pt 2):311–9.

Magown P, Ko AL, Burchiel KJ. The spectrum of trigeminal neuralgia without neurovascular compression. Neurosurgery. 2019;85(3):E553–e559.

Manzoni GC, Torelli P. Epidemiology of typical and atypical craniofacial neuralgias. Neurol Sci. 2005;26(Suppl 2):s65–7.

Marshall K, Chan MD, McCoy TP, et al. Predictive variables for the successful treatment of trigeminal neuralgia with gamma knife radiosurgery. Neurosurgery. 2012;70(3):566–72.

Mathews ES, Scrivani SJ. Percutaneous stereotactic radiofrequency thermal rhizotomy for the treatment of trigeminal neuralgia. Mt Sinai J Med. 2000;67(4):288–99.

Matsushima T, Rhoton AL Jr, de Oliveira E, Peace D. Microsurgical anatomy of the veins of the posterior fossa. J Neurosurg. 1983;59(1):63–105.

Matsushima T, Yamaguchi T, Inoue TK, Matsukado K, Fukui M. Recurrent trigeminal neuralgia after microvascular decompression using an interposing technique. Teflon felt adhesion and the sling retraction technique. Acta Neurochir. 2000;142(5):557–61.

Mazzucchi E, Brinzeu A, Sindou M. Arachnoiditis as an outcome factor for microvascular decompression in classical trigeminal neuralgia. Acta Neurochir. 2019;161(8):1589–98.

Megerian CA, Busaba NY, McKenna MJ, Ojemann RG. Teflon granuloma presenting as an enlarging, gadolinium enhancing, posterior fossa mass with progressive hearing loss following microvascular decompression. Am J Otol. 1995;16(6):783–6.

Mckenzie KG. Trigeminal tractotomy. Clin Neurosurg. 1954;2:50–69; discussion, 69–70. PMID: 13270405.

Messerer M, Dubourg J, Saint-Pierre G, Jouanneau E, Sindou M. Percutaneous biopsy of lesions in the cavernous sinus region through the foramen ovale: diagnostic accuracy and limits in 50 patients. J Neurosurg. 2012;116(2):390–8.

Miller JP, Acar F, Burchiel KJ. Classification of trigeminal neuralgia: clinical, therapeutic, and prognostic implications in a series of 144 patients undergoing microvascular decompression. J Neurosurg. 2009a;111(6):1231–4.

Miller JP, Acar F, Hamilton BE, Burchiel KJ. Radiographic evaluation of trigeminal neurovascular compression in patients with and without trigeminal neuralgia. J Neurosurg. 2009b;110(4):627–32.

Møller AR. The cranial nerve vascular compression syndrome: II. A review of pathophysiology. Acta Neurochir. 1991;113(1–2):24–30.

Mueller HR, Levy A. [On the pathogenesis of trigeminal neuralgia. Study of mechanical factors by means of craniometry]. Acta Neurochir. 1963;11:385–97.

Mullan S, Lichtor T. Percutaneous microcompression of the trigeminal ganglion for trigeminal neuralgia. J Neurosurg. 1983;59(6):1007–12.

Noorani I, Lodge A, Vajramani G, Sparrow O. Comparing percutaneous treatments of trigeminal neuralgia: 19 years of experience in a single centre. Stereotact Funct Neurosurg. 2016;94(2):75–85.

Nugent GR. Surgical treatment: radiofrequency gangliolysis and rhizotomy. In: Fromm GH, Sessle BJ, editors. Trigeminal neuralgia: current concepts regarding pathogenesis and treatment. Stoneham: Butterworth-Heinemann; 1991. p. 159–84.

Obersteiner H, Redlich E. Uber Wessen und Pathogenese der tabischen Hinterstrangsdegeneration. Arb Nuerol Inst Wien Univ. 1884;1–3:158–72.

Oesman C, Mooij JJ. Long-term follow-up of microvascular decompression for trigeminal neuralgia. Skull Base. 2011;21(5):313–22.

Olivecrona H. Tractotomy for relief of trigeminal neuralgia. Arch Neurol Psychiatry. 1942;47(4):544–64.

Olson S, Atkinson L, Weidmann M. Microvascular decompression for trigeminal neuralgia: recurrences and complications. J Clin Neurosci. 2005;12(7):787–9.

Parise M, Ribeiro CT, Vincent M, Gasparetto E. Small cerebellopontine angle cisterns inpatients with trigeminal neuralgia. J Neurosurg. 2010;112(4):900–1. author reply 901

Parise M, Acioly MA, Ribeiro CT, Vincent M, Gasparetto EL. The role of the cerebellopontine angle cistern area and trigeminal nerve length in the pathogenesis of trigeminal neuralgia: a prospective case-control study. Acta Neurochir. 2013;155(5):863–8.

Parise M, Kubo TT, Doring TM, Tukamoto G, Vincent M, Gasparetto EL. Cuneus and fusiform cortices thickness is reduced in trigeminal neuralgia. J Headache Pain. 2014;15(1):17.

Park KJ, Kondziolka D, Berkowitz O, Kano H, Novotny J Jr, Niranjan A, Flickinger JC, Lunsford LD. Repeat gamma knife radiosurgery for trigeminal neuralgia. Neurosurgery. 2012;70(2):295–305; discussion 305. https://doi.org/10.1227/NEU.0b013e318230218e. PMID: 21811188.

Peker S, Kurtkaya O, Uzün I, Pamir MN. Microanatomy of the central myelin-peripheral myelin transition zone of the trigeminal nerve. Neurosurgery. 2006;59(2):354–9. discussion 354-359

Peris-Celda M, Graziano F, Russo V, Mericle RA, Ulm AJ. Foramen ovale puncture, lesioning accuracy, and avoiding complications: microsurgical anatomy study with clinical implications. J Neurosurg. 2013;119(5):1176–93.

Pierpaoli C, Basser PJ. Toward a quantitative assessment of diffusion anisotropy. Magn Reson Med. 1996;36(6):893–906.

Pierpaoli C, Jezzard P, Basser PJ, Barnett A, Di Chiro G. Diffusion tensor MR imaging of the human brain. Radiology. 1996;201(3):637–48.

Pollock BE. Radiosurgery for trigeminal neuralgia: is sensory disturbance required for pain relief? J Neurosurg. 2006;105(Suppl):103–6.

Pollock BE, Schoeberl KA. Prospective comparison of posterior fossa exploration and stereotactic radiosurgery dorsal root entry zone target as primary surgery for patients with idiopathic trigeminal neuralgia. Neurosurgery. 2010;67(3):633–8. discussion 638–639

Pollock BE, Phuong LK, Gorman DA, Foote RL, Stafford SL. Stereotactic radiosurgery for idiopathic trigeminal neuralgia. J Neurosurg. 2002;97(2):347–53.

Pollock BE, Foote RL, Link MJ, Stafford SL, Brown PD, Schomberg PJ. Repeat radiosurgery for idiopathic trigeminal neuralgia. Int J Radiat Oncol Biol Phys. 2005;61(1):192–5.

Polo G, Fischer C, Sindou MP, Marneffe V. Brainstem auditory evoked potential monitoring during microvascular decompression for hemifacial spasm: intraoperative brainstem auditory evoked potential changes and warning values to prevent hearing loss—prospective study in a consecutive series of 84 patients. Neurosurgery. 2004;54(1):97–104. discussion 104–106

Poole J, Mercadante V, Singhota S, Nizam K, Zakrzewska JM. Exploring patient satisfaction of a joint-consultation clinic for trigeminal neuralgia: enabling improved decision-making. Br J Pain. 2022;16(2):237–42.

Premsagar IC, Moss T, Coakham HB. Teflon-induced granuloma following treatment of trigeminal neuralgia by microvascular decompression. Report of two cases. J Neurosurg. 1997;87(3):454–7.

Provost J, Hardy J. [Microsurgery of the trigeminal nerve: functional anatomy]. Neurochirurgie. 1970;16(6):459–70.

Rand RW, Jacques DB, Melbye RW, Copcutt BG, Levenick MN, Fisher MR. Leksell Gamma Knife treatment of tic douloureux. Stereotact Funct Neurosurg. 1993;61(Suppl 1):93–102.

Rappaport HZ, Devor M. Trigeminal neuralgia: the role of self-sustaining discharge in the trigeminal ganglion. Pain. 1994;56(2):127–38.

Rappaport ZH, Govrin-Lippmann R, Devor M. An electron-microscopic analysis of biopsy samples of the trigeminal root taken during microvascular decompressive surgery. Stereotact Funct Neurosurg. 1997;68(1–4 Pt 1):182–6.

Rasche D, Kress B, Stippich C, Nennig E, Sartor K, Tronnier VM. Volumetric measurement of the pontomesencephalic cistern in patients with trigeminal neuralgia and healthy controls. Neurosurgery. 2006;59(3):614–20. discussion 614–620

Rasmussen P. Facial pain. I. A prospective survey of 1052 patients with a view of: definition, delimitation, classification, general data, genetic factors, and previous diseases. Acta Neurochir. 1990;107(3–4):112–20.

Rath SA, Klein HJ, Richter HP. Findings and long-term results of subsequent operations after failed microvascular decompression for trigeminal neuralgia. Neurosurgery. 1996;39(5):933–8. discussion 938–940

Régis J. High-dose trigeminal neuralgia radiosurgery associated with increased risk of trigeminal nerve dysfunction. Neurosurgery. 2002;50(6):1401–2. author reply 1402–1403

Régis J, Manera L, Dufour H, Porcheron D, Sedan R, Peragut JC. Effect of the Gamma Knife on trigeminal neuralgia. Stereotact Funct Neurosurg. 1995;64(Suppl 1):182–92.

Régis J, Metellus P, Hayashi M, Roussel P, Donnet A, Bille-Turc F. Prospective controlled trial of gamma knife surgery for essential trigeminal neuralgia. J Neurosurg. 2006;104(6):913–24.

Régis J, Tuleasca C, Resseguier N, Carron R, Donnet A, Yomo S, Gaudart J, Levivier M. The very long-term outcome of radiosurgery for classical trigeminal neuralgia. Stereotact Funct Neurosurg. 2016;94(1):24–32.

Regis J, Tuleasca C, Resseguier N, et al. Long-term safety and efficacy of Gamma Knife surgery in classical trigeminal neuralgia: a 497-patient historical cohort study. J Neurosurg. 2016;124(4):1079–87.

Rhoton AL Jr. The posterior fossa veins. Neurosurgery. 2000;47(3 Suppl):S69–92.

Rose W. Removal of the Gasserian ganglion for severe neuralgia. Lancet. 1890;136(3505). https://doi.org/10.1016/S0140-6736(01)78645-X.

Saini SS. Reterogasserian anhydrous glycerol injection therapy in trigeminal neuralgia: observations in 552 patients. J Neurol Neurosurg Psychiatry. 1987;50(11):1536–8.

Sandel T, Eide PK. Long-term results of microvascular decompression for trigeminal neuralgia and hemifacial spasms according to preoperative symptomatology. Acta Neurochir. 2013;155(9):1681–92. discussion 1692

Sarsam Z, Garcia-Fiñana M, Nurmikko TJ, Varma TR, Eldridge P. The long-term outcome of microvascular decompression for trigeminal neuralgia. Br J Neurosurg. 2010;24(1):18–25.

Schindler WH. Derivatives of iminodibenzyl. Helv Chim Acta. 1954;37:472–3.

Schürmann K, Butz M, Brock M. Temporal retrogasserian resection of trigeminal root versus controlled elective percutaneous electrocoagulation of the ganglion of gasser in the treatment of trigeminal neuralgia. Report on a series of 531 cases. Acta Neurochir. 1972;26(1):33–53.

Shelden CH, Pudenz RH, Freshwater DB, Crue BL. Compression rather than decompression for trigeminal neuralgia. J Neurosurg. 1955;12(2):123–6.

Sheehan J, Pan HC, Stroila M, Steiner L. Gamma knife surgery for trigeminal neuralgia: outcomes and prognostic factors. J Neurosurg. 2005;102(3):434–41.

Siegfried J. Percutaneous controlled thermocoagulation of gasserian ganglion in trigeminal neuralgia: experience with 1000 cases. In: Samii M, Janetta JP, editors. The cranial nerves. Berlin: Springer; 1981. p. 322–30.

Sindou MP. Neurophysiological navigation in the trigeminal nerve: use of masticatory responses and facial motor responses evoked by electrical stimulationof the trigeminal rootlets for RF-thermorhizotomy guidance. Stereotact Funct Neurosurg. 1999;73(1–4):117–21.

Sindou M, Brinzeu A. Névralgie du trijumeau et neurochirurgie. 2018. ISSN 0246-0378. https://doi.org/10.1016/S0246-0378(18)86582-4, http://www.sciencedirect.com/science/article/pii/S0246-0378(18)86582-4.

Sindou M, Brinzeu A. Topography of the pain in classical trigeminal neuralgia: insights into somatotopic organization. Brain. 2020;143(2):531–40.

Sindou M, Dumot C. Planning of Endocranial Supratentorial Basal Cistern and Skull Base Approaches Depending on Venous Patterns Using a Topogram. World Neurosurg. 2020;134:365–71.

Sindou M, Keravel Y. [Trigeminal neuralgia. Percutaneous thermocoagulation of the trigeminal nerve (author's transl)]. Neurochirurgie. 1979;25(3):166–72.

Sindou M, Keravel Y. [Functional neurosurgery in the cranial nerve hyperactivity syndromes: conclusions]. Neurochirurgie. 2009;55(2):291–2.

Sindou M, Mercier P. Microvascular decompression for hemifacial spasm: surgical techniques and intraoperative monitoring. Neurochirurgie. 2018;64(2):133–43.

Sindou M, Tatli M. [Treatment of trigeminal neuralgia with thermorhizotomy]. Neurochirurgie. 2009;55(2):203–10.

Sindou M, Brinzeu A, Laurent B. Aspects cliniques et thérapeutiques des névralgies des nerfs trijumeau et glossopharyngien. 2020. ISSN 0246-0351. https://doi.org/10.1016/S0246-0351(20)44471-X, http://www.sciencedirect.com/science/article/pii/S0246-0351(20)44471-X.

Sindou M, Keravel Y, Abdennebi B, Szapiro J. [Neurosurgical treatment of trigeminal neuralgia. Direct approach of percutaneous method?]. Neurochirurgie. 1987;33(2):89–111.

Sindou M, Fobe JL, Ciriano D, Fischer C. Hearing prognosis and intraoperative guidance of brainstem auditory evoked potential in microvascular decompression. Laryngoscope. 1992;102(6):678–82.

Sindou M, Fobe JL, Berthier E, Vial C. Facial motor responses evoked by direct electrical stimulation of the trigeminal root. Localizing value for radiofrequency thermorhizotomy. Acta Neurochir. 1994;128(1–4):57–67.

Sindou M, Chavez JM, Saint Pierre G, Jouvet A. Percutaneous biopsy of cavernous sinus tumors through the foramen ovale. Neurosurgery. 1997;40(1):106–10. discussion 110–101

Sindou M, Howeidy T, Acevedo G. Anatomical observations during microvascular decompression for idiopathic trigeminal neuralgia (with correlations between topography of pain and site of the neurovascular conflict). Prospective study in a series of 579 patients. Acta Neurochir. 2002;144(1):1–12. discussion 12–13

Sindou M, Leston J, Howeidy T, Decullier E, Chapuis F. Micro-vascular decompression for primary Trigeminal Neuralgia (typical or atypical). Long-term effectiveness on pain; prospective study with survival analysis in a consecutive series of 362 patients. Acta Neurochir. 2006;148(12):1235–45. discussion 1245

Sindou M, Leston J, Decullier E, Chapuis F. Microvascular decompression for primary trigeminal neuralgia: long-term effectiveness and prognostic factors in a series of 362 consecutive patients with clear-cut neurovascular conflicts who underwent pure decompression. J Neurosurg. 2007;107(6):1144–53.

Sindou M, Leston JM, Decullier E, Chapuis F. Microvascular decompression for trigeminal neuralgia: the importance of a noncompressive technique—Kaplan-Meier analysis in a consecutive series of 330 patients. Neurosurgery. 2008;63(4 Suppl 2):341–50. discussion 350–341

Sindou M, Messerer M, Alvernia J, Saint-Pierre G. Percutaneous biopsy through the foramen ovale for parasellar lesions: surgical anatomy, method, and indications. Adv Tech Stand Neurosurg. 2012;38:57–73.

Sjoqvist O. Studies on pain conduction in the trigeminal nerve. Helsingfors: Mercators Tryckeri; 1938.

Skinner HA. Some histologic features of the cranial nerves. Arch Neurol Psychiatry. 1931;25(2):356–72.

Skirving DJ, Dan NG. A 20-year review of percutaneous balloon compression of the trigeminal ganglion. J Neurosurg. 2001;94(6):913–7.

Smith KJ, McDonald WI. Spontaneous and mechanically evoked activity due to central demyelinating lesion. Nature. 1980;286(5769):154–5.

Smith ZA, Gorgulho AA, Bezrukiy N, McArthur D, Agazaryan N, Selch MT, De Salles AA. Dedicated linear accelerator radiosurgery for trigeminal neuralgia: a single-center experience in 179 patients with varied dose prescriptions and treatment plans. Int J Radiat Oncol Biol Phys. 2011;81(1):225–31. https://doi.org/10.1016/j.ijrobp.2010.05.058. Epub 2011 Jan 13. PMID: 21236592.

Son BC, Kim HS, Kim IS, Yang SH, Lee SW. Percutaneous radiofrequency thermocoagulation under fluoroscopic image-guidance for idiopathic trigeminal neuralgia. J Korean Neurosurg Soc. 2011;50(5):446–52.

Spiller W, Frazier CH. The division of the sensory root of the trigeminus for the relief of tic douloureux; an experimlental pathological and clinical study, with a preliminary report of one surgically sucessful case. Phila Med J. 1901;8:1039–49.

Steiger HJ. Prognostic factors in the treatment of trigeminal neuralgia. Analysis of a differential therapeutic approach. Acta Neurochir. 1991;113(1–2):11–7.

Stomal-Słowińska M, Słowiński J, Lee TK, Uitti RJ, Deen HG, Reimer R, Cheshire WP Jr, Herzog-Bryan G, Wharen RE Jr. Correlation of clinical findings and results of percutaneous balloon compression for patients with trigeminal neuralgia. Clin Neurol Neurosurg. 2011;113(1):14–21.

Sweet WH. Treatment of trigeminal neuralgia by percutaneous rhizotomy. In: Youmans JR, editor. Neurological surgery. Philadelphia: WB Saunders; 1990. p. 3888–921.

Sweet WH, Wepsic JG. Controlled thermocoagulation of trigeminal ganglion and rootlets for differential destruction of pain fibers. 1. Trigeminal neuralgia. J Neurosurg. 1974;40(2):143–56.

TaarnhØJ P. Decompression of the trigeminal root and the posterior part of the ganglion as treatment in trigeminal neuralgia; preliminary communication. J Neurosurg. 1952;9(3):288–90.

Taarnhøj P. Decompression of the posterior trigeminal root in trigeminal neuralgia. a 30-year follow-up review. J Neurosurg. 1982;57(1):14–7.

Tanaka BS, Zhao P, Dib-Hajj FB, Morisset V, Tate S, Waxman SG, Dib-Hajj SD. A gain-of-function mutation in Nav1.6 in a case of trigeminal neuralgia. Mol Med. 2016;22:338–48.

Tang YZ, Wu BS, Yang LQ, Yue JN, He LL, Li N, Ni JX. The long-term effective rate of different branches of idiopathic trigeminal neuralgia after single radiofrequency thermocoagulation: a cohort study. Medicine (Baltimore). 2015;94(45):e1994.

Taptas N. Les injections d' alcool dans Ie ganglion de Gasser a travers Ie trou ovale. Press Med. 1911;19:798.

Tarlov IM. Structure of the nerve root: I. Nature of the junction between the central and the peripheral nervous system. Arch Neurol Psychiatry. 1937a;37(3):555–83.

Tarlov IM. Structure of the nerve root: II. Differentiation of sensory from motor roots; observations on identification of function in roots of mixed cranial nerves. Arch Neurol Psychiatry. 1937b;37(6):1338–55.

Tatli M, Sindou M. Anatomoradiological landmarks for accuracy of radiofrequency thermorhizotomy in the treatment of trigeminal neuralgia. Neurosurgery. 2008;63(1 Suppl 1):ONS129–37. discussion ONS137–128

Tatli M, Satici O, Kanpolat Y, Sindou M. Various surgical modalities for trigeminal neuralgia: literature study of respective long-term outcomes. Acta Neurochir. 2008;150(3):243–55.

Tempel ZJ, Chivukula S, Monaco EA 3rd, Bowden G, Kano H, Niranjan A, Chang EF, Sneed PK, Kaufmann AM, Sheehan J, Mathieu D, Lunsford LD. The results of a third Gamma Knife procedure for recurrent trigeminal neuralgia. J Neurosurg. 2015;122(1):169–79.

Terrier L-M, Zemmoura I, Amelot A, Destrieux C, François P, Velut S. New insights into the trigeminal nerve somatotopy: lessons from partial sensory rhizotomy. Morphologie. 2017;101(335):195.

Terrier LM, Amelot A, François P, Destrieux C, Zemmoura I, Velut S. Therapeutic failure in trigeminal neuralgia: from a clarification of trigeminal nerve somatotopy to a targeted partial sensory rhizotomy. World Neurosurg. 2018;117:e138–45.

Tew JM, Taha JM. Percutaneous rhizotomy in the treatment of intractable facial pain (trigeminal, glossopharyngeal, and vagal nerves). In: Schmidek HH, Sweet WH, editors. Operative neurosurgical techniques. Philadelphia: WB Saunders; 1995. p. 1469–84.

Thiry S, Hotermans J. Traitement de la névralgie essentielle du trijumeau par stéréotaxie et électrocoagulation partielle selective du ganglion de Gasser. Neurochirurgie. 1974;20:55–60.

Tronnier VM, Rasche D, Hamer J, Kienle AL, Kunze S. Treatment of idiopathic trigeminal neuralgia:

comparison of long-term outcome after radiofrequency rhizotomy and microvascular decompression. Neurosurgery. 2001;48(6):1261–7. discussion 1267-1268

Tuleasca C, Carron R, Resseguier N, Donnet A, Roussel P, Gaudart J, Levivier M, Régis J. Patterns of pain-free response in 497 cases of classic trigeminal neuralgia treated with Gamma Knife surgery and followed up for least 1 year. J Neurosurg. 2012;117(Suppl):181–8.

Tuleasca C, Carron R, Resseguier N, Donnet A, Roussel P, Gaudart J, Levivier M, Régis J. Repeat Gamma Knife surgery for recurrent trigeminal neuralgia: long-term outcomes and systematic review. J Neurosurg. 2014;121(Suppl):210–21.

Tuleasca C, Régis J, Sahgal A, De Salles A, Hayashi M, Ma L, Martínez-Álvarez R, Paddick I, Ryu S, Slotman BJ, Levivier M. Stereotactic radiosurgery for trigeminal neuralgia: a systematic review. J Neurosurg. 2018;130(3):733–57.

Tuleasca C, Paddick I, Hopewell JW, Jones B, Millar WT, Hamdi H, Porcheron D, Levivier M, Régis J. Establishment of a therapeutic ratio for gamma knife radiosurgery of trigeminal neuralgia: the critical importance of biologically effective dose versus physical dose. World Neurosurg. 2020;134:e204–13.

Tyler-Kabara EC, Kassam AB, Horowitz MH, Urgo L, Hadjipanayis C, Levy EI, Chang YF. Predictors of outcome in surgically managed patients with typical and atypical trigeminal neuralgia: comparison of results following microvascular decompression. J Neurosurg. 2002;96(3):527–31.

Uryvaev MY, Sudarikova TV, Trufanov IN, Gorskaya TV, Tsybul'kin AG. The fine branches of the human trigeminal nerve. Neurosci Behav Physiol. 2008;38(2):157–60.

Urgosik D, Liscak R, Novotny J, Vymazal J, Vladyka V. Treatment of essential trigeminal neuralgia with gamma-knife surgery. J Neurosurg. 2005;102:29–33.

Verheul JB, Hanssens PE, Lie ST, Leenstra S, Piersma H, Beute GN. Gamma Knife surgery for trigeminal neuralgia: a review of 450 consecutive cases. J Neurosurg. 2010;113(Suppl):160–7.

Villavicencio AT, Lim M, Burneikiene S, Romanelli P, Adler JR, McNeely L, Chang SD, Fariselli L, McIntyre M, Bower R, Broggi G, Thramann JJ. Cyberknife radiosurgery for trigeminal neuralgia treatment: a preliminary multicenter experience. Neurosurgery. 2008;62(3):647–55; discussion 647–55. https://doi.org/10.1227/01.neu.0000317313.46826.dc. PMID: 18425011.

Vitali AM, Sayer FT, Honey CR. Recurrent trigeminal neuralgia secondary to Teflon felt. Acta Neurochir. 2007;149(7):719–22. discussion 722

Waltz TA, Dalessio DJ, Copeland B, Abbott G. Percutaneous injection of glycerol for the treatment of trigeminal neuralgia. Clin J Pain. 1989;5(2):195–8.

White JC, Sweet WH. Pain and the neurosurgeon; a forty-year experience. Springfield, IL: C. C. Thomas; 1969.

Wieser HG, Yaşargil MG. ["Selective amygdalo-hippocampectomy" as a surgical treatment of mesiobasal limbic epilepsy (author's transl)]. Neurochirurgia (Stuttg). 1982;25(2):39–50.

Yadav S, Sonone RM, Jaiswara C, Bansal S, Singh D, Rathi VC. Long-term follow-up of trigeminal neuralgia patients treated with percutaneous balloon compression technique: a retrospective analysis. J Contemp Dent Pract. 2016;17(3):263–6.

Yang Y, Wang Y, Li S, Xu Z, Li H, Ma L, Fan J, Bu D, Liu B, Fan Z, Wu G, Jin J, Ding B, Zhu X, Shen Y. Mutations in SCN9A, encoding a sodium channel alpha subunit, in patients with primary erythermalgia. J Med Genet. 2004;41(3):171–4.

Ying X, Wang H, Deng S, Chen Y, Zhang J, Yu W. Long-term outcome of percutaneous balloon compression for trigeminal neuralgia patients elder than 80 years: a STROBE-compliant article. Medicine (Baltimore). 2017;96(39):e8199.

Young RF. Glycerol rhizolysis for treatment of trigeminal neuralgia. J Neurosurg. 1988;69(1):39–45.

Young B, Shivazad A, Kryscio RJ, St Clair W, Bush HM. Long-term outcome of high-dose gamma knife surgery in treatment of trigeminal neuralgia. J Neurosurg. 2013;119(5):1166–75.

Younis S, Maarbjerg S, Reimer M, Wolfram F, Olesen J, Baron R, Bendtsen L. Quantitative sensory testing in classical trigeminal neuralgia—a blinded study in patients with and without concomitant persistent pain. Pain. 2016;157(7):1407–14.

Zakrzewska JM, Thomas DG. Patient's assessment of outcome after three surgical procedures for the management of trigeminal neuralgia. Acta Neurochir. 1993;122(3–4):225–30.

Zakrzewska JM, Chaudhry Z, Nurmikko TJ, Patton DW, Mullens LE. Lamotrigine (lamictal) in refractory trigeminal neuralgia: results from a double-blind placebo controlled crossover trial. Pain. 1997;73(2):223–30.

Zakrzewska JM, Lopez BC, Kim SE, Coakham HB. Patient reports of satisfaction after microvascular decompression and partial sensory rhizotomy for trigeminal neuralgia. Neurosurgery. 2005;56(6):1304–11. discussion 1311–1302

Zakrzewska JM, Palmer J, Bendtsen L, Di Stefano G, Ettlin DA, Maarbjerg S, Obermann M, Morisset V, Steiner D, Tate S, Cruccu G. Challenges recruiting to a proof-of-concept pharmaceutical trial for a rare disease: the trigeminal neuralgia experience. Trials. 2018;19(1):704.

Zhang H, Lei D, You C, Mao BY, Wu B, Fang Y. The long-term outcome predictors of pure microvascular decompression for primary trigeminal neuralgia. World Neurosurg. 2013;79(5–6):756–62.

# Index





M. Sindou, A. Brinzeu, *Trigeminal Neuralgias: A Neurosurgical Illustrated Guide*,
https://doi.org/10.1007/978-3-031-25113-9

GPSR Compliance

*The European Union's (EU) General Product Safety Regulation (GPSR) is a set of rules that requires consumer products to be safe and our obligations to ensure this.*

*If you have any concerns about our products, you can contact us on ProductSafety@springernature.com*

In case Publisher is established outside the EU, the EU authorized representative is:

Springer Nature Customer Service Center GmbH
Europaplatz 3
69115 Heidelberg, Germany

Batch number: 10732801

Printed by Printforce, the Netherlands